Dietary patterns of low overall quality are the single leading predictor of premature mortality and chronic morbidity in the modern world. No nutrient can remedy that. Changing dietary patterns so they routinely promote rather than undermine health means changing food choices, meal selection, daily routines, and the skill sets – especially **cooking** – on which they rely. The emergence of "culinary medicine," where once only biochemistry prevailed, is testimony to this shift in problem, solution, and the primacy of the actionable and pragmatic. **This textbook** - with a focus on cultivating a discrete set of skills to be practiced and paid forward through teaching- **takes its place among the important and promising advances in the vanguard of public health nutrition**. If the potential of diet – to add years to lives, life to years, and help sustain the vitality of our planet – is to be fulfilled, it will owe much to the widespread uptake of the crucial lessons found in the Culinary Medicine Textbook.

David Katz MD, MPH, FACPM, FACP, FACLM

Kudos to Dr. Deb for getting both chefs and nutrition scientists to the table to create a masterpiece. The Culinary Medicine Textbook lists the essential culinary skills that are required to be able to eat and ENJOY a healthy diet. Anyone can learn how to cook; it takes practice and a sense of humor to learn from mistakes. Deliciously eat your way towards health.

Chef Cat Cora

My dad understood that all life begins in the soil and that healthy soil leads to healthy plants, which leads to healthy people and a healthy planet; it is the only way we can literally save ourselves from ourselves! Dr. Deb truly understands this and has put together an incredible work combining nutrition science and the culinary arts by bringing together chefs with nutrition scientists. **Both are pioneers in their own righ**t – helping people to eat healthy plants.

Farmer Lee, author of The Chef's Garden

CULINARY MEDICINE FROM CLINIC TO KITCHEN

A Hands-on Guide to Transforming Nutrition Guidelines into Cooking Skills

THE ESSENTIAL FOODS

Deborah Kennedy PhD

Content Developed by Nutrition Scientists From Around the World and the Expert Chef Panel

CULINARY RꭗEHAB ©

CONTRIBUTORS

FRUIT
Deborah Kennedy, PhD
Natalie Volin, MS
The Expert Chef Panel

VEGETABLES
Betsy Redmond, PhD, MMSc, RDN
Julia Hilbrands, MS, MPH, RD
Deborah Kennedy, PhD
The Expert Chef Panel

GRAINS
Jody L. Vogelzang, PhD, RDN, FADA, CHES
Jasna Robinson-Wright, MSc, RD, CDE, CIEC
Deborah Kennedy, PhD
The Expert Chef Panel

PROTEIN
Deborah Kennedy, PhD
Julia Hilbrands, MS, MPH, RD
The Expert Chef Panel

FATS & OILS
Rima Kleiner, MS, RDL, LDN
Deborah Kennedy, PhD
The Expert Chef Panel

DAIRY
Julia Hilbrands, MS, MPH, RD
Deborah Kennedy, PhD
Jasna Robinson-Wright, MSc, RD, CDE, CIEC
The Expert Chef Panel

THE INCREDIBLE TEAM OF CHEFS

The following are those chefs who participated in The Food Chapters, helping to create culinary competencies and advancing culinary medicine. Some participated in all the chapters, and others in some of them.

Chef Lyndon Virkler (M.Ed., AOS): Senior Core Faculty Member Emeritus and former Dean at New England Culinary Institute. He is co-author of Farm to Table: An Essential Guide to Sustainable Food Systems for Students, Professionals, and Consumers.

Chef Scott Giambastiani: Food at Google Program Manager Video of Chef Scott

Chef Russell Michel (CHC, CWA): Founder of The Culinary Architect LLC

Chef Kate Waters (Dip CNM, mBANT, CNHC): UK chef and nutritional therapist

Chef Cyndie Story (PhD, RDN, SNS, CC): Founder Culinary Solutions Centers LLC

Chef Kelsey Johnson: Previous Owner Café Linnea Edmonton Alberta

Chef Ron Desantis (MBA, CMC): Chief Culinary Officer at the Hungry Planet® and Principle Advisor of CulnaryNXT

Chef Erica Holland-Toll: Culinary Director at The Culinary Edge. Previous Executive Chef at the Stanford Flavor Lab. Executive chef at a university

Chef Dave Barrett: Previous chef at Walt Disney World, owner of Main Street Kitchens in Hanover, NH

Chef Janet Crandall: Head Chef at the Culinary School at the LGBTQ+ Center in Hollywood, CA

Chef Deb Kennedy (PhD): Culinary Medicine expert and nutritional biochemist. Owner of Build Healthy Kids, Build Healthy Seniors and Culinary Rehab LLC.

THE STUDENTS

Natalie Volin (Tufts University): Sustainability sections in the Food chapters

OTHER CONTRIBUTORS

Joy Hutchinson, MSc, RD: Reviewed the Grain chapter

Kelly LeBlanc MLA, RD, LDN: Reviewed The Grain Chapter

Sustainability: Becky Ramsing MPH, RDN (Sustainability)

The Food Coach Academy

The content of this book was transformed into an online cooking school where students both learn how to cook and how to teach others to cook based on their palate, wallet, and cultural heritage. The culinary competencies are brought to life under the guidance of professional chefs. Dr. Kennedy provides mentorship in culinary medicine and behavior change, and students are guided by experts in motivational interviewing in real time.

CULINARY RⱵEHAB ©

ISBN Paperback: #979-8-9907083-0-3
ISBN Electronic: #979-8-9907083-1-0
Library of Congress Control Number: 2024909141

Culinary Rehab© is a copyright owned by Deborah Kennedy

Printed in the United States of America.

Deborah Kennedy PhD
DrDebKennedy.com

Limit of Liability/ Disclaimer of Warranty:
While Culinary Rehab LLC, the authors, chefs, and contributors have used their best efforts in preparing this work/book, they make no representations or warranties with respect to the accuracy or completeness of the content of this book.

Disclaimer:
This book is not a medical manual and in no way should take the place of medical treatment. **It is always best to check with your healthcare provider before embarking on a health and wellness plan**, especially if you are on any medications or currently have any disease or illness. Culinary Rehab LLC, the authors, chef, or contributors, disclaim liability for any medical outcomes that may occur as a result of following the guidance in this book.

HOW TO USE THE BOOK

Throughout this book you will find a QR code like the one below, which will take you to pictures, images, figures, graphs, and videos. Scan the QR code anytime you see one to get access to them all. We wanted to make sure that no matter what format you purchased this book (online or in print) that you would have access to all the tasty bites that accompany it.

If you would like to stay up to date, join our facebook group.
The Food Coach Academy Facebook Group

If you are interested in the Food Coach Academy, you can take a **free** 42-task sample course here:
The Food Coach Academy Sample Course

TABLE OF CONTENTS

FRUIT

GRAINS

PROTEIN

FATS & OILS

DAIRY

PLANT-BASED MILK ALTERNATIVES

FRUIT

~

By Deborah Kennedy PhD
with
Natalie Volin MS and
The Expert Chef Panel

"Knowledge is knowing that a tomato is a fruit;
wisdom is not putting it in a fruit salad."
Quote by Miles Kington

FRUIT IS A SWEET, nutrient-dense food made up of mostly water, making it relatively low in calories. The perfect snack does exist! Nature intended fruit to be very appealing to the taste buds in order for it to survive as a species. The sweet taste and smell of fruit draws animals in to consume its succulent flesh. As the animal moves around and defecates elsewhere, the seeds are scattered away from the mother plant, thus ensuring the plant's reproduction and survival.

Humans have been eating and enjoying fruit for thousands of years, although the fruit of today looks very different than it did back then. Take the peach as an example: today's peach is sweeter, juicier and 16 times larger than the wild peach, which was the size of a cherry and domesticated in China in 4,000 BC (Kennedy, 2014). Modern fruit is the result of thousands of years of selecting and planting seeds from the tastiest and hardiest varieties, and the fruit we grow and eat now barely resembles the wild fruit of years past.

Fruit — which was once an enjoyable treat and a rarity for many, showing up mostly in Christmas stockings and celebratory meals — has now become overthrown by hyper-palatable sweets that can't compete with anything Mother Nature creates. For many, the bar has been raised on the expectations of what we think is enjoyable. Once you enter the world of processed food and consume candy, cakes, and cookies, you train your taste buds to seek and prefer highly sweetened foods, sweeter than any food nature can create. That simple apple will no longer be enough to satisfy an internal craving for something sweet when apple pie or apple-flavored gummy fruit is around.

The good news is that what can be turned up can also be turned down. It can take as little as two to four weeks of not eating processed sweets to reset your taste buds to enjoy naturally sweet foods again. What was once preferred, is now too sweet, and that is great news! Why? Because fruit provides essential nutrients — vitamins, minerals, fiber and phytochemicals – needed to build and maintain a healthy body without the harmful added sugars that are found in processed sweets and treats.

SECTION 1:
FRUIT CHARACTERISTICS

Fruit is the mature ovary of a flowering plant that contains seeds, and its main role is protecting those seeds that are needed to grow into new plants. One can define fruit from both a botanical perspective and a culinary one. While many people think of berries, apples, and oranges as fruit, few think of nuts, green beans, peas, corn, squash, tomatoes, peppers, and eggplant as fruit too. By definition, though, they are. For the purpose of this book, the fruit chapter will not include those fruit varieties that the majority think of as vegetables and instead will include only sweet or sour tasting fruit, or fruit otherwise known as culinary fruit.

Image: Fruit Characteristics

FRUIT SUBGROUPS

Subgroups of fruit and vegetables are determined based on similarities in food composition as well as the part of the plant, its color, total antioxidant capacity, and botanical family. One reason for the development of a classification system was to make it easier for clinicians to make dietary recommendations (Pennington & Fisher, 2010). The following are the subgroups of fruit which were not included in the United States MyPyramid food guide in 2005 or 2010.

Table 1: Subgroups of Fruit

Subgroup	Fruit	Contributing Nutrients	Classification of Nutrients
Deep Orange/ Yellow Fruit	Apricot, cantaloupe, mango, nectarine, peach, papaya	Alpha-carotene, vitamin C, beta-carotene	Highest in alpha-carotene and second highest in beta-carotene
Red Fruit	Cherry, guava, pomegranate, watermelon	Vitamin C, lycopene and anthocyanidins, flavan-3-ols	Highest in lycopene and second highest in anthocyanidins
Citrus Fruit	Clementine, grapefruit (white and pink), kumquat, lemon, lime, orange, tangerine	Vitamin C, flavanones and lycopene and flavones	Highest in flavanones and second highest in flavones and lycopene
Red, Purple, and Blueberries	Cranberry, blackberry, blueberry, boysenberry, cranberry, raspberry, strawberry	Anthocyanidins, flavan-3-ols, total antioxidant capacity, dietary fiber, manganese, and vitamin C	Highest in anthocyanidins and second highest in flavan-3-ols and total antioxidant capacity
Other Fruit	Apple, artichoke, Asian pear, banana, casaba melon, date, fig, grape, honeydew melon, kiwifruit, pear, pineapple, plum, raisins	Vitamin C, fiber, potassium, choline, magnesium isoflavones, fiber, potassium	Variable depending on the fruit

SECTION 2:

RECOMMENDATIONS FOR FRUIT INTAKE

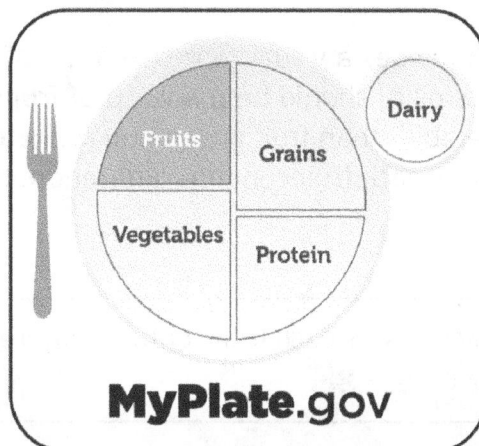

MyPlate.gov

The recommendation for the amount of fruit that one should eat each day to promote good health is usually given alongside a recommendation for vegetable servings as well. While the old adage of "5-a-day" is familiar to many, the following are the recommended daily fruit and vegetable servings from several leading health organizations:

The American Heart Association recommends eating **8 servings of fruits and vegetables** a day (American Heart Association, 2017).

The American Cancer Society recommends **1 ½ to 2 cups of fruits** a day (American Cancer Society, 2017).

Table 2: USDA MyPlate Recommendation for Fruit Per Day

Diets Fruit Table *Daily Recommendation		
Children	2 - 3 years old 4 - 8 years old	1 cup 1 to 1.5 cups
Girls	9 - 13 years old 14 - 18 years old	1.5 cups 1.5 cups
Boys	9 - 13 years old 14 - 18 years old	1.5 cups 2 cups
Women	19 - 30 years old 31 - 50 years old 51+ years old	2 cups 1.5 cups 1.5 cups
Men	19 - 30 years old 31 - 50 years old 51+ years old	2 cups 2 cups 2 cups

Accessed on 1/2020 from https://www.choosemyplate.gov/fruit

The MyPlate guiding system provides a visual representation of these recommendations as it shows that one half of one's plate should be made up of fruits and vegetables, and there should typically be more vegetables than fruit on a plate. MyPlate also recommends eating a variety of fruit in many colors, as each fruit contains different nutrients and therefore varying health benefits.

Eat a variety of fruit in many colors, as each fruit contains different nutrients and therefore varying health benefits.

FRUIT INTAKE AMONG AMERICANS

How are Americans doing with meeting the current guidelines for fruit? Not well. Per capita consumption of fruit decreased from 2004 to 2010, mainly due to a 10% decline in juice intake (Ramsay et al., 2014). Young children start out consuming the recommended amount of fruit set forth by the United States Department of Agriculture (USDA) Dietary Guidelines; however, this is only if juice is counted in total fruit consumption. By the time children reach nine years of age, 75% are not getting the recommended amount of fruit, and intake does not improve as they age.

Graph 1: Fruit Intake in the United States

LIFE STAGE INFLUENCES ON FRUIT INTAKE

Children: Children two to five years of age met and exceeded the daily requirement for fruit (125% to 133% of recommendations) across all socioeconomic groups only if fruit juice was included: without the juice, which accounts for 47% of the recommendation, whole fruit consumption was approximately a half cup per day (Ramsay et al., 2014). Despite an increase in whole fruit consumption by 67% and a decrease in juice by one-third between 2003 and 2010, consumption still remains below recommendations (CDC, 2019).

Teens: A mere 8.5% of high school students aged 14 to 18 years meet the daily recommendations for fruit intake (Moore et al., 2017).

Adults: Only 12.2% of adults met the USDA recommendation for fruit in 2015, and intake was low among all socioeconomic groups. Overall, the groups that did better at meeting the fruit recommendation were women (15.1%), Hispanics (15.7%), and adults 31 to 50 years (13.8%), and the lowest prevalence at meeting the recommendation for fruit was seen in young adults aged 18 to 30 years (9.2%) (Lee-Kwan, 2017).

Graph 2: Percent of Individuals Below Fruit Recommendation in the United States

SECTION 3:

WHY ARE FRUITS SO HEALTHY?

Image: Why Are Fruits so Healthy

Fruit, which is made up of mostly water (from 74% in the banana to 92% in the strawberry), provides more nutrients per calorie than most foods, thus making it a nutrient-dense food. Besides delivering traditional vitamins like vitamin C, and minerals like potassium, fruit also provides phytonutrients, which are plant nutrient powerhouses. Over 100,000 phytonutrients have been discovered to date, and many of them have anti-inflammatory and antioxidant properties. According to the USDA DGA 2015 (2015–2020 Dietary Guidelines for Americans - Health.Gov, 2015), the key contributing nutrients that fruit provides are **vitamin C, potassium, and fiber**, and these are nutrients that are also under-consumed in the U.S. population. Fruits are also healthy because of what they do not have — fruits are naturally low in fat, sodium, and calories, and none have cholesterol.

Figure 1: Fruits High in Fiber, Antioxidants, Potassium, and Nutrient Density

High Fiber	Antioxidant Rich	Most Nutrient-Dense	Potassium Rich
Blackberry	Blackberry	Blackberry	Apricot
Guava	Blueberry	Grapefruit	Banana
Kiwi	Clementine	Lemon	Cantaloupe
Orange	Cranberry	Lime	Cherries
Passion fruit	Kiwi	Orange	Guava
Pear	Orange	Strawberry	Honeydew
Persimmon	Plum		Kiwi
Pomegranate	Raspberry		Melon
Raspberry	Strawberry		Oranges
	Tangerine		Pomegranate

Reference: Antioxidant list created choosing U.S. procured, common, and whole fruit (Carlsen et al., 2010) and Nutrient Density

VITAMINS AND MINERALS IN FRUIT

Fruit is a source of several important vitamins and minerals, especially **vitamin C, vitamin A, potassium, and folate**. It is not surprising that these nutrients are often under-consumed in a Western diet as many individuals fail to meet the recommended intake of fruit each day.

Many people think of Vitamin C as a go-to nutrient when you come down with a cold. While vitamin C does support immune function (though its ability to cure the common cold remains unsubstantiated), it also supports the growth and repair of tissues, promotes healthy gums and teeth, and aids in wound healing. Vitamin C is considered an antioxidant vitamin. Normal metabolic processes create reactive oxygen species (ROS) and free radicals within the body, and high levels of these molecules have been associated with chronic disease. Antioxidants such as vitamin C can neutralize ROS and free radicals, and higher intakes of antioxidants have been associated with lower rates of several chronic diseases (Serafini & Peluso, 2016). Within the fruit category, **good sources of vitamin C include oranges, grapefruit, kiwifruit, strawberries, and cantaloupe**.

Vitamin A is another antioxidant vitamin that works to neutralize damaging free radicals. Vitamin A may also be called retinol or retinal, depending on its form, and the phytochemical beta-carotene can be converted to vitamin A. In addition to its antioxidant capabilities, vitamin A is a crucial component of eye health as well as immune function and reproduction. **Fruits rich in vitamin A include cantaloupe, mangos, and apricots.** In a large multi-year study, researchers found that low serum carotenoid levels (from low vitamin A and beta-carotene intake) along with low physical activity predicted earlier mortality, leading them to conclude that a diet high in vitamin A-rich fruits and vegetables may support longevity (Nicklett et al., 2012).

Folate is a water-soluble B vitamin that is involved in many different processes in the body. Folate helps produce DNA and red blood cells and it is especially important for women of childbearing years. Folate is also important to heart health, and low folate levels have been linked to vascular diseases and other chronic conditions (Institute of Medicine (US) Standing Committee on the Scientific Evaluation of Dietary Reference Intakes and its Panel on Folate, Other B Vitamins, and Choline, 1998). **Good sources of folate in fruit include oranges and orange juice, papaya, banana, and cantaloupe.**

Potassium is a mineral and is one of the main electrolytes in the body. It is involved in just about every process within the body and is required for normal cell function as it helps maintain fluid volume. Potassium also has a strong relationship with sodium, another major electrolyte, and a diet high in potassium can help counteract the hypertensive impact of too much dietary sodium (Torres-Gonzalez et al., 2019). This relationship may be even more pronounced in salt-sensitive individuals. **Fruits that are high in potassium include dried apricots, dried prunes, raisins, bananas, cantaloupe, and apples (with skin on).**

Table 3: Fruit Sources of Select Vitamins and Minerals

Vitamin/Mineral	Recommended Daily Value*	Food Source
Vitamin A	900 µg	Cantaloupe, mangos, dried apricots
Vitamin C	90 mg	Oranges⁺, orange juice⁺, kiwifruit⁺, strawberries⁺, grapefruits⁺, cantaloupe⁺
Folate	400 µg	Oranges, orange juice, papaya, banana, cantaloupe
Potassium	4700 mg	Dried apricots⁺, dried prunes, raisins, bananas, cantaloupe, apple (with skin)

*For adults and children >=4 years of age
⁺Indicates excellent food source that provides >20% Daily Value
https://ods.od.nih.gov/factsheets/list-VitaminsMinerals/

FIBER AND FRUIT

Whole fruit is also an important source of fiber in the diet. Dietary fiber is essentially undigested carbohydrates in the diet, of which there are two types: soluble fiber and insoluble fiber (Slavin & Lloyd, 2012). Soluble fiber, which is found primarily in the flesh or meat of a fruit, attracts water in the gastrointestinal tract and turns into a gel-like substance. This helps slow the rate of digestion, leading to increased satiety. Soluble fiber also plays a role in lowering blood cholesterol levels and maintaining healthy gut microflora. Insoluble fiber is found in the skin and seeds of fruit, and it helps aid in digestion by adding bulk to stool to prevent constipation. Both types of fiber have been found to increase satiety and lower disease risk, both separately and together.

The health benefits of fiber have been studied for centuries. Dietary fiber regulates the digestive system and treats and prevents constipation, decreases blood cholesterol levels, and increases satiety during meals, which aids in weight management. Dietary fiber may also play a role in modulating the immune system by helping to minimize inflammation in the body, and it is well-established that inflammation is involved in the development of chronic diseases such as cardiovascular disease, diabetes, cancer, and obesity (Palmer, 2008).

The recommendation for total dietary fiber intake, which is set by the Institute of Medicine, is 14 grams per 1000 calories consumed, which equates to about **25 grams per day for women**

and 38 grams per day for men (Slavin & Lloyd, 2012). With all the benefits that fiber offers, it is a shame that most Americans only consume an average of about 15 grams of fiber per day, and only about 5% of individuals meet fiber recommendations on a daily basis.

PHYTOCHEMICALS IN FRUIT

The health benefits of vitamins, minerals, and fiber have been well established and fairly well understood for decades, but we are just starting to study and understand the contribution of another component of fruit — phytonutrients. Phytonutrients are responsible for the color, flavor, and odor of plant foods, including fruits. Plants produce phytonutrients as a protective mechanism to ward away pests or to withstand harsh environmental conditions, and just as phytonutrients provide many benefits to the plants that produce them, they are incredibly beneficial to humans who consume them as well. In fact, researchers believe that the phytonutrient content of fruit is largely responsible for their numerous health benefits (Wiseman et al., 2007).

Tens of thousands of phytonutrients have already been identified, and researchers believe there are likely many more that have yet to be discovered. They are grouped into several broad categories, including phenolic acids, lignans, and flavonoids, and all are metabolized slightly differently by the body, thus providing slightly different health effects (Erdman et al., 2007). Research on specific phytonutrients is ongoing and has produced some mixed results thus far, but it is believed that phytonutrients have the potential to stimulate the immune system, prevent toxic substances in the diet from becoming carcinogenic, reduce oxidative damage to cells, slow the growth rate of cancer cells, help regulate hormone signaling and gene expression and activate insulin receptors (Wiseman et al., 2007). There is evidence to suggest that the phytonutrients in fruit may lead to a reduced risk of cardiovascular disease and type 2 diabetes (Dauchet et al., 2006) (González-Castejón & Rodriguez-Casado, 2011). For specific information on the health benefits of various classes of phytonutrients, go to the **Vegetable** chapter.

Given the numerous beneficial components of fruit, what is the relationship between a diet high in fruits and health outcomes? In large population-based epidemiological studies, it's often difficult to separate the effects of eating fruits from the effects of eating vegetables, so these two food categories are often grouped together. However, there are also some studies that have tried to look at the benefit of just fruit in the diet. The findings of both types of studies are summarized in Table 4.

Table 4: Benefits of Diets High in Fruit or High in Fruit and Vegetables

Diets High in Fruit	
Reduce the Risk of Breast Cancer	Women who ate more fruit during adolescence (about three servings per day) had a 25% lower risk of developing breast cancer than those who had less than 0.5 servings of fruit per day (Farvid et al., 2015)
Reduce the Risk of Type 2 Diabetes	Men and women with a greater consumption of whole fruit — especially blueberries, grapes, and apples — experienced a lower risk of type 2 diabetes (Muraki et al., 2013).
	Among female nurses followed for 18 years, an increase of three servings per day of whole fruit was associated with a reduced risk of type 2 diabetes (Bazzano et al., 2008).
	Among European adults, greater fruit variety (but not quantity) was associated with a lower risk of type 2 diabetes (Cooper et al., 2012).
Aid in Weight Loss	Among men and women in the United States, intake of total fruit, berries, and apples/pears was inversely associated with weight change over a four-year period (Bertoia et al., 2015).
Lead to Higher Academic Performance	When almost 300 Australian university students were surveyed, those who had healthier diets, including higher vegetable intake, also had higher Grade Point Averages (Whatnall et al., 2019).
Diets High in Fruits and Vegetables	
Reduce the Risk of Cardiovascular Diseases (CVD)	Higher intake of F&V is associated with a reduced risk of death from CVD, with an average reduction in risk of 4% for each additional serving per day of F&V (Wang et al., 2014).
	Eating eight or more servings of F&V per day resulted in a 30% lower risk of heart attack or stroke compared to eating less than 1.5 servings per day (Hung et al., 2004).
	A large meta-analysis showed that increasing consumption of fruits and vegetables from less than three to more than five servings per day is associated with a 17% reduced risk of coronary heart disease (He et al., 2007).
Lower the Risk of Type 2 Diabetes	In a group of European adults followed for 11 years, a greater quantity of fruit and vegetable intake was associated with a 21% lower risk of type 2 diabetes (Cooper et al., 2012).

Diets High in Fruit	
Increase Happiness, Life Satisfaction, and Well-Being	Among Australian adults, increased fruit and vegetable consumption was predictive of increased happiness, life satisfaction, and overall well-being (Mujcic & J Oswald, 2016).
Reduce the Risk of Age-Related Vision Problems	Among men and women at least 50 years of age, those who had three or more servings of fruit per day had a 36% lower risk of age-related maculopathy than those who had less than 1.5 servings of fruit per day (Cho et al., 2004).

FRUIT AND THE MICROBIOME

The gut microbiome is comprised of trillions of bacterial cells within the gastrointestinal tract, and these bacteria are intricately involved in digestion, intestinal health, and immune function. Research on the gut microbiome is still in its infancy, but we do know there is significant inter-individual variation in the composition of the microbiome. Plus, the composition of the microbiome – the variety and quantity of bacteria residing there – plays a role in health outcomes. Researchers are beginning to discover that the composition of the gut microbiome is influenced by factors like sex, body weight, and diet (Dominianni et al., 2015).

The gut microbiome can be enhanced and supported when probiotics, or foods with live bacterial cultures, are ingested (Fernandez & Marette, 2017). Common probiotic foods include yogurt and other fermented dairy products or fermented vegetables like sauerkraut, kimchi, miso, and natto. Another way the gut microbiome can be enhanced is through the ingestion of prebiotics, and this is where fruit and its fiber content come into play.

Prebiotics are naturally occurring, nondigestible carbohydrates that induce the growth and activity of beneficial bacteria in the colon (Gibson & Roberfroid, 1995). Essentially, prebiotics act as food or fuel for the bacteria in the gut microbiome. The most common prebiotics are the fibers fructo-oligosaccharides, such as inulin, and galacto-oligosaccharides, and there is some research that shows that polyphenols can act as prebiotics as well (Gibson & Roberfroid, 1995). Prebiotics help maintain a good balance of health-promoting bacteria versus disease-promoting bacteria in the large intestines by feeding the beneficial bacteria. Some prebiotic fibers can also be broken down into short-chain fatty acids (SCFA) by the gut microbiota. SCFA has been shown to help maintain a healthy gut barrier to pathogens (Brownawell et al., 2012). **Nectarines, bananas, and raspberries are especially high in fructo-oligosaccharides** (Fernandez & Marette, 2017).

Some recent research has looked at a possible synergistic effect of consuming probiotics and prebiotics together, such as a cup of yogurt topped with prebiotic-rich fruit (Gibson & Roberfroid, 1995). The probiotics in yogurt introduce beneficial bacteria into the gut microbiome, and the prebiotics found in the fruit help provide the necessary fuel for these bacteria to survive and implant in the gastrointestinal tract. This research is still in its infancy and it remains to be seen whether this hypothesized synergistic effect is significant or not.

Much is unknown about prebiotics, but some research suggests that maintaining a healthful balance of gut microbiota may help alleviate symptoms of Irritable Bowel Syndrome, reduce energy intake and markers of insulin resistance, improve body weight management, increase satiety, improve calcium absorption, and reduce the duration, incidence, and symptoms of some forms of diarrhea (Sanders et al., 2014).

SECTION 4:
FRUIT INTAKE AND HEALTH OUTCOMES

When people are asked to think about antioxidant-rich fruits, **blueberries** are often one of the first fruits that come to mind. Indeed, blueberries have high levels of antioxidants, which help to decrease the risk of many diseases caused by oxidative stress (Krikorian et al., 2010). Regular blueberry consumption has also been shown to help reduce blood pressure and arterial stiffness (Johnson et al., 2015).

Other berries can tout similar health benefits. **Blackberries** are packed full of antioxidants, fiber, vitamin C, manganese, and vitamin K. Additionally, they are a good source of folate, and a folate deficiency can lead to megaloblastic anemia, an increased risk of cancer and an increased risk of birth defects (Oregon State University, 2014). **Strawberries** are also an excellent source of vitamin C, and people with higher blood levels of vitamin C have been found to have a lower risk of death from all causes, including cardiovascular disease and cancer (Oregon State University, 2014). **Raspberries** contain the most fiber per gram of any of the berries. The MIND diet (see the chapter on **Brain Health**) prescribes two servings of berries per week to reduce the risk of Alzheimer's and cognitive impairment associated with aging (Morris, 2012; Shishtar et al., 2020).

Fruits outside of the berry family provide numerous health benefits as well. **Peaches** and **nectarines** are excellent sources of vitamin C as well as fiber, vitamin A, potassium, and niacin.

Watermelon is another vitamin C and vitamin A powerhouse. **Apples** are a good source of both soluble and insoluble fiber as well as vitamin C and the antioxidant quercetin, which may help reduce the risk of gout and certain cancers (Fabiani et al., 2016). **Oranges** and other citrus fruits are commonly regarded for their vitamin C content, but they also contain high levels of folate, potassium, and several classes of phytonutrients that have been linked to a reduced risk of cardiovascular disease, cancer, neural tube defects and anemia (Economos & Clay, 1998). **Kiwifruit** contains numerous bioactive materials that have anticancer and antimicrobial activity, as well as good amounts of vitamins A, E, K, lutein, and xanthin (Tyagi et al., 2015). **Bananas** have become synonymous with potassium, but they also contain several bioactive compounds, including phenolics, carotenoids, biogenic amines, and phytosterols, all of which have antioxidant activity (Singh et al., 2016).

Grapes are another class of fruit that has received attention for the potential health benefits they provide, and this is mainly due to the health effects of red wine (explored in greater detail in the **Beverage** chapter). Over 500 antioxidants have been identified in grapes, but the main bioactive components are resveratrol and proanthocyanidins. These compounds are found primarily in the seeds and skin of the fruit and have been found to protect LDL cholesterol from lipid peroxidation, thus attenuating atherosclerosis and ischemic heart disease. They may also act as anti-cancer agents. It is still unknown whether the benefits seen in drinking moderate amounts of wine can also be obtained by eating grapes and what volume of grapes this might amount to. However, like all other fruits, grapes certainly contain valuable phytonutrients that undoubtedly have a positive impact on health outcomes (Bertelli & Das, 2009).

HEALTH BENEFITS OF DIETS HIGH IN FRUITS AND VEGETABLES

As Table 4 shows, researchers have looked at the health impact of eating fruit in general, but we also have good evidence about the nutrient profile and health benefits of specific fruits. Of all fruits, berries have been the most extensively studied. Much of the health benefits of berries are due to their flavonoid content, which is a type of phytonutrient. A recent study by Cassidy and colleagues found that a regular intake of berries (three times per week) can reduce the risk of heart attack by 32% in young and middle-aged women (Cassidy et al., 2013). Other studies have found that berries can also reduce the risk of diabetes and cognitive decline (Calvano et al., 2019; Morris, 2012). Due to their tiny, numerous seeds, berries also yield one of the best fiber-per-calorie bargains in the plant world (Palmer, 2008).

SECTION 5:

WHEN TO LIMIT FRUIT

There are some conditions for which a limitation on the amount or type of fruit consumed is warranted. Below is a summary of those situations.

IRRITABLE BOWEL SYNDROME AND THE LOW FODMAP DIET

Irritable bowel syndrome (IBS) is a catchall term for functional disorders of the gut, including diarrhea and abdominal bloating. Unlike irritable bowel disease (like Crohn's disease and ulcerative colitis), where there are physical abnormalities in the gut, IBS is characterized by strictly functional abnormalities. Because of this, symptoms vary greatly from person to person and are often hard to treat.

One approach that practitioners might suggest for managing IBS is dietary modifications in the form of a low FODMAP diet. FODMAP stands for **F**ermentable **O**ligosaccharides (fructans, galactans), **D**isaccharides (lactose), **M**onosaccharides (fructose), **A**nd **P**olyols (sugar alcohols). These are all types of carbohydrates that individuals may have difficulty digesting, resulting in excess gas, bloating, and diarrhea. The general idea of a FODMAP diet is to cut out foods high in FODMAPs for a period of time and then slowly introduce foods back into the diet to see which cause gastrointestinal (GI) symptoms. See the chapter on **Gastrointestinal Health** for more information.

High FODMAP foods are found in a variety of food groups, but there are certain fruits that fall into the high FODMAP category that should be avoided by individuals following this diet. However, there are also many fruits that are considered low FODMAP that can be included.

Table 5: High and Low FODMAP Fruit

Low FODMAP (Okay to Eat)	High FODMAP (Limit/Avoid)
Unripe bananas	Apples
Blueberries	Apricots
Cantaloupes	Avocados
Cranberries	Ripe bananas
Clementines	Blackberries
Grapes	Grapefruit
Galia melons	Mangoes

Low FODMAP (Okay to Eat)	High FODMAP (Limit/Avoid)
Honeydew melons	Peaches
Kiwi	Pears
Lemons	Plums
Oranges	Raisins
Pineapples	Sultanas
Raspberries	Watermelon
Rhubarb	Dried fruits
Strawberries	Fruit juices and concentrated fruits

KIDNEY DISEASE

The kidneys are responsible for keeping appropriate levels of electrolytes, including potassium in the blood and when they are not working properly, potassium can increase to dangerous levels. Someone with renal disease or on dialysis is often prescribed a low-potassium diet by their clinician to help limit the amount of potassium their sick kidneys need to manage. While fruit is often considered a healthy food, it is high in potassium and must be consumed wisely by individuals prescribed a low-potassium diet. Luckily, there is a wide range of potassium content in fruits, so these individuals should choose fruits that are low in potassium, as shown in Table 6. A patient with kidney disease should be monitored closely by a licensed nutritionist or dietitian to discuss which types of food to eat while their kidneys are not functioning properly.

FRUIT AND THE GLYCEMIC INDEX

Table 6: Fruit High and Low in Potassium

High Potassium Fruit	Low Potassium Fruit
Apricots	Apples, apple juice, and applesauce
Avocados	Blackberries
Bananas	Blueberries
Cantaloupes	Cherries
Dates, dried figs and other dried fruits, raisins	Cranberries
Grapefruit juice	Fruit cocktail
Honeydew melons	Grapes and grape juice
Kiwifruits	Grapefruit
Mangoes	Mandarin oranges
Nectarines	Peaches
Oranges and orange juice	Pears

High Potassium Fruit	Low Potassium Fruit
Papayas	Pineapples and pineapple juice
Pomegranates and pomegranate juice	Plums
Prunes and prune juice	Raspberries
	Strawberries
	Tangerines
	Watermelon

Glucose is the primary sugar in the body and is a component of many foods. The glycemic response refers to how quickly glucose is absorbed after a person eats a carbohydrate-containing food and, in turn, how fast blood glucose rises and then falls. A desirable response is a slow absorption of glucose, leading to a slow and modest rise in blood glucose, followed by a slow return to normal; this is referred to as a low **glycemic response**. A high glycemic response refers to a rapid absorption of glucose which then leads to a spike in blood glucose followed by a plunge. Foods that elicit high glycemic responses may be especially problematic for individuals with diabetes who have difficulty managing their blood sugars.

Different foods elicit different glycemic responses, and they are categorized according to a glycemic index. As one would expect, foods with a high glycemic index will elicit a high glycemic response, and foods with a low glycemic index will elicit a lower glycemic response. Foods with a high glycemic index include white bread and other processed grain products, white rice, russet potatoes, and cornflakes. Foods like whole-wheat products and brown rice have a medium glycemic index, and foods with a low glycemic index include stone-ground wheat products, rolled oats, steel-cut oats, non-starchy vegetables, legumes and lentils.

Diabetics and others concerned about their carbohydrate intake sometimes view fruit with caution because it is thought to have a higher sugar content — albeit naturally occurring sugar — and thus may elicit a higher glycemic response. However, most fruit is considered a low glycemic index food because the fiber and fructose content help to blunt the glycemic response. However, Figure 2 below shows that there are a handful of fruits with a medium or high glycemic index. Additionally, some dried fruits like dates, raisins, and sweetened cranberries have a high glycemic index.

Of note, the glycemic index of a food represents the type of carbohydrate in that food but says nothing about the amount of carbohydrate that is typically eaten. Thus, another measure called the **glycemic load** attempts to take normal portion sizes into account and reflects both the **type** and **amount** of carbohydrate that is typically eaten. Fruits with a low glycemic load are listed in Figure 2.

While glycemic index and glycemic load are terms to be aware of, the American Diabetes Association does not give much weight to these numbers when counseling diabetics and others about healthy meal plans. They also do not want diabetics to shy away from fruits as they are full of vitamins, minerals, and fiber that together provide numerous health benefits. However, because fruits do contain carbohydrates, they do need to be accounted for in one's meal plan if an individual is counting carbohydrates to help manage their blood sugars.

Rather than focusing on the glycemic index or glycemic load, the American Diabetes Association recommends the following principles for healthful eating with or without diabetes Source: http://www.diabetes.org/
- Eat a variety of foods, including vegetables, whole grains, fruits, nonfat dairy foods, healthful fats and lean meats or meat substitutes
- Try not to eat too much food
- Try to not eat too much of one type of food
- Space meals evenly throughout the day
- Don't skip meals

Culinary Tips to lessen the rise in blood sugar after eating fruit:
- Eat fruit with protein (nut or nut butter, cheese, or slice of meat) or oil.
- Add vinegar (Ostman et al., 2005) or cinnamon (Hlebowicz et al., 2007) as it slows gastric emptying, which will blunt the rise in blood glucose levels.
- Select 'just ripe' fruit. Overripe fruit tends to have more simple (instead of complex) sugar strands.

Figure 2: Glycemic Index for Fruit

Table 7 lists fruits with a low Glycemic Load. Note that a Glycemic Load is considered low at 10 or less, medium at 11-19, and high if over 20 (Atkinson et al., 2008)

Table 7: Glycemic Load of Certain Fruits

Fruit	Glycemic Load
Apples	6
Apricots	3
Cherries	9
Kiwifruits	7
Mangoes	8
Nectarines	4
Oranges	3 to 4
Peaches	5 to 6
Pears	5
Pineapple	6
Strawberries	1
Watermelon	4 to 5

ORAL ALLERGY SYNDROME (POLLEN-RELATED FOOD ALLERGY SYNDROME)

Some people who are allergic to pollen may become cross-reactive to certain fruits. This is considered an oral allergy in which the body is tricked into thinking the protein in a piece of fruit is pollen, and the immune system reacts to it by releasing histamine. When histamine is released in the mouth due to eating raw fruit, the lips, tongue, and mouth can feel sore, itchy, burning, or numb. These symptoms may also proceed to the throat and nasal cavity. Below are some examples of cross-reactivity:

Table 8: Cross-Reactivity of Pollen Allergies to Fruit

Pollen Allergy	Reactive Fruit
Ragweed (late summer to fall)	Banana, Cucumber, Cantaloupe, Honeydew, Watermelon, Zucchini
Birch (spring)	Apple, Kiwifruit, Apricot, Cherry, Peach, Pear, Plum
Grass (summer)	Celery, Melon, Orange, Peach, Tomato

Source: Muluk & Cingi, 2018

Cooking fruit may lessen the reactivity as will peeling the fruit or adding lemon to it before consumption. In 1% to 2% of individuals, their oral allergy syndrome (OAS) may become more severe — hives, symptoms lasting more than 15 minutes, trouble swallowing, and reactions to both raw and cooked fruit (Muluk & Cingi, 2018). It is necessary to see a medical professional for the more severe reactions as it can become life threatening.

LATEX-FRUIT SYNDROME

Up to half of individuals who have an allergy to natural rubber latex, can also be allergic to avocado, banana, chestnut, kiwi, peach, tomato, bell pepper and potato (Brophy, 2015).

FRUIT AND DRUG INTERACTIONS

Grapefruit juice interacts with over 85 different medications with half of those reactions being severe or potentially deadly https://www.pharmacytoday.org/article/S1042-0991(15)31392-X/pdf (Tanzi, 2013). In addition, the following are reported interactions between juice and medications that were not severe, but significant enough to be reported in the medical literature (Chen et al., 2018). It is best to avoid grapefruit juice or fresh grapefruit altogether when taking any medication and to exert caution with other juices.

Table 9: Adverse Fruit Juice and Medication Interactions

Fruit Juice	Medication	Effect
Apple juice	Fexofenadine, Atenolol, Aliskiren	Decreased bioavailability
Grape juice	Cyclosporin	Decreased bioavailability
Orange juice	Aliskiren, Atenolol, Celiprolol, Montelukast, Fluoroquinolones, Alendronate	Decreased bioavailability
Orange juice	Aluminum containing antacids	Increased bioavailability
Seville orange juice	Felodipine	Increased bioavailability
Pomelo juice	Sildenafil	Decreased bioavailability
Pomelo juice	Cyclosporin	Increased bioavailability

Beneficial Combinations

Drinking orange juice, or eating a diet high in vitamin C, helps with non-heme (plant-based) iron absorption (Cook & Reddy, 2001). Foods high in beta-carotene, like cantaloupe, apricots, peaches and oranges, can also help with non-heme iron absorption (García-Casal et al., 1998).

SECTION 6:

CLINICAL AND CULINARY RECOMMENDATIONS AND COMPETENCIES

Messaging from the
Menus of Change Annual Report 2020

Think Produce First

Clinical recommendations and competencies are the foundation from which culinary competencies were created. The goal for the culinary medicine practitioner is to help clients and patients develop the skills necessary to meet the clinical recommendations by teaching skill-based learning outlined in the culinary competencies.

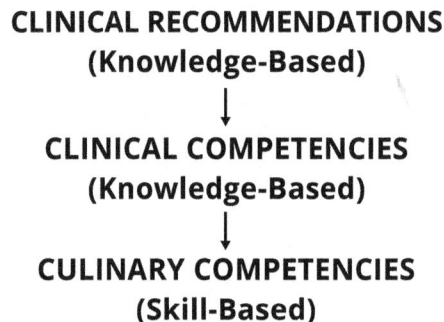

CLINICAL RECOMMENDATIONS
(Knowledge-Based)

↓

CLINICAL COMPETENCIES
(Knowledge-Based)

↓

CULINARY COMPETENCIES
(Skill-Based)

CLINICAL RECOMMENDATIONS (DGA 2020-2025)

1. Depending on total caloric intake, consume 1 to 2 ½ cups of fruit per day
2. At least half of the fruit recommendation should come from whole fruit
3. Eat a variety of fruit
4. Do not consume fruit juice before 12 months of age, and during the second year, juice is not necessary and fruit intake should come from eating whole fruit

CLINICAL COMPETENCIES

1. Define fruit and list the types
2. Recall how many servings of fruit are recommended per day

3. Recall which nutrients for which fruit supply a "good source"
4. List the cohorts at risk of not meeting their daily fruit requirement
5. Relate the importance of fruit in overall health — both prevention and treatment for various diseases
6. Describe fruit's influence on the microbiome
7. Identify fruit low in sugar
8. Identify health conditions that require limiting fruit in one's diet
9. Identify which fruit or juice interacts with certain medications
10. Describe oral allergy syndrome
11. Explain the FODMAP diet

CULINARY COMPETENCIES FOR FRUIT

SHOPPING AND STORING COMPETENCIES

1. Demonstrate how to shop for fresh, frozen, and canned fruit within a budget
2. Describe the two types of ripening in fruit
3. Identify fruits in season
4. Describe what happens to fruit when it freezes and thaws
5. Demonstrate how and when to clean fruit
6. List which fruits are stored in the refrigerator and which ones are left out
7. Describe the method of freezing fruit

Stocking the Kitchen

1. Stock a variety of fruit at home – fresh, frozen, and canned
2. Stock a variety of herbs and spices at home
   a. Fresh basil and mint, for example
   b. Dried cinnamon, chili, tajin, ginger and black pepper, for example
3. Keep fruit sources of acid at home – lemons, limes, and fruit-based vinegars for example

COOKING/PREPARING COMPETENCIES

Knife/Instrument Skills

1. Select the appropriate knife to cut and prepare various sized fruit
2. Demonstrate the use of a peeler
3. Demonstrate making zest using a zester or citrus reamer (optional)
4. Demonstrate use of a melon baller (optional)
5. Utilize a blender to make smoothies

FLAVOR DEVELOPMENT COMPETENCIES

1. Describe how acid affects the flavor of fruit and fruit dishes
2. Describe cooking methods used with fruit to influence the flavor profile
3. Select herbs to use with fruit to add flavor
4. Construct a basic vinegar reduction (optional)
5. Demonstrate how to build flavor without using added sugar

COOKING/PREPARING COMPETENCIES

1. Demonstrate the following cooking/preparation techniques:
2. Prepare a fruit salad
3. Prepare a fruit kebab
4. Construct a healthful smoothie
5. Use frozen fruit in recipes
6. Grill fruit
7. Poach fruit
8. Purée fruit
9. Dehydrate fruit (optional)
10. Prepare frozen fruit treats

SERVING COMPETENCIES

1. Model eating fruit
2. Serve the appropriate number of fruit servings a day
3. Utilize fruit in meals and menu planning
4. Prepare and serve a fruit-based snack
5. Select the best fruit for travel
6. Display the proper serving sizes of fruit

SAFETY COMPETENCIES

1. Demonstrate the prevention of cross-contamination when working with fruit
2. Identify spoilage characteristics of fruit
3. Make use of knife safety skills when preparing fruit
4. Demonstrate washing fruit
5. Demonstrate proper storage of fruit

SECTION 7:

FRUIT AT THE STORE

Purchasing fresh fruit is easy for some, but not for those living in a food desert. Some individuals live in communities with multiple sources of fresh, frozen, and canned fruit from fruit stands, farmer's markets, local co-ops, and large and small grocery store chains, while others only have access to their local convenience store, which provides minimal to no fresh fruit—this is a food desert.

Less than 2% of the population grows their own fruit. The majority of fruit consumed in the United States is purchased outside the home but stored and prepared in the home. Some of that fruit is organic, some is grown in the United States, and some is grown outside the U.S. In-home consumption of fruit consists of fresh fruit (55%), juice (32%), canned (5%), dried (2.4%) and frozen fruit (1.6%) (Produce for Better Health Foundation, 2015).

Today the most commonly purchased fruit are (PMA, 2018):
1. Bananas (73%)
2. Apples (69%)
3. Grapes (62%)
4. Strawberries (62%)
5. Oranges (56%)
6. Watermelon (54%)
7. Lemons (48%)
8. Blueberries (45%)
9. Peaches (42%)
10. Pineapples (42%)

The most commonly consumed fruit juices are orange juice, apple juice, and grape juice.

PESTICIDE RESIDUE ON FRUIT

According to a 2015 Consumer Reports survey, 85% of Americans are concerned about the use of pesticides in produce. The amount of pesticide residue varies greatly between different fruits and vegetables, and levels differ depending on the country of origin (Consumer Reports, 2015). The Consumer Reports Pesticides in Produce Report analyzed 12 years of data from the United States Department of Agriculture (USDA), looking at 48 conventional produce items from 14 different countries. While some of the produce improved over the 12 years of data collection in terms of the amount of pesticide residue, some did not.

When shopping for fruit and vegetables, another great resource to have on hand when deciding to buy organic produce or not is the Environmental Working Group's Clean 15™ and Dirty Dozen™ list that is published every year (Environmental Working Group, 2024). The EWG uses the same data source as the Consumer Reports mentioned above. The USDA Pesticide Data Program analyzes nonorganic produce for pesticide residue after it has been washed and peeled. Those that have the least amount of pesticide residue make the Clean 15™ list, while those with the most amount of pesticide residue make the Dirty Dozen™ list. The goal of these lists is to help consumers limit pesticide exposure by knowing which fruits and vegetables make the most sense to buy organically. It is important to note, however, that the benefits of eating a variety of nonorganic fruits and vegetables far outweigh the risks of pesticide exposure. Fruit on the Environmental Working Group's (EWG) 2024 Clean 15™ and Dirty Dozen™ list are found in Table 10. The full version of each list can be found here: Dirty Dozen, Clean 15.

Table 10: Fruit on the EWG's 2024 Clean 15™ and Dirty Dozen™ Lists

CLEAN 15™ 2024	DIRTY DOZEN™ 2024
Pineapples	Strawberries
Papayas	Grapes
Honeydew melons	Peaches
Kiwifruit	Pears
Mangoes	Nectarines
Watermelon	Apples
	Cherries
	Blueberries

*Note: Raisins have by far the most pesticide residue on them, but because they are considered "processed," they do not appear on the official list.
What clean foods have in common is a thick outer membrane.

Eating more fruits and vegetables, whether organic or not, is so beneficial to one's health that it far outweighs the risk of consuming trace amounts of pesticides in healthy individuals!

WHOLE FRUIT

Nothing is more delicious than biting into a succulent fresh peach. When fruit is ripe, it is at its peak in flavor and sweetness. This is intentional, from an evolutionary perspective, because when a fruit is ripe, its seeds are ready to be spread and begin a new growth cycle.

When selecting fruit, it is important to know which fruits to purchase when they are already ripe and how to identify ripeness, plus which ones will ripen after purchase. The gas ethylene triggers ripening in fruit, which can happen in a burst of gas being released all at once (climacteric fruit) or by a slow release of gas (non-climacteric fruit).

Climacteric fruits continue to ripen after they have been picked, so these fruits can be purchased even when they appear to be under-ripe. After the burst of ethylene to signal the ripening process, these types of fruit convert starch to sugar, which breaks down the cell walls within. All of this leads to the sweetening and softening of the fruit's flesh over time. Examples of climacteric fruits include apples, avocados, bananas, cantaloupes, peaches, pears, plums, tomatoes, papayas, and mangoes.

Non-climacteric fruits ripen only when they are connected to the parent plant because they do not convert starch to sugar and rely on the parent plant for sugar. Examples are blueberries, cherries, grapefruit, lemons, oranges, grapes, melons, pineapples, raspberries, and strawberries. You want to be sure to buy these fruits when they are already ripe, as they will not further ripen off the vine, tree, or bush. Shop for ripe fruit that you will eat in the next four days.

FROZEN FRUIT

Frozen fruit can contain the same nutrient profile as fresh whole fruit. In fact, frozen fruit may have even more nutrients than fresh fruit because the fruit is frozen soon after it is picked, locking in all of the nutrients, while fresh fruit can lose nutrients during transport and while sitting on store shelves. In studies, levels of certain nutrients – vitamins, minerals, total phenols, and fiber - were comparable in the frozen and fresh versions (Bouzari et al., 2015).

Frozen fruit needs to be stored at zero degrees Fahrenheit or lower and eaten within eight to 12 months of storage in the freezer, with the exception of citrus, which is only good for four to six months frozen.

CANNED FRUIT

Consumption of canned fruit has decreased from 15% to a little over 11% between 2000 and 2018 (Shahbandeh, 2019). Canned or jarred fruit can be a healthful choice as long as one is cautious about the other ingredients present (Aubrey, 2013). When fruit is canned or jarred, it needs to soak in a liquid to prevent it from drying out, and a preservative, usually vitamin C (also known as ascorbic acid), is added to prevent spoiling. There are several options for the liquid that can be used to can and jar fruit, and each can vary widely in its sugar content.

Most sugar - Heavy syrup> Light syrup> Fruit juice> No sugar added or packed in water - **least.**

Image: Fruit Canned

Bottom Line: Look for canned and jarred fruit packed in water, or second best, look for fruit packed in 100% fruit juice. If clinically recommended, select fruit with added artificial sweeteners.

DRIED FRUIT

A half cup of dried fruit counts as a one cup USDA serving of fruit. The process of drying fruit involves removing the water present inside. Since the majority of fruit is made up of water, removing it increases the amount of sugar present per unit of weight. Take a look at the difference in fiber and sugar content of the whole fruit versus the dried fruit in Table 11. Natural sugars and fiber increase significantly in the dried version due to the decrease in volume, and oftentimes additional sugar is added in the drying process. It is best to think of dried fruit as nature's candy — focus on whole fruit and have some dried fruit as a treat, making sure to select dried fruit with no added sugar.

Table 11: Sugar and Fiber Content of Fresh Versus Dried Fruit

FRUIT	Sugar per 100 grams of Fruit	Fiber per 100 grams of Fruit
Grapes	15.49	1.4
Raisins	60.00	5
Apricots	9.24	2
Dried Apricots	47.50	7.5

Data taken from the USDA Nutrient Database (USDA, 2018)

JUICE

According to USDA & HHS (2015), one cup of 100% juice counts as a one cup serving of fruit. Since juice is higher in sugar and lower in fiber than whole fruit, it is recommended that no more than half the fruit requirement be satisfied with juice (2015).

Is fruit juice as healthy as whole fruit? The bottom line is NO, for two main reasons:

1. Liquid calories act differently than solid calories: Your body does not compensate for calories that you consume in liquid form the same way it does in solid form. In other words, if you compare drinking 200 calories before a meal to eating 200 calories before the meal, your body would compensate by eating less at the meal only when you ate 200 calories beforehand, not when you drank those 200 calories.

2. Juice provides a larger sugar load without dietary fiber: You are able to drink more servings of fruit at a time than eat the same amount of fruit servings in its whole form. For example, it is easy to consume the juice of four oranges — about one cup of liquid — in a single sitting, whereas most would find it difficult to eat that many oranges at one time. The fiber in the whole fruit increases satiety and thus prevents overconsumption. There is more sugar and zero fiber in a glass of apple juice (28 grams of sugar per cup) than in a medium apple (19 grams of sugar plus 4.4 grams of fiber). Drinking juice (or other sugar-sweetened beverages) with no fiber causes a rapid increase in blood sugar levels, which requires a larger load of insulin to be released. Over time this can stress the body and lead to insulin insensitivity, a precursor of type 2 diabetes.

The science: 71,346 female nurses in the Nurses' Health Study aged 38 years to 63 years were studied prospectively for 18 years. Overall intake of fruits and vegetables was not associated with an increased risk of type 2 diabetes. But, there was a 20% reduction in type 2 diabetes risk with the consumption of three servings of whole fruit and a 10% reduction with each serving of green leafy vegetables. Juice, on the other hand, was an entirely different matter. Drinking an eight ounce glass of juice was associated with an 18% increased risk of developing type 2 diabetes (Bazzano et al., 2008).

SECTION 8:

FRUIT AND SUSTAINABILITY

Growing, transporting, and storing fruit, along with other plant foods, is generally more sustainable than producing animal foods such as dairy and meat. However, several issues must be considered when making the most sustainable choice.

Figure 3: Schematic Supply Chain of Fruit and Vegetable Products (Parajuli et al., 2019)

1. The amount of **water** used to grow fruit varies by type and location, but it is generally lower than grains and other crops that require heavy irrigation. Fruit trees, with their deep roots and long lives, may rely primarily on green water, which is water collected in the soil from rain. However, when fruits are grown in dry, arid regions, they will need more water supplied through irrigation. In terms of processing, whole fruits use less water than juices and fruit products that require more processing. To compare, the combined water footprint (irrigated and groundwater) on average for one orange (150 grams) has a water footprint of 80 liters of water. In contrast, one glass of orange juice (200 ml) costs about 200 liters of water (Mekonnen & Hoekstra, 2010).

Figure 4: Graph: The Average Water Footprint of Fruit (M³/ton)

2. The high demand for a variety of fruits year-round across all seasons has increased the **transportation** of fruit from across and outside the US. More than half of the fresh fruit Americans buy now comes from other countries - bananas from Costa Rica, mangoes from Mexico, and berries from Chile. As a result, the proportion of imported fresh fruit eaten in the United States rose from 23% in 1975 to 53.1% in 2016, according to the Agriculture Department's Economic Research Service.

3. Fruit production accounts for only 1.6% of the **greenhouse gas emissions** (GHGe) from food in the United States. Furthermore, transportation of food, including fruit, only accounts for 5% of the food-related GHGe (Heller et al., 2018). Even with the increased transportation of fruit across the globe, what you eat and how it is grown have a greater impact on the environment than where the fruit came from.

Figure 5: Graph: Contribution of Fruit to Total GHGe From Food

4. Many fruits are susceptible to pests and disease, so farmers often rely on heavy use of pesticides and chemicals to protect crops. Seven fruits are part of the Environmental Working Group's Dirty Dozen™, with strawberries and nectarines topping the list. Studies have shown that children who consume organic produce have lower levels of pesticide metabolites in their blood (Curl Cynthia L et al., 2003).

5. It would be remiss not to mention the workers involved in producing, packaging, and transporting fruit. Workers who pick and manage fruit crops are among the lowest paid for one of the hardest and most strenuous jobs. Work involves long hours with few breaks, heat stress, pesticide exposure, and prolonged squatting or reaching. When purchasing fruit, look for standards that protect the health of food chain workers, such as those promoted by the Food Chain Workers Alliance or the Good Food Purchasing Program.

SECTION 9:
FRUIT IN THE KITCHEN

ON THE TONGUE – THE TASTE OF FRUIT

Most people associate fruit with a sweet taste. In reality, there are many different tastes in fruit: sour (lemon, lime, unripe plum), tangy (lemon and lime flesh), bitter (lemon rind, lime rind, grapefruit, especially those with a yellow rind), and salty (pigface in Australia).

STORING FRUIT

Leave out, even when ripe: Bananas, mangoes, oranges, lemons, limes, melons, papayas, pineapples, and tomatoes

Keep in the refrigerator: Apricots, berries, cherries, figs, grapes, Asian pears

Leave out to ripen, then store in the refrigerator: Apples, avocados, nectarines, peaches, pears, plums (all stone fruit)

When cutting fruit, use a sharp knife. A blunt knife damages more plant cells, and when this happens, more nutrients (like vitamin C) are lost (Portela & Cantwell, 2001). Cut, peeled, and cooked fruit should be refrigerated within two hours of cutting. Cut melons must be refrigerated immediately until served.

Cut fruit will last one to two days in the refrigerator; bananas, apples, and pears will turn brown. Lemon juice, with its acidity, will prevent some of the browning.

IN THE PANTRY

Items to have on hand:
- Fresh fruit
- Frozen fruit
- Dried fruit
- Unsweetened applesauce
- Lemons and limes
- Fresh herbs, like basil, mint, and tarragon. Certain herbs like cilantro, sage, rosemary, and thyme are very strong, so just a little goes a long way.
- Dried herbs and spices – cinnamon, star anise, chili, tajin, ginger
- Local honey
- Himalayan salt
- Black pepper
- Chilies
- Balsamic vinegar and/or flavored vinegars

KNIFE/INSTRUMENT SKILLS AND FRUIT

When preparing dishes with fruit, it is essential to know how to use both a paring knife and a chef knife – for the larger fruit with tough outer skins. Choosing the wrong knife – a paring knife to slice cantaloupe, for example – can lead to injury.

There are several instruments that are not imperative to have but make preparing fruit much easier. They include:
- **Fruit, Knives, and Tools**

Video: Fruit, Knives and Tools

- **Citrus Juicer**
  - Some recipes call for fresh fruit juice, and you can replace water with juice if you want to add extra flavor. You can use your hands to squeeze half of a citrus fruit or use either of the tools shown above.
- **Zester**
  - Zesting fruit provides an intense flavor boost. Zest can be used in baked products, beverages, fruit salads, and even savory dishes.
  - Creating zest, especially fine particles, is difficult with a knife. Various zesters are available, as depicted in the picture above. It is important to avoid zesting the white layer under the skin, as that is very bitter.

FLAVOR DEVELOPMENT

What first attracts us to certain fruit starts with how it looks—the color, the brightness. If one finds the visual attributes of the fruit appealing, it then enters the mouth and becomes all about the flavor, followed by the texture. Since prehistoric times, people have enjoyed eating fruit, not only for pleasure but for the natural sugars that provide quick nutrition and energy. Although the pure taste of raw ripened fruit is enough to provide a pleasurable eating experience, fruit can be cooked for use in either sweet or savory dishes. The simplicity of a fruit salad with various colors, textures, and flavors can be a great dessert or snack, and the preparation options are endless. Grilling, roasting, baking, or broiling fruit will create a caramelized flavor and smoky aroma. A quick sauté of fruit develops a rich flavor and syrupy texture that is made even more complex with the addition of fresh herbs, spices, and/or vinegar.

Whether served hot or cold, cooked or raw, fruit may function as a first course, an accompaniment to protein, or a dessert. From smoothies to salsas, this section explores the cooking methods and ingredients that can not only bring out the best of beloved fruit in its natural state but transform it into delectable dishes the whole family will enjoy.

Combine Textures: Combining fruit with varying textures adds a layer of complexity and enjoyment to a fruit dish. Below are culinary categories of fruit and some examples of fruit within each:

- Pomes: Apple, pear, quince
- Drupes: Apricot, cherry, coconut, date, nectarine, peach, plum
- Citruses: Clementine, lime, lemon, orange, tangerine
- Berries: Blackberry, blueberry, cranberry, gooseberry, red currant, strawberry
- Melons: Cantaloupe, honeydew, watermelon
- Tropical: Banana, cacao, fig, jackfruit, papaya, starfruit

Add Acid: Adding acid to fruit:
- Helps cut the sugar in overly ripe or very sweet fruit while creating a balance of flavor on the tongue to help you crave the next bite
- Acts as a flavor modifier. It helps the fruit's (and other food's) flavor be more pronounced
- Breaks down some fruits and alters their texture slightly
- Stops the oxidation of fruits (turning brown) such as apples when applied to cut surfaces, which helps keep the appearance nice and fresh for serving

Add either vinegar or citrus when serving raw fruit in a fruit salad or a platter of fruit to enhance the flavor profile. Add lemon or lime to a bowl of fruit salad or pour reduced balsamic vinegar over fresh orange slices for a completely different eating experience. (Reduced balsamic vinegar is delicious as it has a stronger, more concentrated flavor.)

Video: Importance of Using a Source of Acid in the Kitchen

Add Herbs and Spices: To create even more depth of flavor, add basil leaves to a watermelon salad or a spicy mix to a fruit salad. The recipe section has many great ideas.

Video: Add Fresh Herbs

Cook Fruit: When you grill, roast, or bake fruit, the sugar tends to caramelize, and the flavor completely changes. Great fruits to grill are peaches, apples, watermelon (with one side dipped in Mexican spices), nectarines, pineapple, pears, grapefruit, and mango.

Pair Sweet with Savory/Salty: Combining the sweetness of fruit with the savory elements and saltiness of the cheese, for example, creates a completely new flavor profile. Below are some examples:
- Cantaloupe with cottage cheese
- Watermelon with feta cheese
- Apple or banana with nut butter

BALSAMIC VINEGAR REDUCTION

Yield: 1 cup

Ingredients
- 2 cups balsamic vinegar (or substitute with red wine, apple cider, or other vinegars)

Instructions

Pour vinegar in a medium-sized saucepan. Bring the vinegar to a boil over medium-high heat, then reduce to a simmer until the liquid has reduced by one-half, about 13 to 15 minutes. The vinegar should be able to coat the back of a spoon. Let cool, then store in an airtight container in the refrigerator for several weeks.

Tip: You may continue to let the liquid reduce further than one-half, but remember it will continue to thicken as it cools.

Video: Balsamic Reduction

Grilled Watermelon with Balsamic Reduction: Drizzle reduced balsamic vinegar on grilled watermelon. It doesn't get tastier than that (actually, it does if you add sliced basil leaves and a dash of salt).

RECIPES & HOW TO

BUILD A HEALTHFUL SMOOTHIE

Smoothies make a great substitute for a standard breakfast or snack. Depending on what you add, it can also be a substitute for lunch or dinner. Smoothies differ from juices as the whole fruit and vegetable are put into the blender, whereas with a juicer, the fiber is shot out the back, and just the juice is collected. The fiber has health-promoting properties of its own, and it also helps blunt the rise in blood sugar after ingesting a drink high in sugar (even if it is a natural sugar).

To build a healthful smoothie, choose an ingredient from each of the categories below. The various chapters throughout this text will discuss smoothie ingredients that can be targeted toward certain cohorts or diseases.

Smoothie Tips
- For a creamy consistency, use avocado, yogurt, soaked nuts, nut butter, or a banana
- To thicken a smoothie, use frozen fruit, nuts or add chia seeds

Ingredients to Build a Smoothie

Image: Build a Smoothie

1 cup Liquid	1 cup Fresh/Frozen Fruit	1 cup Vegetables
Pure Water	Blueberries	Spinach
Milk or Milk Alternative	Kiwi	Leafy Greens e.g. Kale
Coconut Water	Pears	Cucumber
Chilled Herbal Tea	Apples	Carrot
Iced Coffee	Bananas	Beets
Fresh Squeezed Juice	Strawberries	Celery
	Any Favorite Fruit	Cabbage (can be gassy)

1 tbsp Healthy Fats	Herbs (optional)	Additional Boosters
Nut Butter	Basil	Protein Powder
Avocado	Mint	Cacao Powder
Chia Seeds	Parsley	Maca Powder
Flax Seeds	Cilantro	Goji Berries
Tahini	Turmeric Root (+Black Pepper)	Spices: Cinnamon, Vanilla,
Coconut Oil	Ginger Root	Nutmeg, Allspice

Instructions

In the order listed above, add desired ingredients into the blender, then purée until smooth.

Smoothie Bowls:
Instead of drinking the smoothie, pour it into a bowl and top it with sliced fruit, nuts and seeds, granola, and/or nut butter. They are super delicious and very popular.

BUILD A FRUIT SALAD

TASTE → **Sweet / Bitter / Sour-Tart**

TEXTURE → **Soft / Hard and Crunchy**

COLOR → **Red, Orange / Green, Yellow**

ACID → **Lemon / Lime**

- Choose ripe, seasonal fruit in a variety of flavors, from sweet to tart
- Add several textures, from crispy (apples), smooth (melons), crunchy (pomegranate seeds), firm (mango, pineapple), and soft (banana, papaya)
- Wash fruit and cut the same size pieces as it is more appealing to the eye and easier to eat
- Add citrus to enhance the flavor of the fruit, preserve the color, and prevent browning
- Add citrus zest to further add a punch of citrus flavor
  - Lastly, **to turn the flavor up a notch,** you can add a:
  - Balsamic reduction
  - Herbal infusion
  - Small pinch of salt to enhance the sweetness and flavor of the dish

- ○ Optional soft herb garnishes like basil, mint, or tarragon
- ○ A bit of honey if the fruit is sour
- ○ Add a savory and salty element like:
  - ○ Cheese
  - ○ Nuts and seeds

*There is no need to macerate the fruit (draw out the liquid from within the fruit using sugar) as fruit in and of itself, without the use of sugar, makes for a delicious fruit salad. To learn more, go to the chapter on **Sugar**.

Make a Fruit Salad

Video: Make a Fruit Salad

Watermelon, Basil, and Feta Salad: Mix bite-size pieces of watermelon with feta cheese. Add sliced basil and pour a mixture of 1 tablespoon balsamic vinegar, 1/3 cup olive oil, salt, and pepper over the top. Toss gently and eat within an hour. This doesn't keep well as leftovers.

Fish with Mango Salad: Mix together small pieces of mango and peaches (peeled). Whisk together chili, lime zest, ginger, olive oil, and lime juice. Mix the fruit and liquid mixture together and serve with a poached piece of white fish (cod, halibut, or haddock, for example).

Add Fruit to Green Salads: Adding fruit to a green salad adds nutrients, varied textures, and flavors to the dish. The sweetness of the fruit and the bitterness of the greens complement each other.
- **Step 1:** Start with well-washed and dried greens spun in a salad spinner. For maximum flavor, toss the greens in the dressing to be used. (This also reduces the amount of dressing used versus pouring it on.) Greens can range from soft, tender greens like Boston or bibb lettuce to firm-textured and flavorful arugula, spinach, or crunchy romaine.
- **Step 2:** Add fresh and/or dried fruit. If using raw fruits that oxidize, such as apples or pears, toss in lemon juice or vinaigrette after cutting or add at the last minute. Consider different knife cuts to vary texture and eye appeal: julienne or dice apples or pears (leave the skin on for more fiber). Alternate slices of strawberry, kiwi, and orange to add a variety of colors as well as nutrients. Dried cherries pair well with goat cheese on a bed of arugula.

BUILD A FRUIT KEBAB

Ingredients
- Fresh fruit (several different types of fruit)
- Wooden skewers
- Optional soft herb garnishes like basil, mint, or tarragon
- Optional yogurt or melted dark chocolate drizzled on top or used as a dip

Kids and Fruit Kebabs

Video: Kids and Fruit Kebabs

Instructions

Prepare fruit by thoroughly washing it, peeling it if needed, then cutting into bite-sized pieces, if necessary. Thread fruit onto wooden skewers. Top with fresh herbs and/or a drizzle of dark chocolate or yogurt.

BUILD A FRUIT POPSICLE

Ingredients

- 2 cups of fresh fruit of choice (strawberries, watermelon, cantaloupe, etc.)
- Optional add-ins: herbs- basil or mint, Greek Yogurt, 100% fruit juice, lemon juice, lime juice, and pieces of fruit – blueberries and strawberries, for example

Instructions

Purée fresh fruit in a blender until smooth, then add any additional ingredients listed above for flavor or creaminess. Pour mixture into popsicle molds, then freeze for at least two hours or until frozen.
- You can also use the frozen purée as a delicious topping over pancakes, waffles, and yogurt.
- Frozen fruit purée can also be a substitute for sugars and syrup in BBQ sauces

37

COOKING/PREPARATION METHODS

PURÉED FRUIT

Puréeing fruit can be a solution when there is an excess on hand or for processing frozen fruit. When fruit freezes and then thaws, it loses its shape and texture because the cells inside the fruit burst when the water inside of them freezes. When serving thawed fruit, it is best to make a purée or cook with it.

Instructions

- Select your fruit – either frozen or room temperature; any type will work
- Add lemon juice to avoid browning or to brighten red pigments in fruit
  - To add more flavor, add herbs – mint or basil, for example
  - If the fruit is very sour, add a bit of sugar to lessen the sourness
- Purée the entire fruit
- Fruit can be puréed using either an immersion blender or a regular blender

Puréed fruit can be:
- Made into a smoothie bowl
- Made into soup
- Turned into popsicles
- Added to oatmeal or yogurt
- Topped on ice cream, sherbet or sorbet
- Poured on waffles or pancakes
- Added to a seltzer-based drink
- Used in a salad dressing
- And much more

Pear-Apple Sauce: Wash and core apples and pears in a 2:1 ratio (more apple than pear). Place in a large pot. Add 1 tsp cinnamon and 1 cup apple cider for every twelve fruits (you can always add more when cooking if it looks dry). Simmer for 10 minutes. Remove from stove and use either an immersion blender or standing blender to purée and then serve.

Cold Strawberry Summertime Soup: Thaw 2 cups of strawberries (or use fresh). Place in a blender with ½ cup orange or pear juice, 2 sprigs of fresh mint, and (optional) 1 cup yogurt. Blend and serve chilled.

POACHED FRUIT

Poaching fruit adds flavor, tenderizes it, and prevents discoloration of fruits like apples and pears that oxidize once peeled. It is a great alternative to canned fruit that may have too much sugar or other additives. Poaching fruit is a method of capturing the flavor of local fruit at its peak of freshness, and it can also be used as a delicious remedy when fruit is not so ripe and firm.

Instructions

- Select your fruit. The best types are:
  - Pears, apples, and pineapples are peeled and cored, small fruits are left whole, and larger fruits are halved or quartered.
  - Peaches and nectarines: (Peaches and nectarines were peeled by blanching in boiling water, then shocked in cold water, and the skins slipped off.)
  - Apricots, plums, cherries: pits removed, large fruit halved.
- Select the poaching liquid:
  - Water, wine, or fruit juice. Wine can be red or white, depending on the desired color, and can range from slightly sweet to dry. Optional: add lemon or lime juice to the water or fruit juice.
- Select the sweetener: Sugar softens the fiber of the fruit so it is more flexible and helps the fruit to maintain its shape after cooking. It also lengthens the cooking time so the fruit can pick up more of the flavors in the poaching liquid. The amount of sugar depends on the natural sweetness of the fruit and how sweet you wish the dessert to be. It also depends on how firm the fruit is, as softer fruit needs more sugar in the poaching liquid so that the shape can be maintained. Amounts of sugar can range from 5 oz to 1 pound per quart of liquid. Other sweeteners like honey, maple syrup, and brown sugar can be substituted for table sugar for added flavor and a rich caramel color.
  - To limit or avoid adding extra sugar – use fresh squeezed orange juice as the sweetener
- Optional: Choose flavorings:
  - Add a vanilla bean, whole cloves, cinnamon stick, nutmeg, fresh ginger, black peppercorns, star anise, lemon grass, and/or lemon and or orange zest
- Prepare the poaching liquid before peeling the fruit by simmering the liquid with the sweetener and seasonings for 15 minutes to ½ hour; make sure there is enough fluid to immerse the fruit
- Prepare the fruit by peeling, coring, or seeding
- Immerse the prepared fruit in the poaching liquid and simmer gently until just tender, turning halfway through. The fruit is done when a knife can be inserted easily—this may take minutes to an hour.

*Note: If you are using softer fruit or desire a firmer texture, pour the hot poaching liquid over the prepared fruit, cover, and let cool completely overnight. This will preserve the fruit's integrity, shape, and flavor.

- Fruit can be cooled in the poaching liquid if it is firm and removed if the fruit is a softer fruit. In addition – as often occurs – the poaching liquid can be reduced to a syrup that can be drizzled over the fruit.
- Serve the fruit alone or with frozen yogurt or sorbet

Poached fruit can be a dessert, and appetizer or served as a component in another dish such as a salad.

Juniper Berry Poached Pears: The poaching liquid is a red wine, which has Juniper berries and crackled black peppercorns added to it with a touch of honey.

Autumn Poached Apples: The poaching liquid is apple juice, which has cinnamon sticks, ground nutmeg, and a slice of fresh ginger added to it. It can be served with toasted nuts and a dab of sour cream.

Video: Poach Fruit

GRILLED FRUIT

Grilling fruit caramelizes the flavor and adds a smoky flavor, not to mention the appealing grill marks. Grilled fruit can be served as is or topped with yogurt, cheese, honey, balsamic reduction, microgreens, herbs, nuts, or a combination of toppings. Grilled lemon halves are a great garnish for seafood. Grilled fruit, such as grilled pineapple and black bean salsa, also tastes great when added to salsa.

Instructions

- Select fruit that is ripe but firm enough to hold together on the grill.
  - Peaches, nectarines, watermelon, melon, mango, pineapple, and lemon halves keep their shape when grilled
- Cut fruit to uniform size for even cooking. Whole fruit like peaches or nectarines should be halved and pitted. Smaller chunks like diced pineapple or melon can be threaded on skewers for easy handling.

- Optional: Gently marinade fruit before grilling to add some new and intense flavors. For example, adding some chopped chilies, a favorite vinegar, or olive oil
- Optional: add a touch of salt and pepper before grilling
- Preheat the grill to a moderately high temperature. If the fruit has not been marinating beforehand, spray or lightly brush the fruit with a neutral-flavored oil to prevent sticking. Grill the fruit over direct heat until lightly charred on each side, then keep the fruit warm and off to the side.
- Optional: After grilling, dress the fruit with some lemon or lime juice. Add dried spices like Chile powder for an added kick of flavor. Top with yogurt or a bit of cheese. The following are some scrumptious combinations.

Grilled Peaches with Feta: grill peaches, sprinkle with feta cheese and toasted walnuts, and drizzle a balsamic reduction over the top.

Spicy Grilled Watermelon: After the watermelon has been grilled, splash briefly with lime juice and dip the edges in a spicy taco spice mix (Chile powder, cumin, salt and pepper, sweet paprika, dried onion, and garlic). If you don't want to make your own, Skordo has a great taco mix.

Grilled Peaches with Ricotta: Cut peaches in half, remove the pit, and rub with salt and olive oil. Grill cut side down over high heat until slightly softened and charred on the face. Remove from the heat and dress with a splash of lime juice. Fill the cavity where the pit was with ricotta cheese and serve as a base for a green salad alongside some grilled salmon or chicken.

DEHYDRATED FRUIT

Drying fruit is a great way to preserve fruit at its peak of ripeness. It makes a great portable snack and is a delicious addition to granola, oatmeal, and salads. Drying the fruit yourself avoids additives that may be used in commercially dried fruit. While drying methods vary from solar to oven drying to using an electric dehydrator, most fruit dries best at a temperature of 125°F/52°C to 135°F/57°C, so the dehydrator produces the most consistent results.

Instructions

- **Prepare the fruit:** Select fruit that is ripe, unbruised, and free of mold.
  - Wash well and dry
  - Cut into even slices ¼ to ½ inch thick
  - Fruit can be peeled or not, depending on preference (leaving the skin on adds fiber)
  - Fruits with tough skins like cranberries, cherries, or plums should be "cracked" by

blanching briefly in boiling water for 30 to 60 seconds, then shocking in cold water
  - Preheat fruit that will discolor, like bananas, apples, pears, or peaches, by soaking for ten minutes in a solution of lemon juice and water (1 cup per quart of water)
- **Dry the fruit and test for doneness**
  - Place fruit in a single layer on the dehydrator racks following the manufacturer's directions at temperatures between 125°F/52°C to 135°F/57°C
  - Drying time can vary according to humidity, volume, and equipment
  - Fruit is dried when it is leathery and won't stick together when folded over
  - When cut in half, no moisture should be evident
- **Store the fruit:** The University of Colorado Extension Service* recommends "conditioning" the fruit before storage to even out the small amount of remaining moisture in order to reduce spoilage.
  - Cool fruit to room temperature and store fruit in a loosely covered glass jar in a well-ventilated area for four to seven days. Shake daily to avoid fruit sticking together
  - If moisture becomes evident, return it to the food dehydrator and condition it again
  - Store in a tightly covered jar, in a cool dark place, or in a freezer for six to twelve months

*https://extension.colostate.edu/topic-areas/nutrition-food-safety-health/drying-fruits-9-309/

To make fruit roll-ups, use puréed fruit and place in the dehydrator.

Safety Tips: Use a separate cutting board for produce and meats/poultry. Wash the cutting board and utensils with detergent and air dry between uses.

SECTION 10:
SERVING FRUIT

When planning a menu, make sure that whole fruit is served two to three times throughout the day. Breakfast is a great time to serve fresh fruit, as is dessert and snack time, but any time is good. Table 12 lists the number of servings of fruit each day for various age and gender groups. Keep the total daily amount in mind when planning the menu and focus on whole fruit.

Table 12: Fruit Servings per Day

Age (years)	Amount per Day	Serving Size
12 to 23 months	½ to 1 cup	2 to 4 tablespoons
2 to 4	1 to 1 ½ cups	¼ to 1/3 cup juice; 2 inches of a banana cut up in small pieces; ¼ to 1/3 cup applesauce
5 to 8	1 to 2 cups	½ cup juice; 4 inches of a banana; ½ cup applesauce; 16 grapes; ½ small apple; 1 small peach, pear, or orange
Boys 9 to 13	1 ½ to 2 cups	¾ cup juice; 1 cup diced fruit; 1 large orange, peach, or apple; 6 inch banana
Girls 9 to 13	1 ½ to 2 cups	
Boys 14 to 18	2 to 2 ½ cups	1 cup juice; 1 cup diced fruit; 1 large orange, peach, or apple; 8 to 9 inch banana
Girls 14 to 18	1 ½ to 2 cups	
Women 19 to 30	1 ½ to 2 cups	
Women 31 to 59	1 ½ to 2 cups	
Women 60+	1 ½ to 2 cups	
Men 19 to 30	2 to 2 ½ cups	
Men 31 to 59	2 to 2 ½ cups	
Men 60+	2 cups	

Accessed from https://www.myplate.gov/eat-healthy/fruits 4/2022

SECTION 11:

PRACTICAL TIPS TO INCREASE FRUIT CONSUMPTION

1. Keep fruit out on the counter, ready to eat.
2. Prepare a fruit salad close to serving time so it is at its freshest
3. Keep fruit where it is easily seen like near the front of the refrigerator shelf, for example.
4. Make fruit fun and appealing by making kebabs.
5. Teach children (no matter what age) that gummy fruit is not a fruit serving and to think of it as a treat (like a candy bar). They are a concentrated source of sugar. Try the "real food doesn't bounce" experiment where you drop an apple and then bounce a gummy fruit. The message is delivered without nagging.
6. Eat fruit three times a day: at meals and snacks.
7. Serve fruit with cheese for dessert.

8. Mobile produce markets increase fruit consumption, especially if they are located in the right location (Hsiao et al., 2019).
9. School food environmental policies can increase fruit consumption (Micha et al., 2018).
10. Parents' intake of fruits and vegetables is associated with their child's intake (Gasser et al., 2018).

SUMMARY

Fruit is a staple component of healthful diets around the world, and diets high in fruit and vegetable intake have been shown to improve cardiovascular health and reduce the risk of hypertension, diabetes, and cognitive decline. Fruits are an incredibly nutrient-dense food as they are packed full of vitamins and minerals (such as vitamins A and C), fiber, and phytonutrients, many of which have antioxidant and anti-inflammatory properties. Fruits also support a healthy gut microbiome by functioning as a prebiotic.

Despite the numerous nutritional benefits of fruit, less than 15% of adults meet the recommendations for fruit intake each day. Fortunately, there are many ways and opportunities to incorporate a variety of fruits into one's daily eating habits. There is incredible variety within the fruit food group itself, from deep red and yellow fruits like mangos and cantaloupe to red fruits like strawberries to blue or purple fruits like many of the berries. There is an endless assortment of ways to prepare and serve fruit, from fresh to poached to grilled. Regardless of the fruit or preparation method, incorporating fruit into one's diet not only provides a delicious source of flavor and sweetness but also can lead to numerous health benefits.

REFERENCES

2015–2020 Dietary Guidelines for Americans—Health.gov. (2015). https://health.gov/dietaryguidelines/2015/

American Cancer Society. (2017, August 25). It's Easy to Add Fruits and Vegetables to Your Diet. American Cancer Society. https://www.cancer.org/healthy/eat-healthy-get-active/eat-healthy/add-fruits-and-veggies-to-your-diet.html

American Heart Association. (2017). Fruits and Vegetables Serving Sizes. American Heart Association. https://www.heart.org/en/healthy-living/healthy-eating/add-color/fruits-and-vegetables-serving-sizes

Atkinson, F. S., Foster-Powell, K., & Brand-Miller, J. C. (2008). International Tables of Glycemic Index and Glycemic Load Values: 2008. Diabetes Care, 31(12), 2281–2283. https://doi.org/10.2337/dc08-1239

Aubrey, A. (2013). The Salt: Canned Peaches Are As Nutritious As Fresh. Really? NPR.Org. https://www.npr.org/sections/thesalt/2013/05/22/186025393/canned-peaches-are-as-nutritious-as-fresh-really

Bazzano, L. A., Li, T. Y., Joshipura, K. J., & Hu, F. B. (2008). Intake of fruit, vegetables, and fruit juices and risk of diabetes in women. Diabetes Care, 31(7), 1311–1317. https://doi.org/10.2337/dc08-0080

Bertelli, A. A. A., & Das, D. K. (2009). Grapes, wines, resveratrol, and heart health. Journal of Cardiovascular Pharmacology, 54(6), 468–476. https://doi.org/10.1097/FJC.0b013e3181bfaff3

Bertoia, M. L., Mukamal, K. J., Cahill, L. E., Hou, T., Ludwig, D. S., Mozaffarian, D., Willett, W. C., Hu, F. B., & Rimm, E. B. (2015). Changes in Intake of Fruits and Vegetables and Weight Change in United States Men and Women Followed for Up to 24 Years: Analysis from Three Prospective Cohort Studies. PLOS Medicine, 12(9), e1001878. https://doi.org/10.1371/journal.pmed.1001878

Bouzari, A., Holstege, D., & Barrett, D. M. (2015a). Mineral, fiber, and total phenolic retention in eight fruits and vegetables: A comparison of refrigerated and frozen storage. Journal of Agricultural and Food Chemistry, 63(3), 951–956. https://doi.org/10.1021/jf504890k

Bouzari, A., Holstege, D., & Barrett, D. M. (2015b). Vitamin retention in eight fruits and vegetables: A comparison of refrigerated and frozen storage. Journal of Agricultural and Food Chemistry, 63(3), 957–962. https://doi.org/10.1021/jf5058793

Brophy, L. (2015). Geriatric Nutrition: Late-Onset Food Allergies. Today's Dietitian, 17(10), 76.

Brownawell, A. M., Caers, W., Gibson, G. R., Kendall, C. W. C., Lewis, K. D., Ringel, Y., & Slavin, J. L. (2012). Prebiotics and the health benefits of fiber: Current regulatory status, future research, and goals. The Journal of Nutrition, 142(5), 962–974. https://doi.org/10.3945/jn.112.158147

Calvano, A., Izuora, K., Oh, E. C., Ebersole, J. L., Lyons, T. J., & Basu, A. (2019). Dietary berries, insulin resistance and type 2 diabetes: An overview of human feeding trials. Food & Function, 10(10), 6227–6243. https://doi.org/10.1039/c9fo01426h

Carlsen, M. H., Halvorsen, B. L., Holte, K., Bøhn, S. K., Dragland, S., Sampson, L., Willey, C., Senoo, H., Umezono, Y., Sanada, C., Barikmo, I., Berhe, N., Willett, W. C., Phillips, K. M., Jacobs, D. R., & Blomhoff, R. (2010). The total antioxidant content of more than 3100 foods, beverages, spices, herbs and supplements used worldwide. Nutrition Journal, 9, 3. https://doi.org/10.1186/1475-2891-9-3

Cassidy, A., Mukamal, K. J., Liu, L., Franz, M., Eliassen, A. H., & Rimm, E. B. (2013). High anthocyanin intake is associated with a reduced risk of myocardial infarction in young and middle-aged women. Circulation, 127(2), 188–196. https://doi.org/10.1161/CIRCULATIONAHA.112.122408

CDC. (2019, June 5). Children Eating More Fruit, but Fruit and Vegetable Intake Still Too Low. Center for Disease Control. https://www.cdc.gov/nccdphp/dnpao/division-information/media-tools/dpk/vs-fruits-vegetables/index.html

Chen, M., Zhou, S.-Y., Fabriaga, E., Zhang, P.-H., & Zhou, Q. (2018). Food-drug interactions precipitated by fruit juices other than grapefruit juice: An update review. Journal of Food and Drug Analysis, 26(2S), S61–S71. https://doi.org/10.1016/j.jfda.2018.01.009

Cho, E., Seddon, J. M., Rosner, B., Willett, W. C., & Hankinson, S. E. (2004). Prospective study of intake of fruits, vegetables, vitamins, and carotenoids and risk of age-related maculopathy. Archives of Ophthalmology (Chicago, Ill.: 1960), 122(6), 883–892. https://doi.org/10.1001/archopht.122.6.883

Consumer Reports. (2015). Eat the Peach, Not the Pesticide (Pesticides in Produce). https://www.consumerreports.org/cro/produce0515

Cook, J. D., & Reddy, M. B. (2001). Effect of ascorbic acid intake on nonheme-iron absorption from a complete diet. The American Journal of Clinical Nutrition, 73(1), 93–98. https://doi.org/10.1093/ajcn/73.1.93

Cooper, A. J., Forouhi, N. G., Ye, Z., Buijsse, B., Arriola, L., Balkau, B., Barricarte, A., Beulens, J. W. J., Boeing, H., Büchner, F. L., Dahm, C. C., de Lauzon-Guillain, B., Fagherazzi, G., Franks, P. W., Gonzalez, C., Grioni, S., Kaaks, R., Key, T. J., Masala, G., ... InterAct Consortium. (2012). Fruit and vegetable intake and type 2 diabetes: EPIC-InterAct prospective study and meta-analysis. European Journal of Clinical Nutrition, 66(10), 1082–1092. https://doi.org/10.1038/ejcn.2012.85

Curl Cynthia L, Fenske Richard A, & Elgethun Kai. (2003). Organophosphorus pesticide exposure of urban and suburban preschool children with organic and conventional diets. Environmental Health Perspectives, 111(3), 377–382. https://doi.org/10.1289/ehp.5754

Dauchet, L., Amouyel, P., Hercberg, S., & Dallongeville, J. (2006). Fruit and vegetable consumption and risk of coronary heart disease: A meta-analysis of cohort studies. The Journal of Nutrition, 136(10), 2588–2593. https://doi.org/10.1093/jn/136.10.2588

Dominianni, C., Sinha, R., Goedert, J. J., Pei, Z., Yang, L., Hayes, R. B., & Ahn, J. (2015). Sex, Body Mass Index, and Dietary Fiber Intake Influence the Human Gut Microbiome. PLoS ONE, 10(4). https://doi.org/10.1371/journal.pone.0124599

Economos, C., & Clay, W. D. (1998). Nutritional and health benefits of citrus fruits. Twelfth Session of the Intergovernmental Group on Citrus Fruit, Valencia, Spain. http://www.fao.org/3/x2650t/x2650t03.htm

Environmental Working Group. (2021). Dirty Dozen™ Fruits and Vegetables with the Most Pesticides. https://www.ewg.org/foodnews/dirty-dozen.php

Erdman, J. W., Balentine, D., Arab, L., Beecher, G., Dwyer, J. T., Folts, J., Harnly, J., Hollman, P., Keen, C. L., Mazza, G., Messina, M., Scalbert, A., Vita, J., Williamson, G., & Burrowes, J. (2007). Flavonoids and heart health: Proceedings of the ILSI North America Flavonoids Workshop, May 31-June 1, 2005, Washington, DC. The Journal of Nutrition, 137(3 Suppl 1), 718S-737S. https://doi.org/10.1093/jn/137.3.718S

Fabiani, R., Minelli, L., & Rosignoli, P. (2016). Apple intake and cancer risk: A systematic review and meta-analysis of observational studies. Public Health Nutrition, 19(14), 2603–2617. https://doi.org/10.1017/S136898001600032X

Farvid, M. S., Cho, E., Chen, W. Y., Eliassen, A. H., & Willett, W. C. (2015). Adolescent meat intake and breast cancer risk. International Journal of Cancer. Journal International Du Cancer, 136(8), 1909–1920. https://doi.org/10.1002/ijc.29218

Fernandez, M. A., & Marette, A. (2017). Potential Health Benefits of Combining Yogurt and Fruits Based on Their Probiotic and Prebiotic Properties. Advances in Nutrition: An International Review Journal, 8(1), 155S-164S. https://doi.org/10.3945/an.115.011114

García-Casal, M. N., Layrisse, M., Solano, L., Barón, M. A., Arguello, F., Llovera, D., Ramírez, J., Leets, I., & Tropper, E. (1998). Vitamin A and beta-carotene can improve nonheme iron absorption from rice, wheat and corn by humans. The Journal of Nutrition, 128(3), 646–650. https://doi.org/10.1093/jn/128.3.646

Gasser, C. E., Mensah, F. K., Clifford, S. A., Kerr, J. A., & Wake, M. (2018). Parental health behaviour predictors of childhood and adolescent dietary trajectories. Public Health Nutrition, 21(10), 1874–1885. https://doi.org/10.1017/S1368980018000563

Gibson, G. R., & Roberfroid, M. B. (1995). Dietary modulation of the human colonic microbiota: Introducing the concept of prebiotics. The Journal of Nutrition, 125(6), 1401–1412. https://doi.org/10.1093/jn/125.6.1401

González-Castejón, M., & Rodriguez-Casado, A. (2011). Dietary phytochemicals and their potential effects on obesity: A review. Pharmacological Research, 64(5), 438–455. https://doi.org/10.1016/j.phrs.2011.07.004

He, F. J., Nowson, C. A., Lucas, M., & MacGregor, G. A. (2007). Increased consumption of fruit and vegetables is related to a reduced risk of coronary heart disease: Meta-analysis of cohort studies. Journal of Human Hypertension, 21(9), 717–728. https://doi.org/10.1038/sj.jhh.1002212

Heller, M. C., Willits-Smith, A., Meyer, R., Keoleian, G. A., & Rose, D. (2018). Greenhouse gas emissions and energy use associated with production of individual self-selected US diets. Environmental Research Letters, 13(4), 044004. https://doi.org/10.1088/1748-9326/aab0ac

Hlebowicz, J., Darwiche, G., Bjorgell, O., & Almer, L. (2007). Effect of cinnamon on postprandial blood glucose, gastric emptying, and satiety in healthy subjects. Am J Clin Nutr, 85, 1552–1556.

Hsiao, B.-S., Sibeko, L., & Troy, L. M. (2019). A Systematic Review of Mobile Produce Markets: Facilitators and Barriers to Use, and Associations with Reported Fruit and Vegetable Intake. Journal of the Academy of Nutrition and Dietetics, 119(1), 76-97.e1. https://doi.org/10.1016/j.jand.2018.02.022

Hung, H.-C., Joshipura, K. J., Jiang, R., Hu, F. B., Hunter, D., Smith-Warner, S. A., Colditz, G. A., Rosner, B., Spiegelman, D., & Willett, W. C. (2004). Fruit and Vegetable Intake and Risk of Major Chronic Disease. JNCI: Journal of the National Cancer Institute, 96(21), 1577–1584. https://doi.org/10.1093/jnci/djh296

Institute of Medicine (US) Standing Committee on the Scientific Evaluation of Dietary Reference Intakes and its Panel on Folate, Other B Vitamins, and Choline. (1998). Dietary Reference Intakes for Thiamin, Riboflavin, Niacin, Vitamin B6, Folate, Vitamin B12, Pantothenic Acid, Biotin, and Choline. National Academies Press (US). http://www.ncbi.nlm.nih.gov/books/NBK114310/

Johnson, S. A., Figueroa, A., Navaei, N., Wong, A., Kalfon, R., Ormsbee, L. T., Feresin, R. G., Elam, M. L., Hooshmand, S., Payton, M. E., & Arjmandi, B. H. (2015). Daily blueberry consumption improves blood pressure and arterial stiffness in postmenopausal women with pre- and stage 1-hypertension: A randomized, double-blind, placebo-controlled clinical trial. Journal of the Academy of Nutrition and Dietetics, 115(3), 369–377. https://doi.org/10.1016/j.jand.2014.11.001

Kennedy, J. (2014, July 9). Artificial vs Natural Peach [Academic Blog]. James Kennedy. https://jameskennedymonash.wordpress.com/category/infographics/artificial-vs-natural-foods/

Krikorian, R., Shidler, M. D., Nash, T. A., Kalt, W., Vinqvist-Tymchuk, M. R., Shukitt-Hale, B., & Joseph, J. A. (2010). Blueberry supplementation improves memory in older adults. Journal of Agricultural and Food Chemistry, 58(7), 3996–4000. https://doi.org/10.1021/jf9029332

Lee-Kwan, S. H. (2017). Disparities in State-Specific Adult Fruit and Vegetable Consumption—United States, 2015. MMWR. Morbidity and Mortality Weekly Report, 66. https://doi.org/10.15585/mmwr.mm6645a1

Mekonnen, M., & Hoekstra, A. (2010). The green, blue and grey water footprint of farm animals and animal products. American Journal of Hematology - AMER J HEMATOL.

Micha, R., Karageorgou, D., Bakogianni, I., Trichia, E., Whitsel, L. P., Story, M., Peñalvo, J. L., & Mozaffarian, D. (2018). Effectiveness of school food environment policies on children's dietary behaviors: A systematic review and meta-analysis. PloS One, 13(3), e0194555. https://doi.org/10.1371/journal.pone.0194555

Moore, L. V., Thompson, F. E., & Demissie, Z. (2017). Percentage of Youth Meeting Federal Fruit and Vegetable Intake Recommendations, Youth Risk Behavior Surveillance System, United States and 33 States, 2013. Journal of the Academy of Nutrition and Dietetics, 117(4), 545-553.e3. https://doi.org/10.1016/j.jand.2016.10.012

Morris, M. C. (2012). Nutritional determinants of cognitive aging and dementia. Proceedings of the Nutrition Society, 71(1), 1–13. https://doi.org/10.1017/S0029665111003296

Mujcic, R., & J Oswald, A. (2016). Evolution of Well-Being and Happiness After Increases in Consumption of Fruit and Vegetables. American Journal of Public Health, 106(8), 1504–1510. https://doi.org/10.2105/AJPH.2016.303260

Muluk, N. B., & Cingi, C. (2018). Oral allergy syndrome. American Journal of Rhinology & Allergy, 32(1), 27–30. https://doi.org/10.2500/ajra.2018.32.4489

Muraki, I., Imamura, F., Manson, J. E., Hu, F. B., Willett, W. C., van Dam, R. M., & Sun, Q. (2013). Fruit consumption and risk of type 2 diabetes: Results from three prospective longitudinal cohort studies. BMJ (Clinical Research Ed.), 347, f5001. https://doi.org/10.1136/bmj.f5001

Nicklett, E. J., Semba, R. D., Xue, Q.-L., Tian, J., Sun, K., Cappola, A. R., Simonsick, E. M., Ferrucci, L., & Fried, L. P. (2012). Fruit and vegetable intake, physical activity, and mortality in older community-dwelling women. Journal of the American Geriatrics Society, 60(5), 862–868. https://doi.org/10.1111/j.1532-5415.2012.03924.x

Oregon State University. (2014, November 17). Micronutrient Information Center: Dietary Factors. Linus Pauling Institute. https://lpi.oregonstate.edu/mic/dietary-factors

Ostman, E., Granfeldt, Y., Persson, L., & Bjorck, I. (2005). Vinegar supplementation lowers glucose and insulin responses and increases satiety after a bread meal in healthy subjects. EJCN, 59, 983–988.

Palmer, S. (2008). The Top Fiber-Rich Foods List. Today's Dietitian. https://www.todaysdietitian.com/newarchives/063008p28.shtml

Parajuli, R., Thoma, G., & Matlock, M. (2019). Environmental sustainability of fruit and vegetable production supply chains in the face of climate change: A review. Science of The Total Environment, 650, 2863–2879. https://doi.org/10.1016/j.scitotenv.2018.10.019

Pennington, J. A. T., & Fisher, R. A. (2010). Food component profiles for fruit and vegetable subgroups. Journal of Food Composition and Analysis, 23(5), 411–418. https://doi.org/10.1016/j.jfca.2010.01.008

PMA. (2018). Top 20 Fruits and Vegetables Sold in the U.S. 2018. Produce Marketing Association. https://www.pma.com/content/articles/2017/05/top-20-fruits-and-vegetables-sold-in-the-us

Portela, S. I., & Cantwell, M. I. (2001). Cutting Blade Sharpness Affects Appearance and Other Quality Attributes of Fresh-cut Cantaloupe Melon. Journal of Food Science, 66(9), 1265–1270. https://doi.org/10.1111/j.1365-2621.2001.tb15199.x

Produce for Better Health Foundation. (2015). State of the Plate, 2015 Study on America's Consumption of Fruits and Vegetables. Produce for Better Health Foundation. <http://www.PBHFoundation.org>

Ramsay, S. A., Eskelsen, A. K., Branen, L. J., Armstrong Shultz, J., & Plumb, J. (2014). Nutrient Intake and Consumption of Fruit and Vegetables in Young Children. ICAN: Infant, Child, & Adolescent Nutrition, 6(6), 332–344. https://doi.org/10.1177/1941406414549622

Sanders, M. E., Lenoir-Wijnkoop, I., Salminen, S., Merenstein, D. J., Gibson, G. R., Petschow, B. W., Nieuwdorp, M., Tancredi, D. J., Cifelli, C. J., Jacques, P., & Pot, B. (2014). Probiotics and prebiotics: Prospects for public health and nutritional recommendations. Annals of the New York Academy of Sciences, 1309, 19–29. https://doi.org/10.1111/nyas.12377

Serafini, M., & Peluso, I. (2016). Functional Foods for Health: The Interrelated Antioxidant and Anti-Inflammatory Role of Fruits, Vegetables, Herbs, Spices and Cocoa in Humans. Current Pharmaceutical Design, 22(44), 6701–6715. https://doi.org/10.2174/1381612823666161123094235

Shahbandeh, M. (2019). U.S. canned fruit consumption per capita. Statista. https://www.statista.com/statistics/257134/per-capita-consumption-of-canned-fruit-in-the-us/

Shishtar, E., Rogers, G. T., Blumberg, J. B., Au, R., & Jacques, P. F. (2020). Long-term dietary flavonoid intake and risk of Alzheimer disease and related dementias in the Framingham Offspring Cohort. The American Journal of Clinical Nutrition. https://doi.org/10.1093/ajcn/nqaa079

Singh, B., Singh, J. P., Kaur, A., & Singh, N. (2016). Bioactive compounds in banana and their associated health benefits—A review. Food Chemistry, 206, 1–11. https://doi.org/10.1016/j.foodchem.2016.03.033

Slavin, J. L., & Lloyd, B. (2012). Health benefits of fruits and vegetables. Advances in Nutrition (Bethesda, Md.), 3(4), 506–516. https://doi.org/10.3945/an.112.002154

Tanzi, M. (2013). Juice interactions: What patients need to know. https://www.pharmacytoday.org/article/S1042-0991(15)31392-X/pdf

Torres-Gonzalez, M., Cifelli, C., Agarwal, S., & Fulgoni, V. (2019). Sodium and Potassium in the American Diet: Important Food Sources from NHANES 2015–2016 (P18-045-19). Current Developments in Nutrition, 3(Supplement_1). https://doi.org/10.1093/cdn/nzz039.P18-045-19

Tyagi, S., Nanher, A. H., Sahay, S., Kumar, V., Bhamini, K., Nishad, S. K., & Ahmad, M. (2015). Kiwifruit: Health benefits and medicinal importance. 10, 3.

USDA. (2018). FoodData Central. FoodData Central | U.S. Department of Agriculture, Agricultural Research Service. https://fdc.nal.usda.gov/

USDA & HHS. (2015). Dietary Guidelines for Americans 2015-2020. U.S. Department of Health and Human Services and U.S. Department of Agriculture. https://health.gov/dietaryguidelines/2015/guidelines/

Wang, X., Ouyang, Y., Liu, J., Zhu, M., Zhao, G., Bao, W., & Hu, F. B. (2014). Fruit and vegetable consumption and mortality from all causes, cardiovascular disease, and cancer: Systematic review and dose-response meta-analysis of prospective cohort studies. BMJ (Clinical Research Ed.), 349, g4490. https://doi.org/10.1136/bmj.g4490

Whatnall, M. C., Patterson, A. J., Burrows, T. L., & Hutchesson, M. J. (2019). Higher diet quality in university students is associated with higher academic achievement: A cross-sectional study. Journal of Human Nutrition and Dietetics: The Official Journal of the British Dietetic Association, 32(3), 321–328. https://doi.org/10.1111/jhn.12632

Wiseman, M., Cannon, G., Butrum, R., Martin, G., Higginbotham, S., Heggie, S., Jones, C., & Fletcher, M. (2007). Food, Nutrition, Physical Activity and the Prevention of Cancer: A Global Perspective. Summary.

VEGETABLES

~

By Betsy Redmond, PhD, MMSc, RDN,
Julia Hilbrands MS, MPH, RD
and Deborah Kennedy PhD
with
The Expert Chef Panel

"Eat food. Not too much. Mostly plants."
Quote by Micheal Pollal

THE ENCYCLOPEDIA BRITANNICA DEFINES vegetables as "any kind of plant life or plant product," namely "vegetable matter." In common, narrow usage, the term vegetable usually refers to the fresh edible portions of certain herbaceous plants — roots, stems, leaves, flowers, fruit, or seeds (Vegetable, 2020). While fruit is a very specific part of a plant used for reproduction — the mature ovary of a flowering plant — vegetables include many other parts of the plant itself, such as the stems, leaves, and roots. There are some foods that are botanically considered a fruit, but because of their savory element, chefs consider them vegetables — the tomato, bell pepper, and eggplant are examples. The "is it a fruit or a vegetable?" debate has been ongoing for over a century, and in 1893, the Supreme Court stepped in regarding whether or not a tomato was to be taxed as a fruit or a vegetable. Their determination was to use the ordinary definitions of fruit and vegetable, not the official botanical definition and determined that imported tomatoes should be taxed as a vegetable (higher tax) rather than a fruit (lower tax).

For the purpose of this chapter, vegetables will be defined from both a culinary perspective and how these plants are listed in the USDA guidelines. Vegetables that are botanically considered fruits but will be discussed here include avocados, corn, cucumbers, eggplant, okra, olives, legumes (chickpeas and beans), peas, peppers, pumpkin, string beans, tomato and zucchini. For a great read on the classifications of vegetables versus fruit, read Merriam Webster's "Fruit vs. Vegetable.

While the sweetness of most fruits attracts animals for consumption and the spreading of their seeds, vegetables do the opposite with a taste that is typically bitter. A fruit says, "come here" while a vegetable says, "stay away." It has been widely proposed that, from an evolutionary perspective, plants that were sweet were usually healthful, and those that were bitter were poisonous. Our ancient ancestors learned to avoid bitter foods and prefer sweet ones; one reason many parents struggle nightly at the dinner table trying to get their children to eat their vegetables is that they are fighting thousands of years of genetic programming. The good news is that we no longer have to worry about vegetables being poisonous, and we can train our taste buds to like the taste of a variety of vegetables.

SECTION 1:
VEGETABLE CHARACTERISTICS

Image: Vegetable Characteristics

PARTS OF THE PLANT

Vegetables are commonly classified by the part of the plant they come from, such as the root, bulb, fruit, leaf, flower, seed, or stem. The different plant parts offer slightly different tastes, textures, and nutrient profiles. Take roots and leaves: Roots are high in soluble fibers and can be stored for long periods of time, though some contain toxic secondary metabolites, such as the cassava root, which must be soaked in water prior to consumption (Kalala et al., 2018a; Slavin & Lloyd, 2012a), while leafy vegetables, on the other hand, are generally higher in protein and insoluble fiber. Table 1 lists examples of common edible plant parts.

Table 1: Vegetables Divided by Plant Parts

Plant Part	Vegetable Examples
Root and Tubers	Beets, carrots, celeriac, ginger, yams, turnips, parsnips, sweet potatoes, radishes, rutabagas, Jerusalem artichokes
Bulb	Garlic, shallots, fennel, onion
Stem	Asparagus, cardoons

Plant Part	Vegetable Examples
Seed	Fava beans, red kidney beans, white beans, green beans, lentils, corn, peas, chickpeas, soy
Flower	Artichoke, broccoli, cauliflower
Leaf	Chard, celery, Brussels sprouts, green cabbage, endive, spinach, bitter beans, lettuce, parsley, sorrel, leeks, dandelion greens, purslane, arugula
Fruit	Eggplant, avocado, chestnuts, cucumbers, zucchini, gherkins, squash, melons, peppers, tomatoes, pumpkins, peppers (capsicums)
Intermediate form	Button mushrooms, hearts of palm

Ancient fossils of vegetables date back millions of years, and certain vegetable varieties that were cultivated thousands of years ago looked and tasted very differently, and many would be unrecognizable to us today. It is only through selective breeding processes for traits like flavor, size, and color over thousands of years that we have the varieties we are familiar with today.

VEGETABLE SUBGROUPS

Another way vegetables are categorized is by subgroup. Vegetable subgroups were initially introduced in the Dietary Guidelines for Americans (DGA) with the purpose of helping consumers better achieve **vegetable variety** in their diets (U.S. Department of Health and Human Services and U.S. Department of Agriculture, 2005). The Dietary Guidelines for Americans Healthy Eating Pattern categorizes vegetables into five subgroups: dark green, red, and orange, legumes (beans and peas), starchy, and others. The goal is to eat vegetables from each of the subgroups every week in order to consume a full array of nutrients, as each subgroup provides its own unique combination of vitamins, minerals, and phytonutrients. Table 2 reviews each subgroup with vegetable examples and common nutrients found in each.

Table 2: Vegetable Subgroups According to the USDA DGA (USDA DGA 2020-2025)

Subgroup	Vegetable	Common Nutrients
Dark Green Vegetables	Broccoli, spinach, leafy salad greens (including romaine lettuce), collards, bok choy, kale, turnip greens, mustard greens, green herbs (such as parsley or cilantro), beet greens	Vitamin A, vitamin C, folate, vitamin K, potassium, nitrates, sulfur, glucosinolates (a phytochemical), fiber, vitamin B_2, vitamin B_6, lutein and zeaxanthin
Red/Orange	Tomatoes and tomato juice, carrots, sweet potatoes, red peppers (hot and sweet), winter squash, pumpkin	Vitamin A (beta-carotene), vitamin C, potassium, fiber, lycopene

Subgroup	Vegetable	Common Nutrients
Beans, Peas, Lentils	Pinto, white, kidney, and black beans; lentils; chickpeas; lima beans (mature, dried); split peas; edamame (soybeans)	Magnesium, folate, potassium, isoflavones, fiber
Starchy Vegetables	Potatoes, corn, green peas, lima beans (green, immature), cassava	Potassium, fiber, choline, magnesium
Other Vegetables	Lettuce (iceberg), onions, green beans, cucumbers, celery, green peppers, cabbage, mushrooms, avocado, summer squash, zucchini, cauliflower, eggplant, garlic, bean sprouts, olives, asparagus, snow peas, beets, artichokes	Vitamin C, fiber, potassium, choline, magnesium isoflavones, fiber, potassium

SECTION 2:
RECOMMENDATIONS FOR VEGETABLE INTAKE

Clinicians and researchers alike agree that a healthful diet comprises a large quantity and wide variety of vegetables. However, the exact number of vegetable servings one should eat each day differs slightly between leading authorities, such as the Dietary Guidelines for Americans, the National Institutes of Health, and the American Heart Association. The Dietary Guidelines for Americans also went a step further and made specific intake recommendations for each vegetable subgroup.

Official recommendations that combine fruit and vegetable intake range from the low end of at least 400 g/day (five servings/day) to the highest recommendation of 640 to 800 g/day (eight to 10 servings/day) (2015-2020 Dietary Guidelines | Health.Gov; Aune et al., 2017a; Eat Whole Grains, Vegetables, Fruit & Beans, 2018). **One vegetable serving is considered to be a half cup of fresh, frozen, or canned vegetables; one cup of raw leafy green vegetables; or a half-cup of vegetable juice.** Table 3 outlines various recommendations for vegetable intake from leading authorities. For more information on servings and portions, go to the chapter on *Servings and Portions.*

Table 3: Recommended Vegetable Intake from Different Authoritative Sources

Source	Recommended Servings
2015 – 2020 Dietary Guidelines for Americans[a]	2 ½ cup equivalents or 5 servings/day Serving examples: 1 ½ cups/week dark green 5 ½ cups/week red and orange 1 ½ cups/week legumes 5 cups/ week starchy 4 cups/week other
National Institutes of Health DASH* Diet Plan[b]	4 to 5 servings/day Serving examples: 1 cup raw leafy vegetables ½ cup cooked vegetables 6 ounces vegetable juice
American Heart Association[c]	5 servings /day Serving examples: 1 cup raw leafy greens ½ cup cut-up vegetables ½ cup cooked beans or peas ¼ cup 100% vegetable juice
Harvard T.H. Chan School of Public Health: The Healthy Eating Plate[d]	Half of the plate should be vegetables and fruit, with more vegetables than fruit
MIND diet (A combination of the Mediterranean and DASH diet patterns)e	2 or more servings/day, one of which is a green leafy vegetable
Mediterranean Diet	Aim for 7 to 10 servings of fruits and vegetables

*DASH = Dietary Approaches to Stop Hypertension
a) 2015-2020 Dietary Guidelines | Health.Gov
b) DASH Eating Plan | National Heart, Lung, and Blood Institute (NHLBI)
c) Suggested Servings from Each Food Group, 2017
d) Healthy Eating Plate, 2012
e) (Marcason, 2015)

Figure 1: USDA MyPlate Specific Recommendations for Total Vegetable Intake

Daily Vegetable Table		
*Daily Recommendation**		
CHILDREN	2 - 3 years old 4 - 8 year old	1 cup 1 ½ cups
GIRLS	9 - 13 years old 14 - 18 years old	2 cups 2 ½ cups

Daily Vegetable Table		
Daily Recommendation*		
BOYS	9 - 13 years old 14 - 18 years old	2 ½ cups 3 cups
WOMEN	19 - 30 years old 31 - 50 years old 51+ years old	2 ½ cups 2 ½ cups 2 cups
MEN	19 - 30 years old 31 - 50 years old 51+ years old	3 cups 3 cups 2 /12 cups

Source: https://www.choosemyplate.gov/vegetables

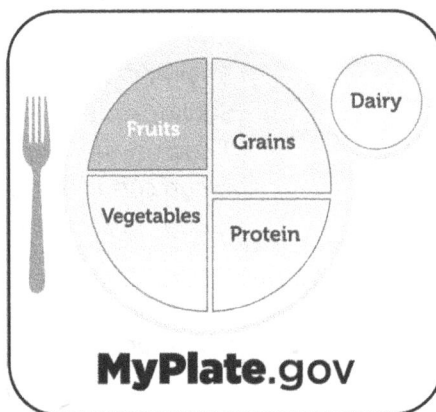

MyPlate.gov

The MyPlate guiding system provides a visual representation of these recommendations. It demonstrates that one half of one's plate should be made up of fruits and vegetables, and there should **be more vegetables than fruit on a plate**. When discussing dietary recommendations, instead of saying "eat more fruits and vegetables" in your instruction, it may be helpful to instead say "**eat more vegetables and fruit**" as your prompt. This is more descriptive of the importance of filling your plate with more vegetables than fruit.

VEGETABLE INTAKE AMONG AMERICANS

Table 4 lists the most commonly purchased vegetables in the United States. Despite frequent purchases of certain vegetables, overall, Americans are falling far short of meeting intake guidelines. Only **9.3% of adults in the United States meet the daily recommendation for total vegetable intake**, and the vast majority fall short of meeting recommendations for individual vegetable subgroups as well (Lee-Kwan, 2017). Research also suggests that when Americans do eat vegetables, they are often consumed with excess fat and sodium (Slavin & Lloyd, 2012).

Table 4: The Most Commonly Purchased Vegetables in the United States

Rank	Vegetable	Percent of Primary Shoppers Purchasing This Food
1	Potatoes	68
2	Onions	66
3	Tomatoes	65
4	Carrots	60
5	Bell peppers	53
6	Lettuce	53
7	Broccoli	51
8	Salad mix	50
9	Cucumbers	49
10	Celery	46

Source: https://www.pma.com/content/articles/2017/05/top-20-fruits-and-vegetables-sold-in-the-us

Figure 2: Average Intakes of Vegetables and Fruit Compared to Recommended Intakes: Age 1 and Older

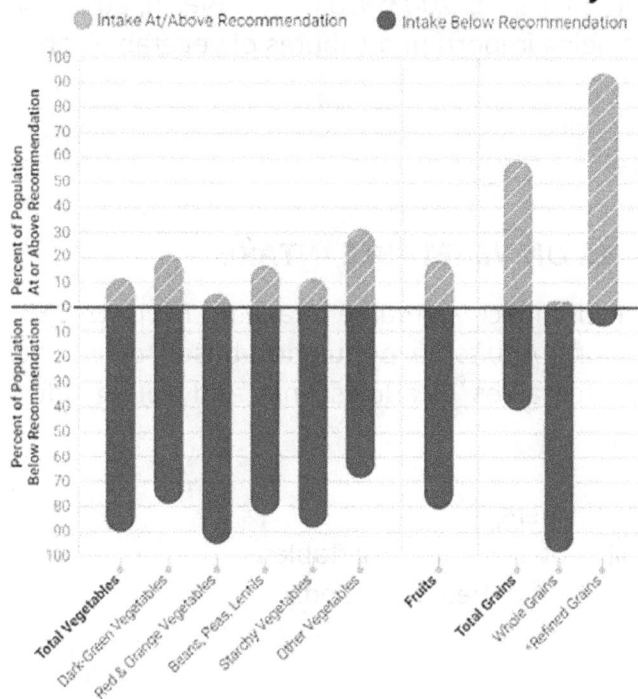

Graphs copied from pages 30 USDA DGA 2020-2025

Based on the What We Eat in America study, which reviewed 2013 – 2016 NHANES data, researchers found that over **80% of Americans do not meet the recommendations for eating vegetables** (2020-2025 Dietary Guidelines | Health.Gov). Plus, **no age or gender group as a whole meets the recommended servings of vegetable groups**. Figure 2 shows the discrepancy between recommendations from the Dietary Guidelines for Americans 2020 – 2025 and actual intake among Americans from the What We Eat in America study referenced above.

ECONOMIC INFLUENCES ON VEGETABLE INTAKE

In a survey of over 1,000 American adults, **cost and access** were the top reasons given for why less than the recommended intake of vegetables and fruits are consumed (2018 Food & Health Survey), and it has been shown that low-income individuals receiving Supplemental Nutrition Assistance Program (SNAP) benefits consume fewer vegetables than those not eligible for SNAP (Wolfson & Bleich, 2015). In economically disadvantaged families, **cooking and preparing one's own food** versus purchasing ready-to-eat food outside the home has been shown to improve the intake of vegetables, and the **frequency and complexity of preparing food at home** has been positively associated with greater consumption of vegetables and fruit (McLaughlin et al., 2003). Additionally, research has shown that SNAP participants who cooked more than six times a week ate more vegetables than those who cooked fewer than two times a week (McLaughlin et al., 2003; Wolfson & Bleich, 2015). SNAP participants report the following reasons as being important attributes of vegetable consumption:
- Price
- Ease of preparation
- How long food keeps

LIFE STAGE INFLUENCES ON VEGETABLE INTAKE

Age and life stage can also impact vegetable intake. In Projects EAT I, II, and III (Eating and Activity in Teens and Young Adults), a population-based cohort study, factors that were predictive of intake of vegetables in adolescents and young adults included (Neumark-Sztainer et al., 2003):
- Taste preferences
- Fewer perceived time barriers
- Higher home availability of fruits and vegetables
- Limited home availability of unhealthful foods
- Home food preparation

Figures 3 and 4: Vegetable Subgroup Intake in the United States

Figure 4-2
Average Intakes of Subgroups Compared to Recommended Intake Ranges: Ages 19 Through 30

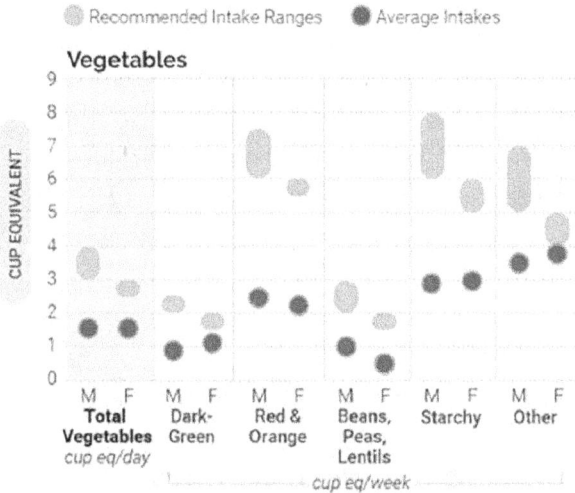

Figure 4-4
Average Intakes of Subgroups Compared to Recommended Intake Ranges: Ages 31 Through 59

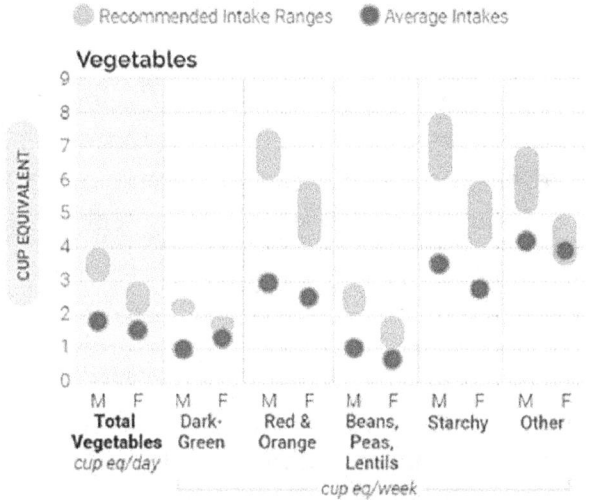

When broken down by the five vegetable subgroups (see Figures 3 and 4), very few met recommendations. There is no age group that met recommendations for dark green vegetables, red/orange vegetables, or starchy vegetables. The intake recommendations for legumes are only met by males ages 1 to 8 years old and females ages 1 to 3 and 9 to 13 years old. The only vegetable group where adults met recommendations were for "other" vegetables, which include lettuce, peppers, celery, and mushrooms. These recommendations were met by males ages 51 to 70 years and females ages 31 to 70 years (National Cancer Institute, 2019).

SECTION 3:

WHY ARE VEGETABLES SO HEALTHFUL?

The only uncontestable food in regard to its healthfulness is the mighty vegetable. Of all the populations studied in nutrition research, a **lower** vegetable intake has never been found to be related to better health, and the healthfulness of vegetables has always been positive and well-established. Because eating more vegetables is essential for the health of individuals, communities, and the planet, you will notice that a **plant-forward** diet is a strong theme throughout this textbook.

Use the correct term: The science unequivocally supports a diet high in vegetables and fruit. However, when you ask clients or patients to follow a plant-based diet or even to become a vegetarian, you are setting people up to fail. Very few individuals will become total vegans, and many will become overwhelmed when being asked to become vegetarian as well. A great strategy is to promote a plant-forward diet and let the client decide how far he, she, or they want to go. Some may go all the way to a full vegetarian or vegan lifestyle, but the majority will not. Setting realistic goals and following the patient's lead is the best strategy for long-term success.

Vegetables are made up of mostly water (~70%) and thus are usually low in calories while being full of nutrients like vitamins, minerals, and phytonutrients. This makes them a **nutrient-dense** food, meaning they have a lot of nutrients per calorie. This is in contrast to processed foods which are typically **energy-dense**, meaning few nutrients per calorie but many calories per gram weight of food. Vegetables are made up of about 3.5% protein and less than 1% fat and are an important source of vitamins and minerals. Legumes are especially high in B vitamins, vitamin C, vitamin K, magnesium, and iron; green leafy vegetables are good sources of vitamin C, folate, carotenoids, calcium, and iron; and root vegetables and tubers contribute significant amounts of vitamin E, carotenoids, iron, potassium and calcium (Jannasch et al., 2017; Slavin & Lloyd, 2012). Additionally, vegetables contain soluble and insoluble fiber and a wide array of phytochemicals, all of which are known to have a beneficial impact on the gut microbiome. However, research in this area is still evolving.

Table 5: Vegetables High in Fiber, Phytonutrients, and Nutrient Density

High Fiber	High Phytonutrients	Especially Nutrient-Dense
Artichokes	Bok choy	Beet greens
Beets	Broccoli	Chard
Broccoli	Brussels sprouts	Chicory
Brussels sprouts	Cabbage	Chinese cabbage
Carrots	Carrots	Collard greens
Green leafy vegetables (Swiss, chard, collard etc.)	Celery	Leaf lettuce
Legumes	Garlic	Parsley

High Fiber	High Phytonutrients	Especially Nutrient-Dense
Potatoes) sweet russet and red)	Kale	Romaine lettuce
Turnips	Lentils	Spinach
	Onions	Watercress
	Spinach	
	Turnips	

VITAMINS AND MINERALS IN VEGETABLES

The Dietary Guidelines for Americans 2015 – 2020 has noted some nutrients are consumed below the recommended levels and thus are considered "nutrients of public concern." These include potassium, fiber, choline, magnesium, calcium, and vitamins A, D, E, and C (2015 – 2020 Dietary Guidelines | Health.Gov; Pikosky et al., 2019). Vegetables are good sources of many of these nutrients, including **potassium, folate, and vitamins A and C**. Specifically, fresh and processed vegetables typically contribute to half of one's vitamin C intake; one-fourth of one's intake of vitamin A, potassium, and dietary fiber; and more than 10% of folate and magnesium intake (Storey & Anderson, 2013).

Potassium and Magnesium

NHANES data (2015 – 2016) found **potatoes to be the top vegetable source of potassium** in the American diet; **other sources include lentils, acorn squash, beet greens, and lima beans** (Office of Dietary Supplements - Potassium; Torres-Gonzalez et al., 2019b). However, only 3% of those included in the NHANES study had usual intakes of potassium greater than the recommended adequate intake (3,400 mg/day for men or 2,600 mg/day for women) (Fulgoni et al., 2011). Potassium works together with **magnesium,** which has been noted to stabilize heart rate and blood pressure and improve endothelial function. **Vegetables that are good sources of magnesium include spinach, Swiss chard, avocado, and potatoes.** Tomatoes are a food that contains both potassium and magnesium, and mixing them with other vegetables that are higher in potassium, like potatoes, and magnesium, like spinach, can help ensure an adequate intake of both nutrients (Krishnaswamy & Gayathri, 2018). Potassium has been noted to counteract the hypertensive effects of increased sodium intake. The Standard American Diet is typically low in potassium and high in sodium, and **increasing the potassium-to-sodium ratio has been shown to decrease hypertension** (Torres-Gonzalez et al., 2019a).

Folate

Excellent vegetable sources of folate include **asparagus, beets, okra, dark green leafy vegetables (spinach, mustard greens, romaine lettuce), black-eyed peas, kidney beans,**

and lentils (Likis, 2016). In a study of Dutch women, vegetables contributed 25% of total dietary folate, making it the main dietary source. Vegetables have been found to be a main dietary source of folate in other countries as well (Looman et al., 2018). A higher intake of fruits and vegetables has been associated with reductions in homocysteine levels (elevated levels are linked to the development of heart disease) due to higher blood levels of folate, along with vitamins C and E and beta-carotene (Mielgo-Ayuso et al., 2017). Conversely, low folate has been linked to vascular disease and other chronic conditions, as well as an increased risk of neural tube defects and other congenital malformations in newborns (Institute of Medicine (U.S.) Standing Committee on the Scientific Evaluation of Dietary Reference Intakes and its Panel on Folate, Other B Vitamins, and Choline, 1998).

Vitamin A and Vitamin C — The Antioxidant Vitamins

Normal metabolic processes generate reactive oxygen species (ROS) and other free radicals, and high levels of ROS have been associated with chronic disease. Antioxidants such as vitamins A and C are known to neutralize ROS and free radicals, and higher intakes of antioxidants have been associated with lower rates of chronic diseases (Willcox et al., 2004). Vegetables are a good source of vitamins A and C, as well as several phytochemicals that act as antioxidants. One of these well-known phytochemicals is beta-carotene, which has a red-orange pigment that is converted into vitamin A. In a review of vegetable intervention studies, researchers found that, in general, a diet high in vegetables was associated with reduced markers of inflammation (Serafini & Peluso, 2016). **Vegetables rich in vitamin A and beta-carotene include sweet potato, pumpkin, carrot, spinach, broccoli, and kale.** In a large study of women over a five-year period, researchers found that the combination of low serum carotenoid levels (e.g., low vitamin A and beta-carotene intake) and low physical activity predicted earlier mortality, leading them to conclude that diets high in fruits and vegetables, especially those with carotenoids, improve longevity (Nicklett et al., 2012). **Vitamin C also functions as an antioxidant** as well as a cofactor in key biosynthesis reactions of collagen, carnitine, and neurotransmitters. **Good vegetable sources of vitamin C include red pepper, broccoli, Brussels sprouts, and cabbage** (Vitamin C: Fact Sheet for Health Professionals).

Vitamin K

Vitamin K in the diet comes in two forms: vitamin K1 (phylloquinone) from plant sources such as **kale, collards, turnips, Swiss chard, parsley, broccoli, spinach, watercress, cabbage and asparagus**; and vitamin K2 (menaquinone) from animal foods such as meat and eggs; fermented foods such sauerkraut, yogurt, or natto (Japanese fermented soybeans); production by gut bacteria; and supplements. Vegetables, specifically green leafy vegetables, are a major dietary source of phylloquinone, the most abundant form of vitamin K in the U.S. diet. Based on NHANES data, vegetables provide 60% of vitamin K for those on a high-vegetable diet and 36% for those on a low-vegetable diet (Harshman et al., 2017). In a large meta-analysis, **higher dietary vitamin K intake was associated with a moderately lower risk of coronary heart disease** (Chen et al., 2019). Some recent research also suggests that vitamin K may be important in maintaining bone structure and avoiding fractures (Schwalfenberg, 2017). A recent meta-analysis found an inverse correlation between a daily dietary vitamin K intake of 50 µg/day and the risk of fracture (Hao et al., 2017). An intake of 50 µg could be met with one ounce of natto, half a cup of raw kale or spinach, one tablespoon of frozen and boiled collards or turnips, or half a cup of roasted soybeans.

Minerals

While **calcium and iron** are not typically found in high amounts in vegetables, plant sources of these minerals become important among those following a vegetarian or especially vegan lifestyle. Calcium is most important for supporting bone structure and function, but it is also required for blood vessel function, nerve transmission, and muscle function. There are no vegetables that are excellent sources of calcium, but green leafy vegetables, including turnip greens, kale, and bok choy, **are considered good food sources of calcium.**

The most important role of iron in the body is as a component of hemoglobin, a protein within red blood cells that carries oxygen from the lungs to the rest of the body. Those with low iron intake, known as iron deficiency anemia, often complain of symptoms such as weakness and fatigue. **Beans and legumes contain significant amounts of iron**, as do potatoes eaten with the skin on.

Table 6: Food Sources of Various Minerals

Vitamin/ Mineral	Daily Value*	Excellent Food Sources (Provides >20% of the Daily Value)	Good Food Sources (Provides 10% to 19% of the Daily Value)
Potassium	4,700 mg	White potatoes	Beet greens, white beans, tomato purée, sweet potato, soybeans, Swiss chard, lima beans, lentils, acorn squash
Magnesium	420 mg	Spinach	Black beans, edamame, avocado, white potato, tomato, acorn squash
Folate	400 µg	Asparagus, beets, okra, dark-green leafy vegetables (spinach, mustard greens, romaine lettuce, turnip greens), black-eyed peas, kidney beans, black beans, navy beans, lentils	Broccoli, Brussels sprouts, green peas, green beans, Swiss chard, kale, carrots, collards, iceberg lettuce, chickpeas

Vitamin/ Mineral	Daily Value*	Excellent Food Sources (Provides >20% of the Daily Value)	Good Food Sources (Provides 10% to 19% of the Daily Value)
Vitamin A	900 µg	Sweet potato, spinach, carrots, red bell pepper, black-eyed peas, broccoli, pumpkin, kale	Tomato juice
Vitamin C	90 mg	Red and green bell pepper, broccoli, Brussels sprouts, tomatoes, cabbage, cauliflower, white potatoes	Spinach, green peas
Vitamin K	120 µg	Green leafy vegetables (kale, collards, turnip greens, Swiss chard, spinach, parsley, watercress), natto, soybeans, broccoli, cabbage, asparagus	Okra, green peas
Calcium	1,300 mg	None	Turnip greens, kale, bok choy
Iron	18 mg	White beans	Lentils, kidney beans, chickpeas, spinach, stewed tomatoes, potatoes with skin

*For adults and children >=4 years of age
Values from https://ods.od.nih.gov/factsheets/list-VitaminsMinerals/

PHYTOCHEMICALS IN VEGETABLES

Phytochemicals or plant chemicals are compounds produced and used by plants that can influence human biochemical and physiologic reactions. From a culinary perspective, phytochemicals give plants their color, odor, and flavor. While there is no official recommendation for the intake of phytochemicals as there is for vitamins and minerals, phytochemicals are the superheroes of the nutrient world as they have been shown to have antioxidant properties, decrease inflammation, modulate hormones and enzymes, aid in detoxification, prevent DNA damage, slow the growth rate of cancer cells and support immune function (Forni et al., 2019). Studies to date include animal studies, laboratory studies, and observational studies; however, intervention studies are lacking, so a cause-and-effect relationship between phytochemicals and disease has not been proven yet.

It is estimated that there are over 5,000 phytochemicals; aside from carotenoids, not much is known about the vast majority of them. The major classes of phytochemicals include polyphenols or phenolics (flavonoids, isoflavonoids), alkaloids, nitrogen-containing compounds (betalains), organosulfur compounds (glucosinolates, allicin), phytosterols and carotenoids (carotenes and xanthophylls such as lutein and zeaxanthin). It is suggested that **>80% of the body's total antioxidant capacity is from polyphenols** (Harasym & Oledzki, 2014). There are some phytochemicals that are found in higher amounts in vegetables, and these include anthocyanins, glucosinolates, carotenoids, and isoflavones; recent research surrounding these phytochemicals will be discussed below. Table 7 outlines the current classification structure of phytochemicals.

Figure 5: Vegetables High in Fiber, Phytonutrients, and Nutrient Density.

Figure 6: Classification of Phytochemicals.

Table 7: Food Sources and Proposed Mechanisms of Various Phytochemicals

Phytochemical Classification			Food Sources	Proposed Mechanism
Phenolics/ Polyphenols	Flavonoids	Anthocyanins (derived from anthocyanidins)	Purple cabbage, red onions, radishes, eggplant, purple cauliflower, purple potatoes	Antioxidant, endothelial protective properties
		Flavonols: Quercetin	Highest in kale; also found in broccoli, red onions, parsley, arugula, spinach, watercress	Antioxidant
		Flavones	Highest in parsley; also found in celery, chili peppers, oregano, peppermint, thyme	Antioxidant
		Isoflavonoids: Daidzein Genistein	Legumes such as soybeans, kudzu, lupine and fava	Anti-cancer mechanisms
	Coumarins		Legumes, clover and soybeans sprouts	Anti-clotting properties

Phytochemical Classification			Food Sources	Proposed Mechanism
Organosulfur Compounds		Sulforaphane	Brussels sprouts, garden cress, mustard greens, turnips, cabbage, kale, watercress, kohlrabi, red cabbage, broccoli, horseradish, cauliflower, bok choy	Antioxidant, possible anti-cancer properties
		Isothiocyanates (derived from glucosinolates)	Broccoli, Brussels sprouts, cabbage, horseradish, kohlrabi, mustard, radish, garden cress, watercress	Reduce oxidative stress
		Indoles	Broccoli, cabbage, cauliflower, Brussels sprouts, collard greens, kale	Anti-cancer mechanisms
		Allylic sulfur compounds (including allicin)	Onion, garlic, scallions, shallots, leeks, chives	Improve lipid profiles
		Betalains	Beets, Swiss chard	Antioxidant
Carotenoids		α-and β-Carotene	Pumpkin, carrot juice, carrots, frozen spinach, sweet potatoes, kale, turnip greens, dandelion greens, winter squash, tomatoes, peas	Antioxidant
		Lycopene	Tomatoes in all forms, parsley, asparagus, baked beans	Antioxidant, anti-cancer properties
		Cryptoxanthin	Pumpkin, sweet red peppers, carrots, yellow corn	Antioxidant
		Lutein and zeaxanthin	Spinach, kale, turnip greens, collards, dandelion greens, mustard greens, summer squash, green peas, avocado	Antioxidant, especially in the macula of the eye
Phytosterols		Sterols and stanols	Raw or boiled soybeans, raw peas, raw Brussels sprouts, sesame oil	Lower LDL cholesterol

One thing that is known about phytochemicals is: "Almost always, benefits are found only when the phytochemical is consumed in food and not pill form." — Eric Rimm of Harvard

Phenolics/Polyphenols

Flavonoids are purple, red, or black polyphenols. They have been shown to have antioxidant capacity as well as the ability to reduce proinflammatory mediators and decrease inflammation (Flavonoids, 2014). There are 12 major subclasses, and the ones most related to vegetables include anthocyanins, flavonols, flavones, and isoflavones. **Flavonoids have been associated with protection against diabetes, cancer, cognitive decline, and cardiovascular disease** (Flavonoids, 2014).

- **Anthocyanins** (derived from anthocyanidins) include cyanidin, delphinidin, malvidin, pelargonidin, peonidin, and petunidin. They are highest in **purple cabbage but are also found in red onions, radishes, eggplant, purple cauliflower, and purple potatoes**, as well as many autumn leaves. Anthocyanins have aromatic rings that can accept singlet oxygen, thereby reducing oxidative damage (Bhagwat et al., 2014). **Diets rich in anthocyanins have been associated with reduced rates of cardiovascular disease** in population studies (Hidalgo et al., 2012). Molecular research has noted anthocyanins to also have endothelial protective properties (Krga et al., 2018).
- **Flavonols** include kaempferol, myricetin, and quercetin. They are **highest in kale** and are also found in **broccoli, red onions, parsley, arugula, spinach, and watercress** (Bhagwat et al., 2014). **Flavones** include apigenin and luteolin and are **highest in parsley** as well as in **celery, chili peppers, oregano, peppermint, and thyme** (Slavin & Lloyd, 2012). Both of these flavonoids have antioxidant properties and help to reduce oxidative damage caused by free radicals in the body (Flavonoids, 2014).
- **Isoflavones/isoflavonoids** include daidzein, genistein, glycitein, and formononetin. Dietary sources of isoflavones include soy and soy products, fava beans, red wine, and flaxseeds (Carotenoids, 2014a; USDA Database for the Isoflavone Content of Selected Foods, Release 2.0). Isoflavones are phytoestrogens, which are plant-derived compounds with structural similarity to 17-β-oestradiol (E2), giving them estrogenic-like activity. Isoflavones have been **noted to be protective against breast, prostate, and other types of cancers**, and their intake may also lead to improved brain function, aid in the management of menopausal symptoms, reduce cardiovascular risk, and help maintain bone density. There is some concern with their excess use, primarily as supplements, since some research suggests they may function as endocrine disrupters and affect fertility and cancer risk (Rietjens et al., 2017). Isoflavones that reach the colon are metabolized by intestinal bacteria, which influence their bioavailability and physiological activity. The metabolites that are produced are based on individual gut bacterial composition (Landete et al., 2016).

Organosulfur Compounds

- **Glucosinolates are found in cruciferous vegetables** such as Brussels sprouts, garden cress, mustard greens, turnip, cabbage, kale, watercress, kohlrabi, red cabbage, broccoli, horseradish, cauliflower, and bok choy (listed in order of glucosinolate content) (McNaughton & Marks, 2003). Glucosinolate metabolites include sulforaphane and isothiocyanates. Sulforaphane is thought to have **anti-cancer and cardiovascular benefits** and may also be helpful in preventing osteoporosis (Vanduchova et al., 2019). They may work by reducing oxidative stress (Bai et al., 2015; Higdon et al., 2007).
  - **Sulforaphane** is easily denatured by heat or acid; see the section In the Kitchen below for more information. One caution to keep in mind is that very high intakes of cruciferous vegetables can lead to insufficient thyroid hormone production.
  - **Indole-3-carbinol** is a product of the breakdown of glucosinolates, which are catalyzed to 3,3'-diindolylmethane (DIM) in the stomach. While considerable work has been done on its association with reducing the risk of hormone-sensitive cancers, newer research is also looking at its ability to decrease the risk of cardiovascular disease, obesity, and diabetes (Licznerska & Baer-Dubowska, 2016).
- **Allicin**, a phytonutrient primarily found in garlic, is another source of organosulfur, a compound which has been noted to offer modest improvements in lipid profiles. Researchers have noted that garlic could "be considered as an alternative option with a higher safety profile than conventional cholesterol-lowering medications" (Ried et al., 2013). Allicin is also heat-sensitive; see the section below, In the Kitchen, for more information.
- **Betalains** are indole-derived yellow and red pigments and are found in **beets and Swiss chard**. They are believed to have antioxidant properties. Betalains are also thought to induce phase II enzymes which help to metabolize drugs, and they may also lower blood pressure and prevent LDL cholesterol oxidation (Esatbeyoglu et al., 2015).

Carotenoids

Carotenoids impart yellow, orange, and red colors to vegetables and fruits and include alpha and beta-carotene, beta-cryptoxanthin, lutein, zeaxanthin, and lycopene. All of these carotenoids act as antioxidants, primarily by terminating damaging chain reactions in the cell membrane by scavenging radicals and quenching singlet oxygens. Overall, carotenoids have a low bioavailability because they are associated with proteins, though **cooking increases their bioavailability** because it helps to weaken this association (Moody et al., 1991; van Het Hof et al., 2000). Additionally, they are better absorbed in the presence of dietary fat. Fat-blocking medications and proton pump inhibitors have both been shown to reduce carotenoid absorption. However, the impact is not thought to be significant (Welcome to the Natural Medicines Research Collaboration). Interestingly, researchers found a synergistic effect in antioxidant and anti-inflammatory action with the co-digestion of carotenoid-rich baby spinach and anthocyanin-rich red cabbage (Phan et al., 2019).

- **Alpha- and beta-carotene** from **carrots, winter squash, and spinach,** and **beta-cryptoxanthin** from **pumpkin, papayas, and sweet red peppers** are considered provitamin A, meaning they can be converted to active vitamin A in the body (USDA, 2018). Large observational studies have shown **reduced risks of cardiovascular disease and cancers** with increasing vitamin A intake, though using supplements that provide a megadose of vitamin A has been associated with increased cancer rates in some populations (Carotenoids, 2014b).
- **Lutein and zeaxanthin** are xanthophylls that are taken up by and **protect the macula of the eye. Xanthophylls** have alternating double and single bonds, and this chemical structure allows them to absorb a lot of blue light, protecting the eye from oxidative damage (Bian et al., 2012). Food sources include **frozen spinach** (the highest source), **frozen kale, frozen turnips, frozen collards,** and **cooked mustard greens** (Krinsky et al., 2003; USDA, 2018).
- **Lycopene** also acts as an antioxidant as it has pairs of electrons that can pick up single oxygen radicals. It is generally found in bright red vegetables, though sometimes the red color of lycopene is blocked by green chlorophyll. Food sources of lycopene include **tomato paste** (the highest source), **tomatoes, sweet potatoes, parsley, and baked beans** (USDA, 2018). Lycopene intake has been associated with **lower rates of breast and prostate cancer**, and a large meta-analysis found a lower rate of prostate cancer in men with the lightest lycopene intake (Etminan et al., 2004). Lycopene levels are higher in processed and/or cooked tomato products (Fielding et al., 2005).

Phytosterols

Phytosterols have been shown to have a significant impact on cholesterol metabolism. Though much of the research on this relationship has examined purified extracts from dietary sources and not whole foods, observational studies have consistently linked higher dietary intake of phytosterols to reduced levels of LDL cholesterol. **Vegetables and legumes high in phytosterols include soybeans, green peas, sesame oil, kidney beans, lentils, and Brussels sprouts** (Racette et al., 2009, 2015).

Nitrogen-Containing Compounds

Research is also looking at synergistic impacts of phytochemicals and other compounds, such as flavonoid- and nitrate-rich foods, which show promising effects on vascular function (Lovegrove et al., 2017). **Food sources of nitrate** include **arugula or rocket, Boston and Bibb lettuce, Swiss chard, celery, fennel, beetroot, kale, spinach, and cabbage.** Some emerging evidence is linking dietary intake of inorganic nitrates and health, focusing on an association with **lowered blood pressure, reduced risk of cardiovascular disease, and increased exercise performance**. Nitrates contribute to the production of nitric oxide (NO), which can lead to vasodilation, resulting in lowered blood pressure (Pikosky et al., 2019).

VEGETABLES AND DIETARY FIBER

Dietary fiber is a nondigestible carbohydrate found in vegetables (plus fruits and whole grains), as well as naturally occurring fiber, such as lignin, inulin, cellulose, and hemicelluloses. Functional fibers, which are isolated nondigestible carbohydrates that are added to foods by manufacturers, include oligosaccharides, fructans, cellulose, hemicelluloses, pectins, beta-glucans, and starch. **The Institute of Medicine recommends a daily fiber intake of 25 g for women and 38 g for men**. However, Americans overall consume an average of only ~15 g of fiber per day (Slavin, 2008). Intake of functional fibers specifically is difficult to quantify in the American diet due to inadequate nutrient databases.

Vegetables that are especially high in fiber include **kidney beans, carrots, artichoke hearts, spinach, Brussels sprouts, squash, turnips, celery, and broccoli.** There are two broad categories of fiber found in vegetables: soluble fiber (especially high in sweet potatoes, Brussels sprouts, asparagus, and parsley) and insoluble fiber (especially high in cauliflower, green beans, and carrots) (Thalheimer, 2013).

The dietary fiber content of vegetables is one of the key reasons why vegetable intake is associated with countless health benefits. Dietary fiber is known to increase stool bulk and reduce the transit time of feces through the bowels, increase excretion of bile acid, thereby lowering serum cholesterol, slow glucose absorption and improve insulin sensitivity, lower blood pressure, inhibit lipid peroxidation, and have anti-inflammatory properties (Thalheimer, 2013). These mechanisms all help explain why increased fiber intake has been associated with a lower risk of coronary heart disease, infectious and respiratory diseases, diabetes, some cancers, and premature death (McRae, 2018; Park et al., 2011). Soluble and insoluble fibers act slightly differently once consumed. Soluble fibers dissolve in water to create a gel-like substance and are more responsible for the cholesterol-lowering and slowed glucose absorption mechanisms of fiber. In contrast, insoluble fibers do not dissolve in water but promote the movement of material through the digestive tract by increasing stool bulk.

Animal experiments, epidemiological data, and clinical trials clearly indicate that higher fiber intake is associated with less weight gain than lower fiber intake. **Intake of fiber tends to delay gastric emptying and delays the return of hunger** (Benini et al., 1995). Increased fiber intake is associated with an increase in satiating gut hormones. The limited number of clinical trials comparing high-fiber foods with low-fiber foods have not provided consistent data indicating that these diets are more efficacious for weight loss than low-fiber control diets; however, randomized, placebo-controlled clinical trials have clearly documented that fiber supplements are accompanied by significantly more weight loss than use of placebos. Thus, the weight of clinical evidence strongly indicates that consumption of dietary fiber, especially from fiber supplements, has beneficial effects on weight management (McRorie, 2015).

An NIH–AARP study that followed over 388,000 adults for nine years found that high dietary fiber intake significantly lowered the risk of death from cardiovascular, infectious, and respiratory diseases in men and women, and fiber intake from just vegetables and beans was weakly associated with lower mortality risk (Park et al., 2011). Another study within the European Prospective Investigation into Cancer and Nutrition (EPIC) cohort found that the risk of colorectal cancer was inversely associated with intakes of fruit, vegetables, and total fiber, and the risk of liver cancer was also inversely associated with total fiber intake (Bradbury et al., 2014).

Though cooking may impact fiber, there is not currently enough research to make targeted cooking recommendations for each fiber type. In a review of 29 vegetables, researchers found **steaming improved the function of fermentable soluble fiber**, while peeling or juicing vegetables dramatically reduced their fiber content (Kalala et al., 2018b).

VEGETABLE PROTEIN

Plant protein and vegetable protein are terms that are sometimes used interchangeably; however, they refer to protein from slightly different groups of foods. Plant protein is considered protein from vegetables as well as from anything that is not meat or dairy, including nuts, beans, legumes, grains, algae (spirulina), seeds, and all soy products. In contrast, vegetable protein refers specifically to protein from vegetables, beans, and legumes, including soy. The 2015 – 2020 Dietary Guidelines for Americans encourage the intake of more plant-based foods and less meat due to several factors, including reduced carbon emissions and water utilization (Katz et al., 2019; McGuire, 2016).

With a growing interest in plant-based diets, numerous studies published recently have looked at the comparison between plant-based or vegetable-based proteins and proteins from animal sources. Though vegetables are not as high in protein per serving as meat, some have as much protein per calorie as meat. One key difference between animal-based and plant-based proteins is that while proteins from animal sources contain all nine essential amino acids and are thus considered complete proteins, proteins from plant sources are typically lacking in at least one essential amino acid; the exception to this is **soy buckwheat, amaranth, and quinoa**. Because most plant sources of protein are not considered complete proteins, it is important to consume a variety of plant-based proteins to ensure all essential amino acids are still being consumed. You can read more about complete and incomplete proteins in the *Vegetarian Diet* chapter.

Research on the effects of plant-based protein on skeletal muscle mass is mixed. A recent review by van Vliet and colleagues concluded that soy protein does not induce muscle protein synthesis to the same extent as protein from animal sources (van Vliet et al., 2015). In contrast, a cross-sectional study by Miki and colleagues found that vegetable protein intake was associated with higher skeletal muscle mass in elderly patients (A. Miki et al., 2017). Other reviews have found that a diet high in plant-based proteins can reduce the risk of cardiovascular disease and that soy protein is just as advantageous to bone health as animal-based protein (van Vliet et al., 2015).

VEGETABLES AND THE MICROBIOME

The composition of gut bacteria is influenced by many factors, such as age, environment, health, and genetics. Diet has also been shown to play a significant role, and a healthful diet and lifestyle have been shown to improve the health and diversity of gut microbes living in the colon (Klinder et al., 2016). The relationship between vegetables and the microbiome is twofold. First, vegetable components – primarily fibers – feed gut bacteria and allow them to proliferate. Second, as a result of being fed, gut bacteria produce metabolic compounds, such as short-chain fatty acids (SCFA) like butyrate, propionate, and acetate, that can be absorbed and used by the body as energy. Soluble fibers are fermented by gut bacteria to a greater extent than insoluble fibers. The increase in bacterial fermentation of soluble fibers can lead to a rise in gut bacteria and a beneficial change in bacterial composition and diversity (Mudgil & Barak, 2013).

Research on the influence of dietary fiber and the gut microbiome has historically looked at the reactions of concentrated fibers rather than fibers from whole foods, so results are often not directly translatable to real-world scenarios. However, there is some evidence emerging on how the intake of whole foods with intact dietary fiber impacts the gut microbiome. Following are some examples:
- Supplementation with inulin derived from chicory was found to support the growth of the microbes Anaerostipes and Bifidobacterium and impair the growth of Bilophila. Lower levels of Bilophila have been linked with improved constipation (Vandeputte et al., 2017). Inulin is also found in onions and Jerusalem artichokes.
- Significant associations have been found between the consumption of plant-based diets and increased levels of Prevotella in the gut (De Filippis et al., 2016; Ruengsomwong et al., 2014). However, the health implications of increased levels of Prevotella are not yet elucidated.

- Cruciferous vegetables (also called brassica) include broccoli, cabbage, mustard greens, turnips and kale, and are rich in sulfur-containing compounds. One of these compounds is glucosinolate, which gut bacteria metabolize into bioactive isothiocyanates (ITCs). Higher circulating levels of ITCs have been associated with lower cancer rates (Fahey et al., 2012).
- A short-term cruciferous vegetable-rich diet has also been associated with a reduction of sulfate-reducing bacteria (SRB). This is notable because SRB has potentially negative impacts on gastrointestinal health primarily due to an increased production of the compound hydrogen sulfide, which has been seen in cases of ulcerative colitis and irritable bowel syndrome (IBS) (Kellingray et al., 2017).
- There is a strong link between dietary polyphenols and the microbiome. Colonic gut bacteria influence the bioavailability of polyphenols by modifying their structure prior to absorption (Kawabata et al., 2019). As discussed in a previous section, polyphenols have the ability to act as antioxidants.

The way vegetables are processed can affect their impact on the gut microbiota. **Steaming** vegetables may ensure better preservation and extraction of glucosinolates and other phytonutrients more than other cooking methods (Palermo et al., 2014). Fermented cruciferous vegetables, such as sauerkraut, contain high levels of lactic acid bacteria, and some research has found intakes of these prebiotic **fermented** foods can lead to significant changes in gut bacteria, resulting in an improvement in symptoms of irritable bowel syndrome (Nielsen et al., 2018).

SECTION 4:
VEGETABLE INTAKE AND HEALTH OUTCOMES

While the optimal vegetable intake is not known, higher intakes of vegetables have been consistently associated with a reduced risk of several chronic diseases. Intake of fruits and vegetables together, vegetables alone, and plant-based diets as a whole have all been studied in association with a long list of health conditions and have been associated with lower rates of all-cause mortality, cancer, cardiovascular disease, coronary heart disease, metabolic conditions, hypertension, type 2 diabetes, age-related macular degeneration, chronic obstructive lung disease, IBD, osteoporosis, asthma, cognitive impairments, mood disorders, and others (Appel et al., 1997; Aune et al., 2017; Jannasch et al., 2017; Kaluza et al., 2017; Kang et al., 2005; Lee & Park, 2017; M. G. Miller et al., 2017; Neville et al., 2014; Rautiainen et al., 2014; Slavin & Lloyd, 2012; Walda et al., 2002). Vegetable intake is also a key contributor to the health benefits of several dietary patterns, including the Mediterranean and DASH dietary patterns (Trichopoulou et al., 2009).

In a meta-analysis of 95 studies, Aune and colleagues looked at the relative risk (RR) of cardiovascular disease, cancer, and all-cause mortality based on varying levels of fruit and vegetable intake. At a vegetable intake of 200 g per day (about two and a half servings), researchers found an 8% lower risk for coronary heart disease (RR 0.92), a 13% lower risk of stroke (RR 0.87), a 10% lower risk of cardiovascular disease (RR 0.90) and a 4% lower risk of cancer (RR 0.96) compared with no vegetable intake. Additionally, a vegetable intake of 500 g per day reduced the risk of stroke by 28%, an intake of 550 g to 600 g per day reduced the risk of cancer by 12% and the risk of coronary heart disease by 30%, and a vegetable intake of 600 g per day reduced the risk of all-cause mortality by 25%. For all disease states except cancer, the risk continued to decline up to a vegetable intake of 800 g per day (10 servings per day). Generally speaking, the reduction in disease risk was most significant at the lower end of intake, identifying that **increasing one's intake of vegetables at all has a positive impact on health, even if total vegetable intake is still low** (Aune et al., 2017).

The Aune et al. meta-analysis also looked at the relationship between disease risk and specific groups of vegetables:
- Green leafy vegetables were inversely associated with coronary heart disease, stroke, cardiovascular disease, and all-cause mortality in a high versus low intake analysis.
- Cruciferous vegetables were inversely associated with risk of cardiovascular disease, cancer, and all-cause mortality in a high versus low intake analysis.
- Beta-carotene-rich vegetables, included in both the dark green and red-orange groups, showed an inverse association with coronary heart disease and cardiovascular disease in a high versus low intake analysis.
- Intake of tomatoes (red-orange group) was inversely correlated with coronary heart disease, cardiovascular disease, and stroke (Aune et al., 2017).

They also found that a high potato intake was associated with lower rates of all-cause mortality compared with a low intake. Table 7 below summarizes even more research on the relationship between vegetable intake and various health conditions.

Table 8: Health Outcomes of Diets High in Vegetables and Diets High in Fruits and Vegetables

DIETS HIGH IN VEGETABLES ARE ASSOCIATED WITH	
Disease State	**Clinical Evidence**
Reduced Risk of All-cause Mortality	In a meta-analysis of 19 prospective studies, the risk of all-cause mortality was found to decline with increasing vegetable intake (RR: 0.96; 95% CI: 0.95, 0.98 (Schwingshackl, Schwedhelm, et al., 2017).
Reduced Risk of Type 2 Diabetes	Based on 13 studies, the risk of T2D decreased by 9% with increasing intake up to 300 g/day (Schwingshackl, Hoffmann, et al., 2017).
	In a group of European adults followed for 11 years, green leafy vegetable intake was inversely associated with diabetes (RR: 0.84 95% CI: 0.74-0.94) (Cooper et al., 2012).
Reduced Risk of Coronary Heart Disease	Vegetable variety and amount were inversely associated with coronary heart disease, based on 1999 – 2014 NHANES data (Conrad et al., 2018).
DIETS HIGH IN VEGETABLES ARE ASSOCIATED WITH	
Aid in Weight Loss	Increasing vegetable consumption was found to result in weight loss, reduced risk of weight gain and overweight/obesity, and reduced waist circumference in women in a systematic review of cohort studies (Nour et al., 2018).
	In a study of Danish women, each additional daily vegetable serving was associated with a reduction in waist circumference of 0.36 cm (Halkjaer et al., 2009).
Lower Odds of Depression	In the Women's Health Initiative, higher intake of vegetables was significantly associated with lower odds of depression, with an odds ratio of 0.62 comparing the highest and lowest quintile of intake (Gangwisch et al., 2015).
DIETS HIGH IN FRUITS AND VEGETABLES ARE ASSOCIATED WITH	
Disease State	**Clinical Evidence**
Reduced Risk of Cardiovascular Diseases	Higher intake of fruits and vegetables (F&V) is associated with a reduced risk of death from CVD, with an average reduction in risk of 4% for each additional serving per day of F&V (Wang et al., 2014).

DIETS HIGH IN FRUITS AND VEGETABLES ARE ASSOCIATED WITH	
	Eating eight or more servings of F&V per day resulted in a 30% lower risk of heart attack or stroke compared to eating less than 1.5 servings per day (Hung et al., 2004).
	A large meta-analysis showed that each additional daily serving of fruits or vegetables provided increased protection against all-cause mortality and cardiovascular mortality; however, additional benefits were not achieved beyond five servings per day (Wang et al., 2014).
	Another large meta-analysis showed that increasing fruit and vegetable consumption from less than three to more than five servings per day is associated with a 17% reduced risk of coronary heart disease (He et al., 2007).
	Combined fruit and vegetable intake is associated with a relative risk of 0.92 (95% CI: 0.90-0.95) for cardiovascular disease risk per 200 g per day consumed (Wang et al., 2014).
Reduced Risk of Type 2 Diabetes	In a group of European adults followed for 11 years, a greater quantity of fruit and vegetable intake was associated with a 21% lower risk of type 2 diabetes (Cooper, 2012).
Reduced Risk of Stroke	Combined fruit and vegetable intake is associated with a relative risk of 0.92 (95% CI: 0.90-0.95) for cardiovascular disease risk per 200 g per day consumed (Aune et al., 2017).
Increased Happiness, Life Satisfaction, and Well-being	Among Australian adults, increased fruit and vegetable consumption was predictive of increased happiness, life satisfaction, and overall well-being (Mujcic & J Oswald, 2016).
	In a cross-sectional survey of 422 young adults, intake of raw fruits and vegetables significantly predicted higher mental health outcomes (Brookie et al., 2018).
	In a dietary intake study of 1,977 employees, fiber intake from vegetables and fruits was significantly inversely associated with depressive symptoms (T. Miki et al., 2016).
Reduced Risk of Age-related Vision Problems	Among men and women at least 50 years of age, those who had three or more servings of fruit per day had a 36% lower risk of age-related maculopathy than those who had less than 1.5 servings of fruit per day (Cho et al., 2004).

DIETS HIGH IN FRUITS AND VEGETABLES ARE ASSOCIATED WITH	
Reduced Risk of Non-cardiovascular Death Events	Higher fruit, vegetable, and legume consumption was associated with a lower risk of non-cardiovascular death events. Maximum benefits were seen at three to four servings per day (equivalent to 375 – 500 g/day) (V. Miller et al., 2017).
Reduced Risk of Cancer	For combined fruit and vegetable intake, the summary RR per 200 g per day was 0.97 (95% CI: 0.95-0.99) for total cancer incidence (Aune et al., 2017).
Reduced Risk of All-cause Mortality	Higher fruit, vegetable, and legume consumption was associated with a lower risk of total mortality. Maximum benefits were seen at three to four servings per day (equivalent to 375 – 500 g per day) (V. Miller et al., 2017).
	For combined fruit and vegetable intake, every 200 g consumed per day resulted in a summary RR of 0.90 for all-cause mortality (95% CI: 0.87-0.93) (Aune et al., 2017).

An analysis of three large prospective cohort studies (N=133,468) from 1986 to 2010 looked at the intake of fruits and vegetables and weight gain over time and found that high vegetable intake was associated with a decrease in weight. The vegetables with both more fiber and a lower glycemic load had the strongest inverse association with weight change compared to low-fiber, high-glycemic-load vegetables (Bertoia et al., 2015). High-fiber, low-glycemic vegetables include soy, cauliflower, summer squash, string beans, pepper, broccoli, Brussels sprouts, and green leafy vegetables, whereas low-fiber, high-glycemic vegetables include peas, corn, and potatoes (Bertoia et al., 2015).

SECTION 5:

WHEN TO LIMIT VEGETABLES

IRRITABLE BOWEL SYNDROME AND THE LOW-FODMAP DIET

Irritable bowel syndrome is a functional gastrointestinal condition that is often accompanied by abdominal pain, bloating, diarrhea and/or constipation. One treatment often used to address these symptoms is a low-FODMAP diet. FODMAP stands for fermentable oligosaccharides, disaccharides, monosaccharides, and polyols, all of which are carbohydrates that are found in everyday foods, including vegetables. The diet takes a two-phase approach. In the first phase, an individual eliminates all foods that contain FODMAPs from the diet for a period of two to six weeks. In the second phase, different groups of FODMAPs are slowly reintroduced to determine if any particular FODMAPs are triggering IBS symptoms. Table 9 outlines foods that are allowable on a low-FODMAP diet and foods that should be avoided. Go to the FOD-MAP diet in the chapter on **Gastrointestinal Health** for more information.

Table 9: Low- and High-FODMAP Vegetables

Low-FODMAP (Allowed)	High-FODMAP (Limit/Avoid)	Type of FODMAP
Bamboo shoots	Garlic	Oligosaccharides (fructans)
Bean sprouts	Onions	Oligosaccharides (fructans)
Broccoli	Asparagus	Fructose
Cabbage — both common and red	Beans — black, broad, kidney, lima, soya	Oligosaccharides (galactans)
Carrots	Cauliflower	Polyols
Celery (less than a 5-cm stalk)	Cabbage, savoy	Polyols
Chickpeas (1/4 cup maximum)	Mange tout (snow pea)	Polyols
Corn (1/2 cob maximum)	Mushrooms	Polyols
Cucumber	Peas	Fructose, polyols
Eggplant	Scallions/spring onions (white part)	Oligosaccharides (fructans)
Green beans		
Green pepper		
Kale		
Lettuce — butter, iceberg, arugula		
Parsnip		
Potato		
Pumpkin		
Red peppers		
Scallions/spring onions (green part)		
Squash		
Sweet potato		
Tomatoes		
Turnip		
Zucchini		

Source: https://www.ibsdiets.org/wp-content/uploads/2016/03/IBSDiets-FODMAP-chart.pdf

KIDNEY DISEASE

The kidney is responsible for maintaining appropriate levels of electrolytes, including potassium, in the blood. When someone has kidney disease and the kidneys are not working properly, potassium levels in the blood can increase to dangerous levels. Someone with kidney disease or on dialysis is often prescribed a low-potassium diet by their doctor to help limit the amount of potassium that their lower-functioning kidneys need to manage. While vegetables are often considered a healthful food, some are high in potassium and need to be consumed in moderation by individuals prescribed a low-potassium diet. Table 10 outlines vegetables that are both high and low in potassium.

Table 10: Vegetables High and Low in Potassium

High-Potassium Vegetables	Low-Potassium Vegetables
Acorn squash	Alfalfa sprouts
Artichoke	Asparagus (limit to 6 spears)
Bamboo shoots	Beans, green, or wax
Baked beans	Broccoli, raw or cooked from frozen
Butternut squash	Cabbage, green or red
Refried beans	Carrots, cooked
Beets	Cauliflower
Black beans	Celery (limit to 1 stalk)
Broccoli, cooked from raw	Corn (½ fresh ear or 1 cup frozen)
Brussels sprouts	Cucumber
Chinese cabbage (bok choy)	Eggplant
Carrots, raw	Kale
Dried beans and peas	Lettuce
Greens (except kale)	Mixed vegetables
Hubbard squash	White mushrooms, raw (limit to ½ cup)
Kohlrabi	Onions
Lentils	Parsley
Legumes	Peas, green
White mushrooms, cooked	Peppers
Okra	Radish
Parsnips	Rhubarb
Potatoes, white and sweet	Water chestnuts
Pumpkin	Watercress

High-Potassium Vegetables	Low-Potassium Vegetables
Rutabagas	Yellow squash
Spinach, cooked	Zucchini
Tomatoes and tomato products	
Vegetable juice	

Source: https://www.kidney.org/atoz/content/potassium

Culinary Methods for Leaching Potassium Out of Vegetables

For those following a low-potassium diet, there are certain cooking methods that can help remove some potassium from vegetables. The process of leaching will pull some, but not all, of the potassium out of vegetables. It also removes water-soluble vitamins. Even if they are using potassium-leaching cooking methods, a patient with kidney disease should be monitored closely and discuss what types of food to eat with their dietitian or clinician.

For potatoes, sweet potatoes, carrots, beets, winter squash and rutabagas:
1. Peel and place the vegetable in cold water
2. Slice the vegetable very thin (e.g., 1/8 inch)
3. Rinse in warm water for a few seconds
4. Soak for a minimum of two hours in a lot of warm water
5. Rinse under warm water again for a few seconds
6. Cook vegetables with five times the amount of water to the amount of vegetable
7. Discard the water, and the vegetable is ready to consume

One recent study showed that leaching cubed potatoes can reduce the potassium content by 50%, while leaching shredded potatoes reduced potassium content by up to 75% (Bethke & Jansky, 2008; Potassium and Your CKD Diet, 2016).

ORAL-ALLERGY SYNDROME (POLLEN FOOD ALLERGY SYNDROME)

Some people who are allergic to pollen may become cross-reactive to certain fruits and vegetables. This is considered an oral allergy in which the body is tricked into thinking the protein in food is pollen, and the immune system reacts to it by releasing histamine. When histamine is released in the mouth due to eating raw fruits or vegetables, the lips, tongue, and mouth can feel sore, itchy, burning, or numb. These symptoms may also proceed to the throat and nasal cavity. Below are some examples of cross-reactivity:

Table 11: Pollen and Vegetable Protein Cross-Reactivity

Pollen Allergy	Vegetables That May Cause a Reaction
Ragweed (late summer to fall)	Cucumber, white potatoes, and zucchini
Birch (spring)	Carrot, celery, parsley and legumes (peanut and soybean)
Grass (summer)	White potato
Mugwort (fall)	Bell pepper, broccoli, cabbage, cauliflower, chard, garlic, onion, parsley

Mulik and Cigni (2018)

Cooking fruits and vegetables may lessen the reactivity, as will removing the peel or adding lemon to them before consumption. In 1% to 2% of individuals, their oral allergy syndrome (OAS) may become more severe and lead to hives, symptoms that last more than 15 minutes, trouble swallowing, and reactions to both raw and cooked fruit (Muluk & Cingi, 2018). **It is necessary to see a medical professional for the more severe reactions as OAS can become life-threatening.**

VEGETABLE-DRUG INTERACTIONS

There is little to no data showing that various vegetables and their phytochemicals have an influence on enzymes that are used to metabolize medications. Theoretically, if a patient is consuming a large number of vegetables and phytochemicals through juicing or an extreme diet with a large number of vegetables, there is the potential that their diet could influence drug metabolism. It is best to be cautious and not consume medications and large amounts of vegetable juices at the same time.

One drug class that deserves attention is warfarin, or Coumadin®. Warfarin is an anti-clotting medication prescribed to patients with heart disease, and it works by creating a partial deficiency in the active form of vitamin K. One of the main functions of vitamin K in the body is to aid in blood clotting, and warfarin works against this function. Thus, the effectiveness of warfarin is affected by an individual's intake of dietary vitamin K. Rather than avoid dietary vitamin K, the American Heart Association (AHA) recommends that patients taking warfarin eat a **consistent** amount of vitamin K each day (A Patient's Guide to Taking Warfarin). For example, this may mean eating one serving of a food high in vitamin K and two servings of a food low in vitamin K each day. If a patient on warfarin eats too much vitamin K, their blood will be more prone to clotting. Table 12 outlines vegetables that are high and low in vitamin K, according to the American Heart Association.

Table 12: Foods High and Low in Vitamin K

Vegetables High in Vitamin K (50+ mcg/serving)		Vegetables Low in Vitamin K (Less than 35 mcg/serving)	
Asparagus (144 µg/ 1 cup frozen, cooked)	Beet greens (152 µg/ 1 cup raw)	Potatoes (13 µg/ 1 cup mashed; 6 µg baked)	Cabbage, Chinese (32 µg/ 1 cup raw)
Broccoli (162 µg/ 1 cup frozen, cooked)	Spinach (152 µg/ 1 cup raw)	Sweet potato (5.1 µg/ 1 cup)	Onions (.6 µg/ 1 cup raw)
Brussels sprouts (155 µg /1 cup raw)	Broccoli rabe (89 µg/ 1 cup raw)	Carrots (16.9 µg/ 1 cup raw)	Peas (24 µg/ 1 cup raw)
Turnip greens (676 µg/ 1 cup frozen & boiled)	Soybeans (66 µg/ 1 cup sprouted & cooked)	Cauliflower (13 µg/ 1 cup raw)	Pumpkin seeds (5.3 µg/ 1 cup roasted)
Endive (58 µg / 1/2 cup)	Cabbage, Chinese (57 µg/ 1 cup cooked)	Tomato (6.2 µg/ 1 cup canned)	Radish (1.5 µg/ 1 cup raw)
Garden cress (270 µg/ 1 cup raw)	Green beans (51 µg/ 1 cup frozen and boiled)	Chickpeas (6.6 µg/ 1 cup canned)	Red cabbage (34.4 µg/ 1 cup raw)
Kale (81 µg/ 1 cup raw)	Mustard greens (144 µg / 1 cup raw)	Cilantro (12.4 µg/ ¼ cup raw)	Summer squash (3.7 µg/ 1 cup raw)
Radicchio (102 µg/ 1 cup shredded)	Swiss chard (299 µg / 1 cup raw)	Corn (0.5 µg/ 1 cup raw)	Turnips (0.1 µg/ 1 cup raw)
		Cucumber (19.7 µg/ 1 cup raw)	Mushrooms (0 µg/ 1 cup raw)
		Green peppers (11.1 mcg / 1 cup raw)	

USDA National Nutrient Database for Standard Reference Legacy, 2018

SECTION 6:

CLINICAL & CULINARY RECOMMENDATIONS AND COMPETENCIES

Messaging from the Menus of Change Annual Report 2020

Think Produce First, and *Limit Potatoes*

CLINICAL RECOMMENDATIONS (USDA DGA 2015-2020, USDA DGA 2020-2025)

1. Eat more vegetables in both raw and cooked form
2. Eat a variety of vegetables – dark green, red, orange, beans, peas, lentils, starchy and other vegetables
3. Focus on vegetables that support nutrients of concern: potassium, folate, vitamins A and C, fiber, antioxidants
4. Vegetables should be consumed in a nutrient-dense form, with limited additions such as salt, butter, or creamy sauces

CLINICAL COMPETENCIES

1. Define a vegetable and list the types
2. Recall which nutrients for which vegetable supply a "good source"
3. Recall how many servings of vegetables are recommended per day
4. Identify which cohorts are most at risk of not meeting their daily vegetable requirement
5. Relate the importance of consuming vegetables for overall health
6. Identify health conditions that may require limiting vegetable intake
7. List vegetable's influence on the microbiome
8. Determine which vegetables interact with certain medications
9. Describe oral-allergy syndrome
10. Describe a low FODMAP diet

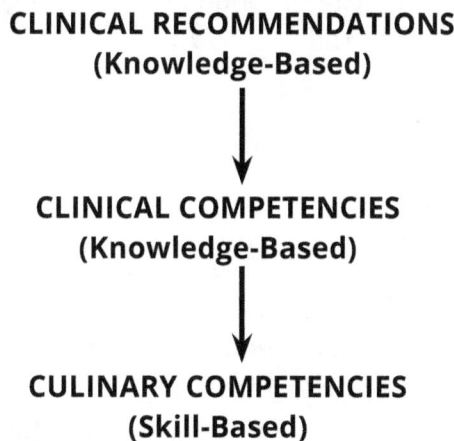

CLINICAL RECOMMENDATIONS
(Knowledge-Based)

↓

CLINICAL COMPETENCIES
(Knowledge-Based)

↓

CULINARY COMPETENCIES
(Skill-Based)

SHOPPING COMPETENCIES

1. Demonstrate how to shop for vegetables — fresh, frozen, canned — within a budget
2. Describe ripening

3. Select vegetable products with healthful ingredients
4. Identify vegetables in season
5. Distinguish between starchy and non-starchy vegetables
6. Classify vegetables into their subgroups and list the weekly requirement for each
7. Demonstrate how to best clean vegetables
8. Demonstrate freezing vegetables
9. Define organic produce

Stocking the Kitchen

1. Stock a variety of vegetables at home – fresh, frozen, fermented and canned
2. Stock vegetable flavor enhancers
   a. A variety of herbs and spices
   b. Food sources of acid – citrus and vinegars
   c. Umami ingredients – tomato paste, mushrooms, and soy sauce, for example
   d. Capers
   e. Oils and flavored oils
   f. Salty foods – anchovies and soy sauce, for example

COOKING/PREPARING COMPETENCIES
Knife/Instrument Skills

1. Model the use of the proper knife skills when preparing vegetables
2. Demonstrate the use of a paring knife
3. Demonstrate the use of a chef's knife
4. Demonstrate the use of a peeler
5. Demonstrate the use of a blender

FLAVOR DEVELOPMENT COMPETENCIES

1. Describe how acid affects the flavor of vegetables
2. Create a vegetable dish using complementary herbs and spices
3. Display cooking techniques to reduce bitterness
4. Describe how the various cooking methods used with vegetables influence the flavor profile
5. Explain salt's impacts on vegetables
6. Demonstrate how to add flavor with a minimal amount of salt

COOKING COMPETENCIES

1. Describe how various cooking methods affect nutrient bioavailability
2. Prepare a raw vegetable and green salad
3. Steam vegetables
4. Roast vegetables
5. Sauté vegetables
6. Microwave vegetables
7. Cook a vegetable-based soup
8. Blend a vegetable-based smoothie
9. Braise vegetables
10. Grill vegetables
11. Make a vegetable slaw
12. Ferment vegetables
13. Blanch vegetables

SERVING COMPETENCIES

1. Model eating vegetables
2. Serve the appropriate number of vegetable servings a day
3. Describe how to make vegetables the center of the plate
4. Plan and serve a vegetarian meal
5. Display the correct serving size of vegetables on a dinner plate
6. Use vegetables to bulk up and extend leftovers
7. Prepare and serve a vegetable-based snack
8. Pack an assortment of vegetables suitable for travel
9. Utilize vegetables in meals and in menu planning
10. Pre-prepare raw vegetables in batches for the week

SAFETY COMPETENCIES

1. Demonstrate washing vegetables
2. Demonstrate storing cooked vegetables safely
3. Demonstrate storing raw vegetables safely
4. Demonstrate the prevention of cross-contamination when working with vegetables
5. Identify spoilage characteristics of vegetables
6. Make use of knife safety skills when preparing vegetables

SECTION 7:
VEGETABLES AT THE STORE

Over half of grocery trips involve the purchase of produce, which is why this section is in the front of the store. Fruits and vegetables are perishable, and grocery chains strategically have customers entering the store through the produce department to increase sales. This is a helpful design because, as of 2015, only 9.3% of Americans were shown to eat enough vegetables, and the location of the produce aisle prompts the consumer to buy fresh produce (Lee-Kwan, 2017).

Produce is a $60 billion industry, with 50% of consumers surveyed purchasing vegetables primarily at a full-service grocery store (New FMI Analysis Suggests Produce in Retail Needs a Fresh Look, 2019). Millennials, however, are purchasing less from grocery stores (34%), instead preferring to look at alternate channels such as farmers' markets, online retailers, dollar stores, and convenience stores.

Selecting a mixture of vegetables from various plant parts and subgroups will ensure that individuals are ingesting the full array of vitamins, minerals, and phytonutrients required for optimal health.

ORGANIC DEFINED

Organic farming in the United States began in the 1940s, and today, over 40 organizations and agencies certify organic foods (US EPA, 2015). The National Organic Program is a USDA marketing program and it sets standards for 'organic' practices. The Organic Foods Production Act passed in 1990 set standards for producing, handling, and processing of organically grown agriculture products.

Produce can be labeled organic if (Organic | Agricultural Marketing Service; Organic 101, p. 101):
- It is not genetically modified or has had ionizing radiation
- It is grown in soil that has no prohibited substances applied to it in the previous three years prior to harvest
  - Prohibited substances include – most synthetic fertilizers and pesticides, and sewage sludge

For more on crop standards: https://www.ams.usda.gov/grades-standards/organic-standards.

A list of allowable and prohibited substances in organic farming practices is sure to surprise you https://www.ecfr.gov/current/title-7/part-205/subpart-g.

Products Made with Organic Ingredients

There are several "levels" of Organic that can appear on a label and it is based on the percent of organic ingredients in the product. The following are U.S definitions, check other countries regulations as they may differ.

100% Organic: The products contain 100% organically produced ingredients and processing aids, not counting added water and salt.

Organic: The product must contain at least 95% organic ingredients, not counting added water and salt, and have no added sulfites. Up to 5% of it may be from non-organic ingredients.

Made with Organic Ingredients: The product must contain at least 70% organic ingredients, not counting added water and salt, and have no added sulfites except for wine. Up to 30% of it may be from non-organic ingredients.

Product has some Organic Ingredients: This is for products with less than 70% organic ingredients.

Organic production, organic food information, and access tools from the USDA https://www.nal.usda.gov/farms-and-agricultural-production-systems/organic-production

The Organic Foods Production Act (OFPA) and the National Organic Program (NOP) oversees agricultural products that are sold and labeled, in the United States as Organic. The exception for this is small operations (sales totals $5,000 or less).

PESTICIDE RESIDUE ON VEGETABLES

Eighty-five percent of Americans are concerned about pesticide residue that might be left on produce. The amount of pesticide residue varies greatly between different fruits and vegetables, and levels also differ depending on the country of origin. A 2015 Pesticide Report published by Consumer Reports analyzed 12 years of data from the USDA's Pesticide Data Program, which analyzes nonorganic produce for pesticide residue after it has been washed and peeled. In this specific report, researchers looked at 48 conventional produce items from 14 different countries (Pesticides in Produce, 2015). While the level of pesticides on some of the produce improved over the 12 years of data collection, other produce varieties did not see improvements. You can read the full Pesticide Report.

The Environmental Working Group (EWG) is a nonprofit organization whose mission is to empower people to live more healthful lives, and every year they publish Clean 15™ and Dirty 12™ lists to help consumers decide which variety of organic vegetables and fruits to buy in order to minimize their exposure to synthetic pesticide residue (Clean Fifteen™ Conventional Produce with the Least Pesticides; Environmental Working Group, 2019). The EWG also uses data from the USDA's Pesticide Data Program, and produce that has the least amount of synthetic pesticide residue makes the Clean 15™ list, while those with the most amount of pesticide residue make the Dirty 12™ list. The EWG suggests that consumers purchase the organic variety of produce that is on the Dirty Dozen™ list so as to limit synthetic pesticide exposure. It is important to note, however, that **the benefits of eating a variety of fruits and vegetables (organic or not) far outweigh the risks of pesticide exposure.**

Table 13: Vegetables on the EWG'S 2024 Clean 15™ and Dirty 12™ Lists

Clean 15™	Dirty Dozen™
Avocados	Spinach
Sweet corn	Kale, collard, mustard greens
Onions	Bell and hot peppers
Sweet peas (frozen)	Green Beans
Asparagus	
Cabbage	
Mushrooms	
Sweet potatoes	

The full version of each list can be found here: Dirty Dozen, Clean 15

Eating more fruits and vegetables, whether they are organic or not, is so beneficial to one's health that it far outweighs the risk of consuming trace amounts of pesticides in healthy individuals.

WHOLE VEGETABLES

When selecting vegetables at the store or farmers market, look for an even color and firmness and avoid soft spots or cracking. With artichokes, asparagus, and cauliflower, ensure that the leaves or florets are compact. Unlike fruit, vegetables do not ripen, and they do not get sweeter with age. Rather, they grow from a small size to a larger size. Carrots are sweeter and tastier when young and tend to get woody when they are too large. Vegetables can bolt when they are overripe — that is, put up a vertical shoot for a flower and go to seed, and the resulting taste can be bitter and off-putting. For leafy vegetables, look for crisp leaves and stalks with little to no browning, yellowing, or wilting. This guide will help when harvesting and buying vegetables: Farmer's Almanac: Learn How and When to Pick Vegetables and Fruit. https://www.almanac.com/when-harvest-vegetables-and-fruit-best-flavor

FROZEN VEGETABLES

Frozen vegetables can be a great option for consumers, especially when access to fresh produce is limited. The nutrient content of frozen vegetables is comparable to, and sometimes greater than, their fresh counterparts (Bouzari et al., 2015). Both varieties lose some nutrients due to conditions of harvesting and transport, but in the end their nutrient profile is similar.

Once a vegetable is harvested, it continues to undergo chemical changes due to the enzymes present within it. Freezing soon after harvesting halts this enzymatic activity, helping to preserve the color, flavor, and most of the nutrient profile. The one characteristic that is not maintained through freezing is texture. With freezing, water contained within the plant cells expands and causes the cell walls to burst, making the produce much softer when thawed as a result of losing most of its structure. High-starch vegetables such as corn, lima beans, and peas are not as affected by this softening and loss of texture.

Blanching after harvesting also helps to halt the enzymatic activity, preserve color, and remove unwanted microorganisms. Blanching involves either putting the vegetables in a quick steam bath or submerging them in boiling water, followed by a rapid cooling off in ice water. Some water-soluble vitamins like vitamins B and C will be lost in this process. Frozen vegetables need to be stored at 0°F/-18°C or lower and, for the best quality, eaten within eight to 12 months of frozen storage.

CANNED VEGETABLES

Canned vegetables can be just as nutritious as frozen or fresh varieties as long as there is no added salt, fat, or sugar (S. R. Miller & Knudson, 2014). However, they are prone to lose some of their water-soluble vitamin content — the B vitamins and vitamin C — due to heat that is used in the canning process.

There are three steps involved in the canning process:
- Processing:
  - Vegetables are usually picked at their peak and washed, most are peeled, and then they are cut/diced/chopped if needed.
  - Water and sometimes other ingredients are then added to the can to displace the air.
- Sealing: Once the can is sealed,, no oxygen is present, protecting the vegetables from losing nutrients due to oxidation.
- Heating: Each can is heated to a certain temperature to kill any bacteria present. The heat causes some of the water-soluble vitamins to degrade.

From a culinary perspective, it is always better to work with fresh produce, but from a health and wellness perspective, **any type of produce a client can afford and access is the best choice for them.** One job of the chef is to teach clients how to transform canned and frozen varieties into tasty dishes.

Some tips when using canned vegetables:
- If any salt is added to the can, rinse the vegetables thoroughly under cold water to remove some of the sodium.
- Do not overheat canned vegetables, as that will cause more water-soluble vitamins to be lost.
- Avoid purchasing cans that are bulging, have cracks, or are leaking as this can be a sign of the bacteria that causes botulism.

SECTION 8:

VEGETABLES AND SUSTAINABILITY

In the last 20 years, global fruit and vegetable production has increased by about 60% per person, which is good news for health and chronic disease prevention (FAOSTAT). Across the vegetable supply chain, sustainability is impacted in many areas, from the production methods and raw material inputs to the post-harvest management, yield, quality, and transportation — see Figure 7 (Karlsson Potter & Röös, 2021). Growing, transporting, and storing vegetables are generally more sustainable than producing animal foods, such as dairy and meat. There are several issues to consider when making the most sustainable choice for vegetables, which may differ from individual to individual depending on their priorities.

Greenhouse gas emissions (GHGe): Agriculture contributes 30% to 40% of all human-related greenhouse gas (GHG) emissions, but it is also highly affected by climate change. Vegetables are especially vulnerable because of their seasonality and timely water requirements. Vegetable production accounts for only 2.6% of the **greenhouse gas emissions** (GHGe) from food in the United States. As a group, vegetables have among the lowest greenhouse gas footprints — even when transport, packaging, and processing are accounted for. In fact, emissions from most plant-based products are 10 to 50 times lower than animal-based products (Poore & Nemecek, 2018).

Transportation: Environmental impacts related to the production phase of vegetables are mostly associated with fertilizers, diesel use, and emissions due to land use change. However, within this group, there is huge variation. For example, vegetables grown in heated greenhouses use more energy than those transported across the country on a truck. In one study, importing lettuce from Spain to the U.K. during winter produced three to eight times lower emissions than producing it locally during the winter, as heating greenhouses to grow out of season in cold areas uses significant amounts of energy (Hospido et al., 2009). Conversely, vegetables transported by air, such as asparagus, which is often air-freighted from South America, have a much higher GHGe footprint than the snap peas grown by the local farmer. It should be noted that less than 1% of our food travels by air; most of it travels by rail or sea. If a vegetable is marked with a distant country of origin and is highly perishable, such as green beans or asparagus, it is more likely to have been airfreighted.

Water: Water usage can vary by location and the type of vegetable grown, but as a whole, water usage is much lower for vegetables in general than for animal products and crops, such as rice and wheat (Poore & Nemecek, 2018). Vegetables, including starchy root vegetables, on average, require less than half the water per kilogram of producing fruit and 43 times less than beef. However, vegetables that are grown in dry areas require more irrigation and rely on scarce water. Water scarcity is perhaps one of the most crucial issues facing agriculture, and climate change may alter the methods and inputs needed to produce vegetables in the future.

While processing vegetables typically uses more water and energy, produce is usually processed as soon as possible and close to where it was grown. This may decrease waste and energy needed for storage and transportation. The following table compares the water footprints of different tomato products with several other foods.

Figure 9: The Average Water Footprint of Tomato Products (M3/ton).

Land and biodiversity: Similar to GHGe and water, growing vegetables requires less land per kilogram of product than animal-based foods. Growing a diverse mix of crops on the land enhances soil health and biodiversity, which is defined as the variety and diversity of life on Earth — from animals to microorganisms. Farming practices such as the use of cover crops and crop rotation build soil structure, moisture, and nutrients. These practices also promote better weed, pest, and disease management; reduce the need for fertilizers; and result in higher yields. For this reason, purchasing vegetables from farmers who are using these integrative farming practices ensures a more sustainable product (Nair et al., 2014).

Pesticides: Many vegetables are prone to insects and disease, thus requiring the use of pesticides and other chemicals, some of which may have harmful effects. The Environmental Working Group has a free tool – Clean 15™ and Dirty Dozen™ lists, which were discussed earlier– that consumers can use to help decide when it might be best to splurge for an organic product.

Labor: Many vegetables require high labor input from farm to fork, and food system workers, including seasonal farm workers, are often paid low wages and experience poor working conditions. When purchasing vegetables, look for standards that protect the health of food chain workers, such as those promoted by the Food Chain Workers Alliance or the Good Food Purchasing Program.

In summary, to make the most sustainable vegetable choices:
- Buy local, grown in season when possible.
- Avoid vegetables that are transported by air if possible.
- Avoid vegetables grown in heated greenhouses.
- Rinse and scrub vegetables and fruit before eating.
- Eat what you purchase. If you can't, try freezing or pickling them to increase their storage life. You can also chop or purée a mix of vegetables and toss them into soups or sauces for added nutrition and flavor.
- Consider the type of packaging. Less plastic is always better.
- Keep eating your vegetables! They're always a great choice!

SECTION 9:

VEGETABLES IN THE KITCHEN

ON THE TONGUE — THE TASTE OF VEGETABLES

From an evolutionary perspective, fruit draws eaters in with its sweet taste and aroma in order to spread its seeds and reproduce, but vegetables try to avoid being eaten because they are part of the plant itself. They do this by secreting natural pesticides and toxins which tend to have a bitter taste to the human tongue. Given that less than 10% of adults and as few as 2% of children meet the daily vegetable requirement, this is an effective way to avoid being eaten (Lee-Kwan, 2017; Moore et al., 2017)! One explanation for this low intake is the evolutionary theory that humans are genetically wired to avoid bitter taste because bitter foods are often poisonous while sweet foods are not (Drewnowski & Gomez-Carneros, 2000a; Glendinning, 1994).

Much of the bitter taste in vegetables comes from the phytonutrients within them: phenols, terpenoids, alkaloids, flavonoids, glucosinolates, and isothiocyanates. While phytonutrients provide numerous health benefits that were described in the previous chapter and will be explored later in this chapter, they often leave a bitter, astringent, and/or acrid taste. The bitter **taste of vegetables is a barrier to adequate intake** for many individuals, especially for those who are supertasters (Dinehart et al., 2006; Drewnowski & Gomez-Carneros, 2000a). Cruciferous vegetables are especially high in glucosinolates and are often perceived as very bitter vegetables. Interestingly, these vegetables, which include cabbage, kale, broccoli, cauliflower, Brussels sprouts, kohlrabi, collards and Chinese cabbage, were all selectively bred from the wild cabbage. There is also some evidence to suggest that calcium content in vegetables may contribute to the bitter taste, and vegetables with higher calcium content — bitter melon, watercress, collards, mustard greens, Chinese broccoli and kale — are often rated very bitter (Tordoff & Sandell, 2009).

The food industry has been 'debittering' the food supply for years by removing these health-promoting chemicals through breeding plants to contain fewer phytonutrients, and as a result, fewer people are being exposed to the bitter taste of vegetables (Drewnowski & Gomez-Carneros, 2000b). While preferring or even liking bitter taste is not an innate preference for many, one can "train" their taste buds to tolerate and even enjoy eating vegetables. It can take up to a dozen attempts for a child to like a new food. There is also much that can be done in the kitchen to decrease the bitterness and bring out the best features in vegetables.

STORING VEGETABLES

Do not wash produce before storing it, and if the vegetable or fruit is peeled or sliced, always refrigerate it. Adding an acid like lemon juice on exposed cut areas will help to prevent browning from oxidation. Since most fruits produce ethylene gas as they age, it is **best to store fruits and vegetables separately** as the ethylene gas will cause vegetables to spoil quickly. Here is a list of ethylene-producing and ethylene-sensitive produce. See Table 14 for a guide to storing vegetables.

Table 14: Where to Store Vegetables

Leave Out	Cool, Dark, Dry Place	Refrigerate
Avocado Cucumbers (can be refrigerated for 1 to 3 days) Eggplant Peppers (can be refrigerated for 1 to 3 days) Tomatoes	Garlic Onions Potatoes Squash	Beets Broccoli Carrots Cauliflower Celery Green beans Radishes Mushrooms (do not wash first or they will become slimy) Leafy greens (store in a sealed bag with paper towels to prevent excess moisture loss, causing leaves to wilt)

PREPARING VEGETABLES

1. **Preparing a batch of raw vegetables for the week** helps to save time, and convenience encourages consumption, helping one to meet one's daily requirements.
   a. Wash and cut up vegetables
      i. Carrots, broccoli, cauliflower, cabbage, celery and peppers make a great combination
         1. Do not wash or tear leafy vegetables, as they will degrade quickly
2. Place in a container or large plastic bag with a paper towel at the bottom to collect the excess moisture
3. Tearing lettuce preserves more vitamin C (ascorbic acid) than slicing it with a sharp knife (Barry-Ryan & O'Beirne, 1999).
4. As soon as a vegetable is cut, enzymes start to degrade the plant. To minimize degradation, salad preparation should be done last minute.

IN THE PANTRY

It is great to have these items on hand to make delicious vegetables that can be crave-able!

1. Fresh vegetables
2. Frozen vegetables
3. The following adds an umami flavor:
    a. Dried or fresh mushrooms
    b. Soy sauce or tamari
    c. Sun-dried tomatoes
    d. Nutritional yeast
    e. Nori flakes
4. Herbs and spices to enhance flavor, like ginger, garlic, paprika, turmeric, dill, oregano, and more (for example: dill on carrots, oregano on zucchini)
5. Onion and garlic
6. Tomato paste
7. Lemon or lemon zest to enhance the flavor profile
8. Salt and pepper
9. Extra-virgin olive oil
10. Flavored oils (for example: clementine olive oil on green beans)
11. Olive and capers
12. Nuts and seeds
13. Anchovies
14. Fermented foods like sauerkraut, pickled vegetables, and kimchi

FLAVOR DEVELOPMENT

The challenge when cooking with vegetables is dealing with the often-present bitter taste. Knowing what flavors to add to counterbalance the bitter taste, the cooking methods to bring out the sweetness in vegetables, and how to enhance the flavor profile of vegetables using acid, herbs, and spices will help transform a dreaded dish for some into a scrumptious one.

Most people tend to overcook their vegetables, drown them in heavy sauces and butter, or turn what can be a healthful salad into a calorie-laden dish. No one can blame them, as they are actually just trying to transform a taste they dislike into one they like in the only way they know how. Teaching the cooking techniques in this section will give them the tools to transform vegetables into at least tolerable and, at times, craveable food. One just needs to try Cat Cora's Caramelized Brussels Sprouts to understand falling in love with a vegetable (The authors recommend replacing half of the butter with olive oil and decreasing salt in this recipe.)

To decrease the bitterness of certain vegetables:
- Pair a bitter vegetable with a sweeter one to counterbalance the bitterness, for example, pairing radicchio with roasted sweet potato.
- Use umami flavors — Parmesan cheese, mushrooms, tomato, miso — to counterbalance the bitterness, for example adding miso onto steamed Brussels sprouts.
- A dash of salt will decrease the bitterness, for example, adding soy sauce to steamed broccoli.

To brighten a vegetable dish:
- Add an acid like lemon or lime juice to the finished dish. Acid will affect the color of vegetables, causing a dulling of the vibrant hues, so add it at the very end.

Sugar, salt, and fat:
- To decrease the amount of fat added to a vegetable dish, cook in a small amount of liquid — water or broth — and add a dash of oil at the end.
- To decrease the amount of salt needed to enhance the flavor of vegetables, add salt throughout the cooking process. If you wait until the end of the cooking process, you will need to add more salt to get the same taste. In addition, adding umami flavors will decrease the need for salt.
- To avoid adding any sugar to a vegetable dish, grill, roast, or caramelize the vegetable to bring out its natural sweetness.

Raw versus cooked vegetables — which is more healthful? The answer to this complicated question is best answered by Dr. Liu, a Cornell University researcher who studies lycopene. In an interview, he stated, "We cook them so they taste better. If they taste better, we're more likely to eat them. And that's the whole idea.*" Don't focus too much on raw versus cooked but rather on what your patient/client will consume.

For specific information on the effect of cooking on certain nutrients, refer to the chapter on Cooking and Bioavailability. (*Fact or Fiction: Raw Veggies Are Healthier than Cooked Ones - Scientific American, 2009.)

COOKING TECHNIQUES TO SAVE NUTRIENTS

It is important to preserve the nutrients in vegetables when preparing them for consumption.

In order to preserve nutrients:

- Cook vegetables quickly: Steam over a small amount of water for three to four minutes, or stir-fry in a hot pan with a small amount of heated oil.
- Save boiling for soups or stews as the liquid causes nutrients to be leached out of the vegetable cells into the surrounding liquid, which can then be consumed.
- For cruciferous vegetables, chop and wait up to an hour for the myrosinase enzyme to act on glucoraphanin to produce the powerhouse bioactive nutrient — sulforaphane. After the waiting period, the cruciferous vegetable can be cooked quickly or eaten raw.
- Avoid peeling vegetables before cooking as this leads to greater nutrient loss (due to cooking) and fiber loss (due to peeling) (Shahnaz et al., 2003).
- To preserve allicin, a compound with major health benefits in garlic, crush or chop garlic cloves and leave them for 10 minutes before heating.

Pre-cooking Techniques/Preserving Vegetables

Blanching Vegetables

Blanching kills harmful bacteria found on the outer surface of vegetables. It also stops enzymatic reactions that cause a loss of flavor, color, and texture after picking.

For blanching, place vegetables in boiling water for a short amount of time — time differs depending on the vegetable — and then shock them straight into ice-cold water to preserve the color.

Freezing Vegetables

Freezing allows for preserving vegetables for a long period — from eight to 12 months. This allows for growing and buying in bulk when vegetables are plentiful and storing them for later on, which saves time and money.

To freeze vegetables, follow the process below:

WASH $\longrightarrow$ BLANCH $\longrightarrow$ CUT $\longrightarrow$ FREEZE

- Only freeze vegetables that are at the height of their flavor.
- Vegetables that do not freeze well include cabbage, celery, cress, cucumbers, endives, Irish potatoes, lettuce, parsley and radishes.
- For instructions on how to freeze, the best containers to use, packaging and labeling techniques, plus freezer management techniques, Clemson's Cooperative Extension has lots of great advice. https://hgic.clemson.edu/factsheet/freezing-basics/

Knife Skills and Vegetables

It is essential to choose the right tool for the job, and with knives, knowing what size and shape are best to use when preparing different types of vegetables helps to prevent accidents in the kitchen.

Cutting Vegetables

Video: Cutting Vegetables

Build a Salad

There are limitless varieties of salads ranging from a side dish to an entire meal depending on what is put into it. Table 14 lists the five categories that go into building a meal-salad.

Table 15: Build a Super Salad

Pre-Washed Greens	Grains	Protein	Salad Dressing	Additions
Arugula	Barley	Cheese	Oil + lemon juice	Avocado
Kale	Couscous	Eggs	Vinaigrette	Dried fruit
Lettuce – all types	Quinoa	Fish – canned salmon, tuna, etc.	Avoid low-fat and added sugar dressings	Nuts
Mesclun/ Spring mix	Rice – all types	Legumes – beans, lentils, chickpeas etc.		Precut vegetables – all types
Spinach		Meat – chicken, turkey etc..		Seeds
Watercress		Tofu, tempeh, seitan		Tomatoes

For a side salad, you can leave out or reduce the amount of protein and grains in the salad. It all depends on what is going to accompany the salad, like rice and beans or fish and quinoa.

Add the dressing right before serving, as the liquid will wilt the greens, and the acid from the vinegar will "cook" the vegetables and leaves. Make sure to dry the leaves thoroughly after washing so that they can pick up more of the salad dressing.

Salad dressings do not need to be elaborate. In fact, the simple varieties are often the best. The basic formula is:

1 PART VINEGAR OR OTHER ACID LEMON OR LIME JUICE	3 to 4 PARTS OIL

- 1 part sauerkraut juice as the acid and 3 parts olive oil
- Lemon juice and virgin olive oil
- Flavored oil (orange-infused oil) with champagne vinegar
- For more on delicious salad dressings, go to the Fats/Oils chapter

Steaming Vegetables

Steaming is one of the best cooking methods for retaining nutrients. The most important part of steaming vegetables is to avoid overcooking them, as this will degrade some of the nutrients found in them. The second tip is to make sure that the water in the pot is low enough to steam and not high enough to touch the vegetables, as this will lead to boiling, which will leach nutrients from the vegetables.

Steam for a short period of time (under five minutes, depending on the vegetable). You are looking for firmness but also the ability to poke a fork or knife into the vegetable. You know you have cooked for too long if:
- The vibrant color has dulled
- The vegetable has lost all its firmness

Steaming Vegetables

Video: Steaming Vegetables

Sautéing/Stir-Frying

The secret to stir-frying is to cook over high heat for a brief amount of time using an oil that has a high smoke point. Making a stir fry is a great way to introduce more vegetables into the diet. For a meal, add a source of protein – either animal or vegetable.

Choose an oil: Peanut, safflower, canola, grape seed and sunflower (See the chapter on Fats and Oils for further information).

Prepare the ingredients into bite-size pieces: It is very important to have all ingredients ready to go because once the cooking process starts, it happens quickly.
- Cut vegetables into thinner, longer pieces (see the picture above) of the same size so that they cook at the same time.

Identify the cooking time: Separate ingredients into groups with similar cooking times. For animal sources of protein, cook them first then transfer to a bowl. For vegetables, separate those that are harder and take more time to cook (carrots, broccoli, and green beans for example) from those that cook quickly (bean sprouts, and mushrooms for example).

Heat the wok or cast iron pan and then add the oil: Once the oil is glimmering, it is ready.
- Cook the aromatics quickly, making sure they do not burn. Once you can smell them, add the vegetables.
- If cooking with meat – chicken, shrimp, pork, beef – cook it after the aromatics, scoop it out into a bowl and then add back in at the end.
- Cook the harder vegetables first, and when almost ready, add the quicker-cooking vegetables (and tofu, seitan, and tempeh). Stir often.

Add flavor: Choose any of the following and/or add your own favorites: Add, then taste, then add again if desired. If a thick sauce is desired (not necessary), mix 1 tablespoon of cornstarch with 3 to 4 tablespoons of water and add to the stir fry.
- Soy sauce
- Fish sauce, oyster sauce
- Asian wine (Shaoxing)
- Rice vinegar
- Curry paste
- Stock –vegetable
- Toasted sesame oil

Garnish (optional): Garnish with cashews, peanuts, scallions, cilantro, basil, and/or sesame seeds

Table 15 lists four categories of food that go into making a stir fry. The columns include examples, but feel free to make your own based on what you have on hand.

Table 16: Build a Stir Fry

Protein	Aromatics	Hard Vegetables	Quick Cooking Vegetables
Beef, pork	Garlic	Broccoli	Asparagus
Chicken	Ginger	Carrots	Bean sprouts
Fish, shellfish	Onions	Cabbage	Leafy greens – kale, spinach etc..
Tofu, tempeh	Shallots	Cauliflower	Mushrooms
Seitan		Celery	Sugar snap peas
		Green beans	

Roasted Vegetables

Roasting vegetables is the best way to get even the pickiest of eaters to try new varieties. It brings out the vegetable's sweetness by caramelizing the sugars. The varieties are endless depending on the type of vegetable you select.

Step 1: Select a variety of vegetables in various colors
- Root vegetables — beets, carrots, parsnips, potatoes, sweet potatoes
- Cruciferous vegetables — cabbage, Brussels sprouts, broccoli, cauliflower
- Softer vegetables — zucchini, summer squash, mushrooms, peppers
- Other — onions

Step 2: This is an important step to ensure that the vegetables cook at the same time. In the mix, you may have hard root vegetables and softer types like zucchini. Cut the root vegetables in similar sizes and cut soft vegetables in larger pieces than the hard vegetables so they cook at the same time.

Step 3: Toss the cut-up vegetables with olive oil in a bowl. Add enough to coat lightly using your hands to spread the oil over the entire surface of the cut vegetable. You don't want your vegetables swimming in oil.

Step 4: Add salt and pepper plus any hardier spices of your choosing (save fresh herbs to sprinkle on the end product). Examples include dried garlic, oregano, thyme, and rosemary. Don't use fresh garlic, as the pieces will burn in the oven, causing a burnt and unpleasant flavor.

Step 5: Cook in a hot preheated oven 400°F/204°C for 30 to 45 depending on the size of your pieces. Turn the vegetables every 15 to 20 minutes to make sure the pieces cook evenly. For doneness, you are checking for a fork to be inserted easily in the harder varieties especially and to see brown edges (not black).

Step 6: Remove from the oven and top with fresh herbs like parsley, basil, sage and/or Parmesan cheese. (Don't add a lot of salt when cooking if you are adding the cheese at the end because it adds saltiness to the dish.)

Roasting Vegetable

Video: Roasting Vegetables

Cooking with Acid

- Vegetables that can be made into noodles include:
- Zucchini or other squash (remove the core as that is where most of the water comes from)
- Carrots
- Cucumber
- Daikon
- Kohlrabi
- Beets
- Sweet potatoes and butternut squash can be spiralized, but they need to be sautéed over heat in oil for two to three minutes
    - Spiralize the vegetables into noodles.
    - Cook vegetable noodles with lemon juice 10 minutes before serving. Add lemon juice, first pressed olive oil, and a dash of salt to the noodles. This will not only soften the vegetables but add flavor as well.
    - Add scallions, chopped red pepper, nuts, and seeds to the final product.

Love & Lemons has great recipe ideas for vegetable noodles. https://www.loveandlemons.com/veggie-noodles/

Build a Soup with Vegetables

When creating soup, always think about layering flavors. Whatever you add, you want it to be at its fullest flavor. For example, why add diced carrots when roasted carrots would amp up the flavor tremendously?

Step 1: Sauté aromatics in oil
- Four tablespoons of a neutral oil — olive oil, grapeseed oil, canola oil, peanut oil
- Aromatics: Build your own aromatic using the following formula or by using the ingredients listed in Table 16: **2 parts onion + 1 part sweet vegetable + 1 part other vegetable**

Table 17: Aromatic Ingredients

Onion	Sweetness	Other Vegetable	Additional Ingredients
Leek	Carrot	Celery	Bacon, pancetta
Onions – various types (vedalia, purple, etc.)	Fennel	Celery root	Cumin
Shallot	Peppers	Parsnip	Garlic
			Ginger
			Other spices
			Tomato or tomato paste
			Turmeric

Below are some common ingredients for various aromatics:
- Mirepoix: Onion, carrot, celery
- White mirepoix: Leeks, parsnip
- Italian soffritto (also known as battuto): Red onion, carrot, celery + garlic and parsley
- Spanish soffritto: Bell peppers + garlic, tomato paste
- German: Leek, carrots, celery root
- Cajun: Bell pepper, onion, and celery
- Mexican: Onions, garlic, dried oregano, chipotle or other pepper
- Asian: Shallots and ginger
- Indian: Onion, garlic, cumin and turmeric

Step 2: Select at least three kinds of vegetables to go into the soup and some dried spices (save leafy greens until the end). To the aromatics, add dried spices (curry, oregano, thyme, etc.), bloom them (heat them briefly until you can smell them strongly), and then add fresh garlic (garlic can burn quickly, so make sure you add the rest of the vegetables and broth quickly before that happens).

Step 3: Add broth to the vegetable mixture

Step 4: (Optional) Add protein if desired — chicken, lamb, chickpeas, beans, lentils, etc.

Step 5: Cook the soup mixture on a low simmer for one hour. Low and slow is the way to go in order to develop the flavors.

Step 6: (Optional) For a creamy soup either add blended cashews, coconut milk, or dairy and cook to thicken (do not boil).

Step 7: Add leafy greens during the last five minutes of cooking

Step 8: Toppings — this step adds a pop of flavor right before serving. Many people omit this step, but it is quick and easy. Examples of toppings include:
- Herbs — cilantro, parsley, and basil, for example, either in whole herb form or as a pesto
- Crunchy — toasted onions or shallots, roasted nuts, tortilla chips, baked chickpeas and croutons
- A small dollop of cream (sour cream, cashew cream)

Salting vegetables requires a delicate hand.

Salt will draw water out of produce through a process called osmosis. Salt weakens the indigestible carbohydrate (pectin) in many fruits and vegetables, allowing for a more tender piece of produce. The key, however, is not to oversalt or cook too long, as no one likes a mushy bowl of vegetables. To prevent this:

Salt vegetables just before grilling, frying, or baking.
- Legumes — dried beans and peas — have a very tough outer shell which requires softening. Cooking in salted water helps to dissolve the pectin to create tender legumes.
- When boiling vegetables, add salt to the water beforehand, allowing it to dissolve in the water. The salted water will prevent the vegetable from leaching its nutrients (magnesium and sodium, for example) into the unsalted boiling water through diffusion. This will result in both a nicely seasoned vegetable and one that retains more of its nutrients.
- The exceptions are watery vegetables/fruit like eggplant, tomatoes, and zucchini, which require salting beforehand to allow time for the water to be drawn out before cooking over the grill or frying (about 15 minutes).

SECTION 10:

SERVING VEGETABLES

Make sure when planning a menu that vegetables are front and center. Do not be afraid to make them the focus of the dish. In the chapter on **Protein** you will learn about the protein flip whereby the serving size of protein decreases and vegetable increases without sacrificing taste or appeal.

Vegetables can be served at breakfast (in hash browns, omelets or other egg dishes), lunch (two servings in a soup or a salad for example) and dinner (two servings of a variety of vegetables, steamed, puréed, or roasted). Table 15 lists the number of servings of vegetables each day for various age and gender groups. Keep the total daily amount in mind when planning the menu and serve cravable vegetables without resorting to sugar, fat and salt.

Table 18: Vegetable Servings per Day

Age (years)	Amount per Day	Serving Size
12 to 23 months	2/3 to 1 cup	2 to 4 tablespoons
2 to 4	1 to 2 cups	¼ to 1/3 cup vegetables
5 to 8	1 ½ to 2 ½ cups	½ cup juice; 4 inches of a banana; ½ cup applesauce; 16 grapes; ½ small apple; 1 small peach, pear, or orange
Boys 9 to 13	2 to 3 ½ cups	¾ cup juice; 1 cup diced fruit; 1 large orange, peach, or apple; 6 inch banana
Girls 9 to 13	1 ½ to 3 cups	
Boys 14 to 18	2 ½ to 4 cups	1 cup leafy greens, ½ cup cut-up vegetables, ½ cup cooked beans, or peas
Girls 14 to 18	2 ½ to 3 cups	
Women 19 to 30	2 ½ to 3 cups	
Women 31 to 59	2 to 3 cups	
Women 60+	2 to 3 cups	
Men 19 to 30	3 to 4 cups	
Men 31 to 59	3 to 4 cups	
Men 60+	2 ½ to 3 ½ cups	

Accessed from https://www.myplate.gov/eat-healthy/vegetables 4/2022

SECTION 11:

PRACTICAL TIPS TO INCREASE VEGETABLE CONSUMPTION

1. Keep cut-up vegetables in the refrigerator front and center for snacking. Think beyond just carrot and celery — asparagus, zucchini, and pepper sticks, and radish, broccoli, and cauliflower work well, too.
2. Start dinner with a salad, even if eating takeout
3. Reheat leftovers with steamed vegetables. One cup of leftover Chinese food can be transformed into four cups of dinner with the addition of steamed or sautéed vegetables
4. Have a great dipping sauce on hand for those veggie sticks – hummus for example. Set a trap around dinnertime. Put out veggies and dip while you are cooking dinner. Hungry kids and adults will munch on them while waiting for their meal.
5. Fill up on the healthful food first (vegetables) before dipping into the treats.
6. Eat at least two vegetable servings at lunch and dinner, plus one with each snack.
7. Introduce new vegetables in a peer group. A multi-country trial, "Art on a Plate," tested the liking of salad after a cooking workshop in children aged 4 to 14 years. "Liking" increased in 30% of the participants, which was significant (van der Horst et al., 2019).

SUMMARY

Vegetables really are the superstars of the food world as they are packed full of vitamins, minerals, phytonutrients and fiber. While each food has its place in a healthful diet, vegetables are largely under-consumed by the majority of Americans (over 80%), and the research on their ability to promote health is one of the very few irrefutable facts in nutrition science. The list of health benefits of eating vegetables (along with fruits) is very long. They prevent cardiovascular disease, high blood pressure, diabetes, diverticulosis, certain cancers and age-related eye diseases plus much more; decrease all-cause mortality; increase fertility; and help with weight loss. There is no drug on the planet that has an influence on even a fraction of these benefits.

Since the human condition is one in which a bitter taste is often rejected, it often takes certain culinary skills to transform vegetables into something tasty and desirable. Because the desire for bitter-tasting food is not innate like it is for seeking sweet/sugary tastes, it also takes awareness that it can take up to a dozen attempts or more to train taste buds to like the flavor profile of vegetables. Vegetables can be eaten raw, roasted, steamed, caramelized, or stir-fried, as well as many other methods that can transform "ho-hum" and even "icky" into a craveable dish. Knowing how to transform and bring out the desired flavors in vegetables can produce delicious vegetables that even the biggest vegetable skeptics can enjoy.

REFERENCES

2015-2020 Dietary Guidelines | health.gov. Retrieved March 15, 2020, from https://health.gov/our-work/food-nutrition/2015-2020-dietary-guidelines/guidelines/

2015-2020 Dietary Guidelines | health.gov. Retrieved March 20, 2020, from https://health.gov/our-work/food-nutrition/2015-2020-dietary-guidelines/guidelines/

2018 Food & Health Survey. International Food Information Council Foundation. Retrieved March 22, 2020, from https://foodinsight.org/wp-content/uploads/2018/05/2018-FHS-Report-FINAL.pdf

A Patient's Guide to Taking Warfarin. Www.Heart.Org. Retrieved March 28, 2020, from https://www.heart.org/en/health-topics/arrhythmia/prevention--treatment-of-arrhythmia/a-patients-guide-to-taking-warfarin

Appel, L. J., Moore, T. J., Obarzanek, E., Vollmer, W. M., Svetkey, L. P., Sacks, F. M., Bray, G. A., Vogt, T. M., Cutler, J. A., Windhauser, M. M., Lin, P. H., & Karanja, N. (1997). A clinical trial of the effects of dietary patterns on blood pressure. DASH Collaborative Research Group. The New England Journal of Medicine, 336(16), 1117–1124. https://doi.org/10.1056/NEJM199704173361601

Aune, D., Giovannucci, E., Boffetta, P., Fadnes, L. T., Keum, N., Norat, T., Greenwood, D. C., Riboli, E., Vatten, L. J., & Tonstad, S. (2017a). Fruit and vegetable intake and the risk of cardiovascular disease, total cancer and all-cause mortality-a systematic review and dose-response meta-analysis of prospective studies. International Journal of Epidemiology, 46(3), 1029–1056. https://doi.org/10.1093/ije/dyw319

Bai, Y., Wang, X., Zhao, S., Ma, C., Cui, J., & Zheng, Y. (2015). Sulforaphane Protects against Cardiovascular Disease via Nrf2 Activation. Oxidative Medicine and Cellular Longevity, 2015, 407580. https://doi.org/10.1155/2015/407580

Barry-Ryan, C., & O'Beirne, D. (1999). Ascorbic Acid Retention in Shredded Iceberg Lettuce as Affected by Minimal Processing. Journal of Food Science, 64(3), 498–500. https://doi.org/10.1111/j.1365-2621.1999.tb15070.x

Benini, L., Castellani, G., Brighenti, F., Heaton, K. W., Brentegani, M. T., Casiraghi, M. C., Sembenini, C., Pellegrini, N., Fioretta, A., & Minniti, G. (1995). Gastric emptying of a solid meal is accelerated by the removal of dietary fibre naturally present in food. Gut, 36(6), 825–830. https://doi.org/10.1136/gut.36.6.825

Bertoia, M. L., Mukamal, K. J., Cahill, L. E., Hou, T., Ludwig, D. S., Mozaffarian, D., Willett, W. C., Hu, F. B., & Rimm, E. B. (2015). Changes in Intake of Fruits and Vegetables and Weight Change in United States Men and Women Followed for Up to 24 Years: Analysis from Three Prospective Cohort Studies. PLOS Medicine, 12(9), e1001878. https://doi.org/10.1371/journal.pmed.1001878

Bethke, P. C., & Jansky, S. H. (2008). The effects of boiling and leaching on the content of potassium and other minerals in potatoes. Journal of Food Science, 73(5), H80-85. https://doi.org/10.1111/j.1750-3841.2008.00782.x

Bhagwat, S., Haytowitz, D. B., & Holden, J. M. (2014). USDA Database for the Flavonoid Content of Selected Foods Release 3. 176.

Bian, Q., Gao, S., Zhou, J., Qin, J., Taylor, A., Johnson, E. J., Tang, G., Sparrow, J. R., Gierhart, D., & Shang, F. (2012). Lutein and zeaxanthin supplementation reduces photooxidative damage and modulates the expression of inflammation-related genes in retinal pigment epithelial cells. Free Radical Biology & Medicine, 53(6), 1298–1307. https://doi.org/10.1016/j.freeradbiomed.2012.06.024

Bouzari, A., Holstege, D., & Barrett, D. M. (2015). Vitamin retention in eight fruits and vegetables: A comparison of refrigerated and frozen storage. Journal of Agricultural and Food Chemistry, 63(3), 957–962. https://doi.org/10.1021/jf5058793

Bradbury, K. E., Appleby, P. N., & Key, T. J. (2014). Fruit, vegetable, and fiber intake in relation to cancer risk: Findings from the European Prospective Investigation into Cancer and Nutrition (EPIC). The American Journal of Clinical Nutrition, 100 Suppl 1, 394S-8S. https://doi.org/10.3945/ajcn.113.071357

Brookie, K. L., Best, G. I., & Conner, T. S. (2018). Intake of Raw Fruits and Vegetables Is Associated With Better Mental Health Than Intake of Processed Fruits and Vegetables. Frontiers in Psychology, 9, 487. https://doi.org/10.3389/fpsyg.2018.00487

Carotenoids. (2014a, April 28). Linus Pauling Institute. https://lpi.oregonstate.edu/mic/dietary-factors/phytochemicals/carotenoids

Carotenoids. (2014b, April 28). Linus Pauling Institute. https://lpi.oregonstate.edu/mic/dietary-factors/phytochemicals/carotenoids

Chen, H.-G., Sheng, L.-T., Zhang, Y.-B., Cao, A.-L., Lai, Y.-W., Kunutsor, S. K., Jiang, L., & Pan, A. (2019). Association of vitamin K with cardiovascular events and all-cause mortality: A systematic review and meta-analysis. European Journal of Nutrition, 58(6), 2191–2205. https://doi.org/10.1007/s00394-019-01998-3

Cho, E., Seddon, J. M., Rosner, B., Willett, W. C., & Hankinson, S. E. (2004). Prospective study of intake of fruits, vegetables, vitamins, and carotenoids and risk of age-related maculopathy. Archives of Ophthalmology (Chicago, Ill.: 1960), 122(6), 883–892. https://doi.org/10.1001/archopht.122.6.883

Clean Fifteen™ Conventional Produce with the Least Pesticides. Environmental Working Group. Retrieved March 28, 2020, from https://www.ewg.org/foodnews/clean-fifteen.php

Conrad, Z., Raatz, S., & Jahns, L. (2018). Greater vegetable variety and amount are associated with lower prevalence of coronary heart disease: National Health and Nutrition Examination Survey, 1999-2014. Nutrition Journal, 17(1), 67. https://doi.org/10.1186/s12937-018-0376-4

Cooper, A. J., Sharp, S. J., Lentjes, M. A. H., Luben, R. N., Khaw, K.-T., Wareham, N. J., & Forouhi, N. G. (2012). A Prospective Study of the Association Between Quantity and Variety of Fruit and Vegetable Intake and Incident Type 2 Diabetes. Diabetes Care, 35(6), 1293–1300. https://doi.org/10.2337/dc11-2388

DASH Eating Plan | National Heart, Lung, and Blood Institute (NHLBI). Retrieved March 20, 2020, from https://www.nhlbi.nih.gov/health-topics/dash-eating-plan

De Filippis, F., Pellegrini, N., Vannini, L., Jeffery, I. B., La Storia, A., Laghi, L., Serrazanetti, D. I., Di Cagno, R., Ferrocino, I., Lazzi, C., Turroni, S., Cocolin, L., Brigidi, P., Neviani, E., Gobbetti, M., O'Toole, P. W., & Ercolini, D. (2016). High-level adherence to a Mediterranean diet beneficially impacts the gut microbiota and associated metabolome. Gut, 65(11), 1812–1821. https://doi.org/10.1136/gutjnl-2015-309957

Dinehart, M. E., Hayes, J. E., Bartoshuk, L. M., Lanier, S. L., & Duffy, V. B. (2006). Bitter taste markers explain variability in vegetable sweetness, bitterness, and intake. Physiology & Behavior, 87(2), 304–313. https://doi.org/10.1016/j.physbeh.2005.10.018

Dirty Dozen™ Fruits and Vegetables with the Most Pesticides. (2019). Shopper's Guide to Pesticides in Produce. https://www.ewg.org/foodnews/dirty-dozen.php

Drewnowski, A., & Gomez-Carneros, C. (2000a). Bitter taste, phytonutrients, and the consumer: A review. The American Journal of Clinical Nutrition, 72(6), 1424–1435. https://doi.org/10.1093/ajcn/72.6.1424

Drewnowski, A., & Gomez-Carneros, C. (2000b). Bitter taste, phytonutrients, and the consumer: A review. The American Journal of Clinical Nutrition, 72(6), 1424–1435. https://doi.org/10.1093/ajcn/72.6.1424

Eat wholegrains, vegetables, fruit & beans. (2018, April 24). World Cancer Research Fund. https://www.wcrf.org/dietandcancer/recommendations/wholegrains-veg-fruit-beans

Esatbeyoglu, T., Wagner, A. E., Schini-Kerth, V. B., & Rimbach, G. (2015). Betanin—A food colorant with biological activity. Molecular Nutrition & Food Research, 59(1), 36–47. https://doi.org/10.1002/mnfr.201400484

Etminan, M., Takkouche, B., & Caamaño-Isorna, F. (2004). The role of tomato products and lycopene in the prevention of prostate cancer: A meta-analysis of observational studies. Cancer Epidemiology, Biomarkers & Prevention: A Publication of the American Association for Cancer Research, Cosponsored by the American Society of Preventive Oncology, 13(3), 340–345.

Fahey, J. W., Wehage, S. L., Holtzclaw, W. D., Kensler, T. W., Egner, P. A., Shapiro, T. A., & Talalay, P. (2012). Protection of humans by plant glucosinolates: Efficiency of conversion of glucosinolates to isothiocyanates by the gastrointestinal microflora. Cancer Prevention Research (Philadelphia, Pa.), 5(4), 603–611. https://doi.org/10.1158/1940-6207.CAPR-11-0538

Fielding, J. M., Rowley, K. G., Cooper, P., & O' Dea, K. (2005). Increases in plasma lycopene concentration after consumption of tomatoes cooked with olive oil. Asia Pacific Journal of Clinical Nutrition, 14(2), 131–136.

Flavonoids. (2014, April 28). Linus Pauling Institute. https://lpi.oregonstate.edu/mic/dietary-factors/phytochemicals/flavonoids

Forni, C., Facchiano, F., Bartoli, M., Pieretti, S., Facchiano, A., D'Arcangelo, D., Norelli, S., Valle, G., Nisini, R., Beninati, S., Tabolacci, C., & Jadeja, R. N. (2019). Beneficial Role of Phytochemicals on Oxidative Stress and Age-Related Diseases. BioMed Research International, 2019, 8748253. https://doi.org/10.1155/2019/8748253

Fulgoni, V. L., Keast, D. R., Bailey, R. L., & Dwyer, J. (2011). Foods, fortificants, and supplements: Where do Americans get their nutrients? The Journal of Nutrition, 141(10), 1847–1854. https://doi.org/10.3945/jn.111.142257

Gangwisch, J. E., Hale, L., Garcia, L., Malaspina, D., Opler, M. G., Payne, M. E., Rossom, R. C., & Lane, D. (2015). High glycemic index diet as a risk factor for depression: Analyses from the Women's Health Initiative. The American Journal of Clinical Nutrition, 102(2), 454–463. https://doi.org/10.3945/ajcn.114.103846

Glendinning, J. I. (1994). Is the bitter rejection response always adaptive? Physiology & Behavior, 56(6), 1217–1227. https://doi.org/10.1016/0031-9384(94)90369-7

Halkjaer, J., Tjønneland, A., Overvad, K., & Sørensen, T. I. A. (2009). Dietary predictors of 5-year changes in waist circumference. Journal of the American Dietetic Association, 109(8), 1356–1366. https://doi.org/10.1016/j.jada.2009.05.015

Hao, G., Zhang, B., Gu, M., Chen, C., Zhang, Q., Zhang, G., & Cao, X. (2017). Vitamin K intake and the risk of fractures: A meta-analysis. Medicine, 96(17), e6725. https://doi.org/10.1097/MD.0000000000006725

Harasym, J., & Oledzki, R. (2014). Effect of fruit and vegetable antioxidants on total antioxidant capacity of blood plasma. Nutrition (Burbank, Los Angeles County, Calif.), 30(5), 511–517. https://doi.org/10.1016/j.nut.2013.08.019

Harshman, S. G., Finnan, E. G., Barger, K. J., Bailey, R. L., Haytowitz, D. B., Gilhooly, C. H., & Booth, S. L. (2017). Vegetables and Mixed Dishes Are Top Contributors to Phylloquinone Intake in US Adults: Data from the 2011-2012 NHANES. The Journal of Nutrition, 147(7), 1308–1313. https://doi.org/10.3945/jn.117.248179

He, F. J., Nowson, C. A., Lucas, M., & MacGregor, G. A. (2007). Increased consumption of fruit and vegetables is related to a reduced risk of coronary heart disease: Meta-analysis of cohort studies. Journal of Human Hypertension, 21(9), 717–728. https://doi.org/10.1038/sj.jhh.1002212

Healthy Eating Plate. (2012, September 18). The Nutrition Source. https://www.hsph.harvard.edu/nutritionsource/healthy-eating-plate/

Hidalgo, M., Martin-Santamaria, S., Recio, I., Sanchez-Moreno, C., de Pascual-Teresa, B., Rimbach, G., & de Pascual-Teresa, S. (2012). Potential anti-inflammatory, anti-adhesive, anti/estrogenic, and angiotensin-converting enzyme inhibitory activities of anthocyanins and their gut metabolites. Genes & Nutrition, 7(2), 295–306. https://doi.org/10.1007/s12263-011-0263-5

Higdon, J. V., Delage, B., Williams, D. E., & Dashwood, R. H. (2007). Cruciferous vegetables and human cancer risk: Epidemiologic evidence and mechanistic basis. Pharmacological Research, 55(3), 224–236. https://doi.org/10.1016/j.phrs.2007.01.009

Hung, H.-C., Joshipura, K. J., Jiang, R., Hu, F. B., Hunter, D., Smith-Warner, S. A., Colditz, G. A., Rosner, B., Spiegelman, D., & Willett, W. C. (2004). Fruit and vegetable intake and risk of major chronic disease. Journal of the National Cancer Institute, 96(21), 1577–1584. https://doi.org/10.1093/jnci/djh296

Institute of Medicine (US) Standing Committee on the Scientific Evaluation of Dietary Reference Intakes and its Panel on Folate, Other B Vitamins, and Choline. (1998). Dietary Reference Intakes for Thiamin, Riboflavin, Niacin, Vitamin B6, Folate, Vitamin B12, Pantothenic Acid, Biotin, and Choline. National Academies Press (US). http://www.ncbi.nlm.nih.gov/books/NBK114310/

Jannasch, F., Kröger, J., & Schulze, M. B. (2017). Dietary Patterns and Type 2 Diabetes: A Systematic Literature Review and Meta-Analysis of Prospective Studies. The Journal of Nutrition, 147(6), 1174–1182. https://doi.org/10.3945/jn.116.242552

Kalala, G., Kambashi, B., Everaert, N., Beckers, Y., Richel, A., Pachikian, B., Neyrinck, A. M., Delzenne, N. M., & Bindelle, J. (2018a). Characterization of fructans and dietary fibre profiles in raw and steamed vegetables. International Journal of Food Sciences and Nutrition, 69(6), 682–689. https://doi.org/10.1080/09637486.2017.1412404

Kalala, G., Kambashi, B., Everaert, N., Beckers, Y., Richel, A., Pachikian, B., Neyrinck, A. M., Delzenne, N. M., & Bindelle, J. (2018b). Characterization of fructans and dietary fibre profiles in raw and steamed vegetables. International Journal of Food Sciences and Nutrition, 69(6), 682–689. https://doi.org/10.1080/09637486.2017.1412404

Kaluza, J., Larsson, S. C., Orsini, N., Linden, A., & Wolk, A. (2017). Fruit and vegetable consumption and risk of COPD: A prospective cohort study of men. Thorax, 72(6), 500–509. https://doi.org/10.1136/thoraxjnl-2015-207851

Kang, J. H., Ascherio, A., & Grodstein, F. (2005). Fruit and vegetable consumption and cognitive decline in aging women. Annals of Neurology, 57(5), 713–720. https://doi.org/10.1002/ana.20476

Katz, D. L., Doughty, K. N., Geagan, K., Jenkins, D. A., & Gardner, C. D. (2019). Perspective: The Public Health Case for Modernizing the Definition of Protein Quality. Advances in Nutrition (Bethesda, Md.), 10(5), 755–764. https://doi.org/10.1093/advances/nmz023

Kawabata, K., Yoshioka, Y., & Terao, J. (2019). Role of Intestinal Microbiota in the Bioavailability and Physiological Functions of Dietary Polyphenols. Molecules (Basel, Switzerland), 24(2). https://doi.org/10.3390/molecules24020370

Kellingray, L., Tapp, H. S., Saha, S., Doleman, J. F., Narbad, A., & Mithen, R. F. (2017). Consumption of a diet rich in Brassica vegetables is associated with a reduced abundance of sulphate-reducing bacteria: A randomized crossover study. Molecular Nutrition & Food Research, 61(9). https://doi.org/10.1002/mnfr.201600992

Klinder, A., Shen, Q., Heppel, S., Lovegrove, J. A., Rowland, I., & Tuohy, K. M. (2016). Impact of increasing fruit and vegetables and flavonoid intake on the human gut microbiota. Food & Function, 7(4), 1788–1796. https://doi.org/10.1039/c5fo01096a

Krga, I., Tamaian, R., Mercier, S., Boby, C., Monfoulet, L.-E., Glibetic, M., Morand, C., & Milenkovic, D. (2018). Anthocyanins and their gut metabolites attenuate monocyte adhesion and transendothelial migration through nutrigenomic mechanisms regulating endothelial cell permeability. Free Radical Biology & Medicine, 124, 364–379. https://doi.org/10.1016/j.freeradbiomed.2018.06.027

Krinsky, N. I., Landrum, J. T., & Bone, R. A. (2003). Biologic mechanisms of the protective role of lutein and zeaxanthin in the eye. Annual Review of Nutrition, 23, 171–201. https://doi.org/10.1146/annurev.nutr.23.011702.073307

Krishnaswamy, K., & Gayathri, R. (2018). Nature's bountiful gift to humankind: Vegetables & fruits & their role in cardiovascular disease & diabetes. The Indian Journal of Medical Research, 148(5), 569–595. https://doi.org/10.4103/ijmr.IJMR_1780_18

Landete, J. M., Arqués, J., Medina, M., Gaya, P., de Las Rivas, B., & Muñoz, R. (2016). Bioactivation of Phytoestrogens: Intestinal Bacteria and Health. Critical Reviews in Food Science and Nutrition, 56(11), 1826–1843. https://doi.org/10.1080/10408398.2013.789823

Lee, Y., & Park, K. (2017). Adherence to a Vegetarian Diet and Diabetes Risk: A Systematic Review and Meta-Analysis of Observational Studies. Nutrients, 9(6). https://doi.org/10.3390/nu9060603

Lee-Kwan, S. H. (2017). Disparities in State-Specific Adult Fruit and Vegetable Consumption—United States, 2015. MMWR. Morbidity and Mortality Weekly Report, 66. https://doi.org/10.15585/mmwr.mm6645a1

Licznerska, B., & Baer-Dubowska, W. (2016). Indole-3-Carbinol and Its Role in Chronic Diseases. Advances in Experimental Medicine and Biology, 928, 131–154. https://doi.org/10.1007/978-3-319-41334-1_6

Likis, F. (2016). Folic Acid. Journal of Midwifery & Women's Health, 61(6), 797–798. https://doi.org/10.1111/jmwh.12584

Looman, M., van den Berg, C., Geelen, A., Samlal, R. A. K., Heijligenberg, R., Klein Gunnewiek, J. M. T., Balvers, M. G. J., Leendertz-Eggen, C. L., Wijnberger, L. D. E., Feskens, E. J. M., & Brouwer-Brolsma, E. M. (2018). Supplement Use and Dietary Sources of Folate, Vitamin D, and n-3 Fatty Acids during Preconception: The GLIMP2 Study. Nutrients, 10(8). https://doi.org/10.3390/nu10080962

Lovegrove, J. A., Stainer, A., & Hobbs, D. A. (2017). Role of flavonoids and nitrates in cardiovascular health. The Proceedings of the Nutrition Society, 1–13. https://doi.org/10.1017/S0029665116002871

Marcason, W. (2015). What Are the Components to the MIND Diet? Journal of the Academy of Nutrition and Dietetics, 115(10), 1744. https://doi.org/10.1016/j.jand.2015.08.002

McLaughlin, C., Tarasuk, V., & Kreiger, N. (2003). An examination of at-home food preparation activity among low-income, food-insecure women. Journal of the American Dietetic Association, 103(11), 1506–1512. https://doi.org/10.1016/j.jada.2003.08.022

McNaughton, S. A., & Marks, G. C. (2003). Development of a food composition database for the estimation of dietary intakes of glucosinolates, the biologically active constituents of cruciferous vegetables. The British Journal of Nutrition, 90(3), 687–697. https://doi.org/10.1079/bjn2003917

McRorie J. W., Jr (2015). Evidence-Based Approach to Fiber Supplements and Clinically Meaningful Health Benefits, Part 2: What to Look for and How to Recommend an Effective Fiber Therapy. Nutrition today, 50(2), 90–97. https://doi.org/10.1097/NT.0000000000000089

McRae, Marc P. "Dietary Fiber Intake and Type 2 Diabetes Mellitus: An Umbrella Review of Meta-analyses." Journal of chiropractic medicine vol. 17,1 (2018): 44–53. doi:10.1016/j.jcm.2017.11.002

Mielgo-Ayuso, J., Valtueña, J., Huybrechts, I., Breidenassel, C., Cuenca-García, M., De Henauw, S., Stehle, P., Kafatos, A., Kersting, M., Widhalm, K., Manios, Y., Azzini, E., Molnar, D., Moreno, L. A., & González-Gross, M. (2017). Fruit and vegetables consumption is associated with higher vitamin intake and blood vitamin status among European adolescents. European Journal of Clinical Nutrition, 71(4), 458–467. https://doi.org/10.1038/ejcn.2016.232

Miki, A., Hashimoto, Y., Matsumoto, S., Ushigome, E., Fukuda, T., Sennmaru, T., Tanaka, M., Yamazaki, M., & Fukui, M. (2017). Protein Intake, Especially Vegetable Protein Intake, Is Associated with Higher Skeletal Muscle Mass in Elderly Patients with Type 2 Diabetes. Journal of Diabetes Research, 2017, 7985728. https://doi.org/10.1155/2017/7985728

Miki, T., Eguchi, M., Kurotani, K., Kochi, T., Kuwahara, K., Ito, R., Kimura, Y., Tsuruoka, H., Akter, S., Kashino, I., Kabe, I., Kawakami, N., & Mizoue, T. (2016). Dietary fiber intake and depressive symptoms in Japanese employees: The Furukawa Nutrition and Health Study. Nutrition (Burbank, Los Angeles County, Calif.), 32(5), 584–589. https://doi.org/10.1016/j.nut.2015.11.014

Miller, M. G., Thangthaeng, N., Poulose, S. M., & Shukitt-Hale, B. (2017). Role of fruits, nuts, and vegetables in maintaining cognitive health. Experimental Gerontology, 94, 24–28. https://doi.org/10.1016/j.exger.2016.12.014

Miller, S. R., & Knudson, W. A. (2014). Nutrition and Cost Comparisons of Select Canned, Frozen, and Fresh Fruits and Vegetables: American Journal of Lifestyle Medicine. https://doi.org/10.1177/1559827614522942

Miller, V., Mente, A., Dehghan, M., Rangarajan, S., Zhang, X., Swaminathan, S., Dagenais, G., Gupta, R., Mohan, V., Lear, S., Bangdiwala, S. I., Schutte, A. E., Wentzel-Viljoen, E., Avezum, A., Altuntas, Y., Yusoff, K., Ismail, N., Peer, N., Chifamba, J., ... Prospective Urban Rural Epidemiology (PURE) study investigators. (2017). Fruit, vegetable, and legume intake, and cardiovascular disease and deaths in 18 countries (PURE): A prospective cohort study. Lancet (London, England), 390(10107), 2037–2049. https://doi.org/10.1016/S0140-6736(17)32253-5

Moody, D. E., Reddy, J. K., Lake, B. G., Popp, J. A., & Reese, D. H. (1991). Peroxisome proliferation and nongenotoxic carcinogenesis: Commentary on a symposium. Fundamental and Applied Toxicology: Official Journal of the Society of Toxicology, 16(2), 233–248. https://doi.org/10.1016/0272-0590(91)90108-g

Moore, L. V., Thompson, F. E., & Demissie, Z. (2017). Percentage of Youth Meeting Federal Fruit and Vegetable Intake Recommendations, Youth Risk Behavior Surveillance System, United States and 33 States, 2013. Journal of the Academy of Nutrition and Dietetics, 117(4), 545-553.e3. https://doi.org/10.1016/j.jand.2016.10.012

Mudgil, D., & Barak, S. (2013). Composition, properties and health benefits of indigestible carbohydrate polymers as dietary fiber: A review. International Journal of Biological Macromolecules, 61, 1–6. https://doi.org/10.1016/j.ijbiomac.2013.06.044

Mujcic, R., & J Oswald, A. (2016). Evolution of Well-Being and Happiness After Increases in Consumption of Fruit and Vegetables. American Journal of Public Health, 106(8), 1504–1510. https://doi.org/10.2105/AJPH.2016.303260

Muluk, N. B., & Cingi, C. (2018). Oral allergy syndrome. American Journal of Rhinology & Allergy, 32(1), 27–30. https://doi.org/10.2500/ajra.2018.32.4489

National Cancer Institute. (2019). Usual Dietary Intakes: U.S. Population, 2007-2010. Epidemiology and Genomics Research Program website. https://epi.grants.cancer.gov/diet/usualintakes/national-data-usual-dietary-intakes-2007-to-2010.pdf

Neumark-Sztainer, D., Wall, M., Perry, C., & Story, M. (2003). Correlates of fruit and vegetable intake among adolescents. Findings from Project EAT. Preventive Medicine, 37(3), 198–208. https://doi.org/10.1016/s0091-7435(03)00114-2

Neville, C. E., Young, I. S., Gilchrist, S. E. C. M., McKinley, M. C., Gibson, A., Edgar, J. D., & Woodside, J. V. (2014). Effect of increased fruit and vegetable consumption on bone turnover in older adults: A randomized controlled trial. Osteoporosis International: A Journal Established as Result of Cooperation between the European Foundation for Osteoporosis and the National Osteoporosis Foundation of the USA, 25(1), 223–233. https://doi.org/10.1007/s00198-013-2402-x

New FMI Analysis Suggests Produce in Retail Needs a Fresh Look. (2019, March 8). The Food Industry Association. https://www.fmi.org/newsroom/news-archive/view/2019/03/08/new-fmi-analysis-suggests-produce-in-retail-needs-a-fresh-look

Nicklett, E. J., Semba, R. D., Xue, Q.-L., Tian, J., Sun, K., Cappola, A. R., Simonsick, E. M., Ferrucci, L., & Fried, L. P. (2012). Fruit and vegetable intake, physical activity, and mortality in older community-dwelling women. Journal of the American Geriatrics Society, 60(5), 862–868. https://doi.org/10.1111/j.1532-5415.2012.03924.x

Nielsen, E. S., Garnås, E., Jensen, K. J., Hansen, L. H., Olsen, P. S., Ritz, C., Krych, L., & Nielsen, D. S. (2018). Lacto-fermented sauerkraut improves symptoms in IBS patients independent of product pasteurization—A pilot study. Food & Function, 9(10), 5323–5335. https://doi.org/10.1039/c8fo00968f

Nour, M., Lutze, S. A., Grech, A., & Allman-Farinelli, M. (2018). The Relationship between Vegetable Intake and Weight Outcomes: A Systematic Review of Cohort Studies. Nutrients, 10(11). https://doi.org/10.3390/nu10111626

Office of Dietary Supplements—Potassium. Retrieved December 13, 2020, from https://ods.od.nih.gov/factsheets/Potassium-Health%20Professional/

Palermo, M., Pellegrini, N., & Fogliano, V. (2014). The effect of cooking on the phytochemical content of vegetables. Journal of the Science of Food and Agriculture, 94(6), 1057–1070. https://doi.org/10.1002/jsfa.6478

Park, Y., Subar, A. F., Hollenbeck, A., & Schatzkin, A. (2011). Dietary fiber intake and mortality in the NIH-AARP diet and health study. Archives of Internal Medicine, 171(12), 1061–1068. https://doi.org/10.1001/archinternmed.2011.18

Park, Y., Subar, A. F., Hollenbeck, A., & Schatzkin, A. (2011). Dietary fiber intake and mortality in the NIH-AARP diet and health study. Archives of internal medicine, 171(12), 1061–1068. https://doi.org/10.1001/archinternmed.2011.18

Pesticides in Produce. (2015, March 19). [Consumer Reports]. Https://Www.Consumerreports.Org/Cro/Produce0515. https://www.consumerreports.org/cro/produce0515

Pikosky, M., Cifelli, C., Agarwal, S., & Fulgoni, V. (2019). Do Americans Get Enough Nutrients from Food? Assessing Nutrient Adequacy with NHANES 2013–2016 (P18-040-19). Current Developments in Nutrition, 3(Supplement_1). https://doi.org/10.1093/cdn/nzz039.P18-040-19

Potassium and Your CKD Diet. (2016, January 7). National Kidney Foundation. https://www.kidney.org/atoz/content/potassium

Racette, S. B., Lin, X., Ma, L., & Ostlund, R. E. (2015). Natural Dietary Phytosterols. Journal of AOAC International, 98(3), 679–684. https://doi.org/10.5740/jaoacint.SGERacette

Racette, S. B., Spearie, C. A., Phillips, K. M., Lin, X., Ma, L., & Ostlund, R. E. (2009). Phytosterol-deficient and high-phytosterol diets developed for controlled feeding studies. Journal of the American Dietetic Association, 109(12), 2043–2051. https://doi.org/10.1016/j.jada.2009.09.009

Rautiainen, S., Lindblad, B. E., Morgenstern, R., & Wolk, A. (2014). Total antioxidant capacity of the diet and risk of age-related cataract: A population-based prospective cohort study of women. JAMA Ophthalmology, 132(3), 247–252. https://doi.org/10.1001/jamaophthalmol.2013.6241

Ried, K., Toben, C., & Fakler, P. (2013). Effect of garlic on serum lipids: An updated meta-analysis. Nutrition Reviews, 71(5), 282–299. https://doi.org/10.1111/nure.12012

Rietjens, I. M. C. M., Louisse, J., & Beekmann, K. (2017). The potential health effects of dietary phytoestrogens. British Journal of Pharmacology, 174(11), 1263–1280. https://doi.org/10.1111/bph.13622

Ruengsomwong, S., Korenori, Y., Sakamoto, N., Wannissorn, B., Nakayama, J., & Nitisinprasert, S. (2014). Senior Thai fecal microbiota comparison between vegetarians and non-vegetarians using PCR-DGGE and real-time PCR. Journal of Microbiology and Biotechnology, 24(8), 1026–1033. https://doi.org/10.4014/jmb.1310.10043

Schwalfenberg, G. K. (2017). Vitamins K1 and K2: The Emerging Group of Vitamins Required for Human Health. Journal of Nutrition and Metabolism, 2017, 6254836. https://doi.org/10.1155/2017/6254836

Schwingshackl, L., Hoffmann, G., Lampousi, A.-M., Knüppel, S., Iqbal, K., Schwedhelm, C., Bechthold, A., Schlesinger, S., & Boeing, H. (2017). Food groups and risk of type 2 diabetes mellitus: A systematic review and meta-analysis of prospective studies. European Journal of Epidemiology, 32(5), 363–375. https://doi.org/10.1007/s10654-017-0246-y

Schwingshackl, L., Schwedhelm, C., Hoffmann, G., Lampousi, A.-M., Knüppel, S., Iqbal, K., Bechthold, A., Schlesinger, S., & Boeing, H. (2017). Food groups and risk of all-cause mortality: A systematic review and meta-analysis of prospective studies. The American Journal of Clinical Nutrition, 105(6), 1462–1473. https://doi.org/10.3945/ajcn.117.153148

Scientific Report of the 2015 Dietary Guidelines Advisory Committee. U.S. Department of Health and Human Services and U.S. Department of Agriculture. Part D. Chapter 5: Food Sustainability and Safety, p. 283.

Available from: https://health.gov/sites/default/files/2019-09/Scientific-Report-of-the-2015-Dietary-Guidelines-Advisory-Committee.pdf

Serafini, M., & Peluso, I. (2016). Functional Foods for Health: The Interrelated Antioxidant and Anti-Inflammatory Role of Fruits, Vegetables, Herbs, Spices and Cocoa in Humans. Current Pharmaceutical Design, 22(44), 6701–6715. https://doi.org/10.2174/1381612823666161123094235

Shahnaz, A., Khan, M., Sheikh, M., & Muhammad, S. (2003). Effect of peeling and cooking on nutrients in vegetables. Pakistan Journal of Nutrition, 2, 189–191.

Slavin, J. L. (2008). Position of the American Dietetic Association: Health implications of dietary fiber. Journal of the American Dietetic Association, 108(10), 1716–1731. https://doi.org/10.1016/j.jada.2008.08.007

Slavin, J. L., & Lloyd, B. (2012a). Health benefits of fruits and vegetables. Advances in Nutrition (Bethesda, Md.), 3(4), 506–516. https://doi.org/10.3945/an.112.002154

Storey, M. L., & Anderson, P. A. (2013). Contributions of white vegetables to nutrient intake: NHANES 2009-2010. Advances in Nutrition (Bethesda, Md.), 4(3), 335S-44S. https://doi.org/10.3945/an.112.003541

Suggested Servings from Each Food Group. (2017, January 22). American Heart Association. https://www.heart.org/en/healthy-living/healthy-eating/eat-smart/nutrition-basics/suggested-servings-from-each-food-group

Thalheimer, J. (2013, December). A Soluble Fiber Primer—Plus the Top Five Foods That Can Lower LDL Cholesterol. Today's Dietitian, 15(12), 16.

Tordoff, M. G., & Sandell, M. A. (2009). Vegetable bitterness is related to calcium content. Appetite, 52(2), 498–504. https://doi.org/10.1016/j.appet.2009.01.002

Torres-Gonzalez, M., Cifelli, C., Agarwal, S., & Fulgoni, V. (2019a). Sodium and Potassium in the American Diet: Important Food Sources from NHANES 2015–2016 (P18-045-19). Current Developments in Nutrition, 3(Supplement_1). https://doi.org/10.1093/cdn/nzz039.P18-045-19

Torres-Gonzalez, M., Cifelli, C., Agarwal, S., & Fulgoni, V. (2019b). Sodium and Potassium in the American Diet: Important Food Sources from NHANES 2015–2016 (P18-045-19). Current Developments in Nutrition, 3(Suppl 1). https://doi.org/10.1093/cdn/nzz039.P18-045-19

Trichopoulou, A., Bamia, C., & Trichopoulos, D. (2009). Anatomy of health effects of Mediterranean diet: Greek EPIC prospective cohort study. BMJ (Clinical Research Ed.), 338, b2337. https://doi.org/10.1136/bmj.b2337

U.S. Department of Health and Human Services and U.S. Department of Agriculture. (2005). DGA 2005. https://health.gov/dietaryguidelines/dga2005/document/html/chapter6.htm

USDA. (2018). FoodData Central. FoodData Central | U.S. Department of Agriculture, Agricultural Research Service. https://fdc.nal.usda.gov/

USDA Database for the Isoflavone Content of Selected Foods, Release 2.0. 69.

van der Horst, K., Mathias, K. C., Prieto Patron, A., & Allirot, X. (2019). Art on a Plate: A Pilot Evaluation of an International Initiative Designed to Promote Consumption of Fruits and Vegetables by Children. Journal of Nutrition Education and Behavior, 51(8), 919-925.e1. https://doi.org/10.1016/j.jneb.2019.03.009

van Het Hof, K. H., West, C. E., Weststrate, J. A., & Hautvast, J. G. (2000). Dietary factors that affect the bioavailability of carotenoids. The Journal of Nutrition, 130(3), 503–506. https://doi.org/10.1093/jn/130.3.503

van Vliet, S., Burd, N. A., & van Loon, L. J. C. (2015). The Skeletal Muscle Anabolic Response to Plant- versus Animal-Based Protein Consumption. The Journal of Nutrition, 145(9), 1981–1991. https://doi.org/10.3945/jn.114.204305

Vandeputte, D., Falony, G., Vieira-Silva, S., Wang, J., Sailer, M., Theis, S., Verbeke, K., & Raes, J. (2017). Prebiotic inulin-type fructans induce specific changes in the human gut microbiota. Gut, 66(11), 1968–1974. https://doi.org/10.1136/gutjnl-2016-313271

Vanduchova, A., Anzenbacher, P., & Anzenbacherova, E. (2019). Isothiocyanate from Broccoli, Sulforaphane, and Its Properties. Journal of Medicinal Food, 22(2), 121–126. https://doi.org/10.1089/jmf.2018.0024

Vegetable. (2020, March 12). Encyclopedia Britannica. https://www.britannica.com/topic/vegetable

Vitamin C: Fact Sheet for Health Professionals. National Institutes of Health Office of Dietary Supplements. Retrieved March 28, 2020, from https://ods.od.nih.gov/factsheets/VitaminC-HealthProfessional/

Walda, I. C., Tabak, C., Smit, H. A., Räsänen, L., Fidanza, F., Menotti, A., Nissinen, A., Feskens, E. J. M., & Kromhout, D. (2002). Diet and 20-year chronic obstructive pulmonary disease mortality in middle-aged men from three European countries. European Journal of Clinical Nutrition, 56(7), 638–643. https://doi.org/10.1038/sj.ejcn.1601370

Wang, X., Ouyang, Y., Liu, J., Zhu, M., Zhao, G., Bao, W., & Hu, F. B. (2014). Fruit and vegetable consumption and mortality from all causes, cardiovascular disease, and cancer: Systematic review and dose-response meta-analysis of prospective cohort studies. BMJ (Clinical Research Ed.), 349, g4490. https://doi.org/10.1136/bmj.g4490

Welcome to the Natural Medicines Research Collaboration. Retrieved December 13, 2020, from https://naturalmedicines.therapeuticresearch.com/

Willcox, J. K., Ash, S. L., & Catignani, G. L. (2004). Antioxidants and prevention of chronic disease. Critical Reviews in Food Science and Nutrition, 44(4), 275–295. https://doi.org/10.1080/10408690490468489

Wolfson, J. A., & Bleich, S. N. (2015). Fruit and vegetable consumption and food values: National patterns in the United States by Supplemental Nutrition Assistance Program eligibility and cooking frequency. Preventive Medicine, 76, 1–7. https://doi.org/10.1016/j.ypmed.2015.03.019

GRAINS

~

By Jody L.Vogelzang PhD, RDN, FADA, CHES,
Jasna Robinson-Wright, MSc, RD, CDE, CIEC and
Deborah Kennedy PhD
with
The Expert Chef Panel
Reviewed by Kelly LeBlanc MLA, RD, LDN

"Smiles, rainbows, and a grain of rice. I could survive on that."
Quote by Anthony T. Hinks

GRAINS NOURISH THE WORLD. For thousands of years, grains have been a dietary staple for billions of people. Rice, wheat, and maize are considered the most commonly consumed cereal grains, accounting for over 90% of the world's grain consumption and far surpassing more traditional, small-crop grass grains and pseudo-grains such as millet and sorghum (Whole Grains Council). Because of the large demand for and consumption of these three staple grains, more research has been conducted on maize, rice, and wheat than other small crop grains.

Planting and growing grains began about 14,000 years ago (McGee, 2004).

The Oxford Dictionary defines grains as cultivated cereal crops used as food. Cereals are the fruit or the seed of the grass family. After being harvested, dry grains are more durable than other staple foods such as fruits and vegetables, which makes them well-suited for industrial agriculture, long-term storage, and transporting without temperature control. These factors have made grains an important part of the global food system and they account for much of the caloric intake of many nations.

Historically, the development of grain agriculture allowed excess food to be stored safely without the need for temperature control which provided food to early permanent settlers and contributed to the division of societies into classes (Wessel, 1984). Nutritionally, whole grains provide protein, healthful fats, dietary fiber, minerals such as iron and magnesium, B vitamins, and phytonutrients. Due to the starch content, grains, in general, are the largest source of carbohydrates of any food group (Compare Nutrients in Various Grains | The Whole Grains Council).

SECTION 1:
GRAIN CHARACTERISTICS

Image: Grain Characteristics

Whole grains are technically a complete fruit as they contain the ovary of the plant. They are defined as **intact, ground, cracked or flaked fruit of grains in which all components of the kernel, e.g., the bran, germ, and endosperm, are present in the same relative proportions as in the intact grain**. Examples of whole grains include whole wheat, oats, brown rice, rye, barley and bulgur. Whole grains contain more fiber, fat, and protein than processed grains because of the inclusion of the fibrous bran and the germ, which contains fat and protein.

- Bran: A source of fiber. Also contains B vitamins, iron, zinc, magnesium, antioxidants and phytochemicals.
- Endosperm: A source of starchy carbohydrates, some protein, and small amounts of B vitamins and minerals.
- Germ/Yolk: A source of healthful fats, phytonutrients, B vitamins, vitamin E and antioxidants.

For some fruits and seeds — rice, barley, oats, wheat, einkorn, emmer and spelt — an additional outer layer exists and it is known as the husk (also referred to as chaff). The husk is inedible for humans and must be removed before processing, but livestock with their many stomachs can consume the chaff.

Image: Husk and Bran

There are two main classifications of grains: **cereal grains**, which are part of the grass family, and **pseudo-cereals**, which are not. Ancient grains are grains that appear largely the same as they did in ancient times. Table 1 lists the various types of grains (Ancient Grains | The Whole Grains Council).

Table 1: Grain Classification

Cereals (Poaceae Family)	Pseudo-Cereals
Barley	*Amaranth
*Fonio	*Buckwheat
Maize (corn)	*Quinoa
*Millet	
Oat	
Rice	
Rye	
*Sorghum	
*Teff	
Triticale	
*Wild rice	
Wheat • *Eikorn • *Emmer • *Farro • Freekeh • KAMUT® • *Spelt • Bulgur	

*Ancient grain

PROCESSED GRAINS

The Dietary Guidelines for Americans (DGA) identifies two groups of grains — whole and refined. All grains have to be processed to some degree, whether it is to just remove the inedible husk (dehulling) leaving a whole grain, or **removing the bran and germ (polishing/pearling) leaving a refined grain** (Springmann, 2019). The refining process leaves only the soft starchy endosperm and causes a loss of fiber, vitamins, and minerals. Some refined grain products (such as white flour products, breakfast cereals, etc.) are enriched with vitamins (like niacin, riboflavin, and thiamin) and minerals (such as iron) that were lost during milling. White flour is also fortified in Canada and the U.S. with folic acid. However, refined grain products are still lower in fiber and some other nutrients, such as magnesium, compared to the original whole grains.

Figure 1: Grains Listed by Cooking Times

The processing of grains involves many potential steps and impacts how long the grain must be cooked. The following bullets list grains that take the most cooking time (dehulled grain) to the least cooking time (ground grain). Digestion time also decreases in this manner with the most refined grains being digested and absorbed the quickest.
- Dehulling: Removes the inedible outer hull
- Sprouting: The seed is partially germinated
- Pearling/Polishing: The bran and germ are stripped away
- Cracking: The grain is milled into smaller pieces
- Cutting: The grain is sliced into smaller pieces
- Rolling: The grain is steamed and then rolled flat
- Puffing: High pressure or steam is used to inflate the grain
- Grinding: The grain is pulverized into a meal or flour

Whole grains promote health, while ultra-processed grains do not

---

SECTION 2:

RECOMMENDATIONS FOR GRAIN INTAKE

The DGA recommends at least **half of grains (≥ 50%) consumed be sourced from whole grains**. Similarly, Canada's Food Guide recommends that Canadians choose whole grain foods (Health Canada, 2021). Table 2 lists the exact amounts recommended by the USDA.

Table 2: USDA My Plate Recommendations for Grains

Cohort	Age	Total Grains	Whole Grains, Minimum
Toddlers	12-23 months	1 ¾ to 3 oz-equiv	1 ½ to 2 oz-equiv
Children	2-4 yrs 5-8 yrs	3 to 5 oz-equiv 4 to 6 oz-equiv	1½ to 3 oz-equiv 2 to 3 oz-equiv
Girls	9-13 yrs 14-18 yrs	5 to 7 oz-equiv 6 to 8 oz-equiv	2 ½ to 3 ½ oz-equiv 3 to 4 oz-equiv
Boys	9-13 yrs 14-18 yrs	5 to 9 oz-equiv 6 to 10 oz-equiv	3 to 4 ½ oz-equiv 3 to 5 oz-equiv
Women	19-30 yrs 31-59 yrs 60+ yrs	6 to 8 oz-equiv 5 to 7 oz-equiv 5 to 7 oz-equiv	3 to 4 oz-equiv 3 to 3 ½ oz-equiv 3 to 3 ½ oz-equiv
Men	19-30 yrs 31-59 yrs 60+ yrs	8 to 10 oz-equiv 7 to 10 oz-equiv 6 to 9 oz-equiv	4 to 5 oz-equiv 3½ to 5 oz-equiv 3 to 4 ½ oz-equiv

Source: https://www.myplate.gov/eat-healthy/grains

WHAT IS AN OUNCE EQUIVALENT?

The DGA recommends consuming whole grain foods in "ounce equivalents." **One ounce equivalent is about 28 grams**. Table 3 lists approximate ounce equivalents for a variety of different grain foods.

Table 3: USDA My Plate Examples of Ounce Equivalent of Grains

Food	Amount in 1 ounce-equivalent (oz-equiv) of Grains
Bagels	1" mini bagel
Bagel or pita chips	⅓ cup bagel or pita chips
Barley	½ cup, cooked
Buckwheat	½ cup, cooked
Biscuits	1 small biscuit
Breads	1 regular slice of bread 1 small slice of French bread 4 snack-size slices of rye bread
Bulgur	½ cup, cooked
Challah bread	1 medium or regular slice
Chapati	1 small chapati or roti (6") ½ large chapati or roti (8")

Food	Amount in 1 ounce-equivalent (oz-equiv) of Grains
Cornbread	1 small piece of cornbread
Couscous	½ cup, cooked
Crackers	5 whole wheat crackers 2 rye crispbreads 7 square or round crackers
English muffins	½ English muffin
Muffins	1 small muffin
Oatmeal	½ cup, cooked 1 packet instant 1 ounce (⅓ cup), dry (regular or quick)
Pancakes	1 pancake (4½" diameter) 2 small pancakes (3" diameter)
Pasta - spaghetti, macaroni, noodles	½ cup, cooked 1 ounce, dry
Popcorn	3 cups, popped
Quinoa	½ cup, cooked
Ready-to-eat breakfast cereal	1 cup, flakes or rounds 1¼ cup, puffed
Rice	½ cup, cooked 1 ounce, dry
Tortillas	1 small flour tortilla (6" diameter) 1 corn tortilla (6" diameter)

The Oldways Whole Grains Council recommends looking for the Whole Grain Stamp on the label of grain products. The Stamp states how many grams of whole grain are present in one serving of the food regardless of whether it's 100% whole grain or not, which can help consumers keep track of their whole grain intake (Whole Grains Council).

GRAIN INTAKE AMONG AMERICANS

Figure 2: Contribution of Whole Grains to Total Grain Intake

Whole grain intake is abhorrently low in the United States for all age groups. Most Americans consume mostly refined grains in lieu of whole grains and for others, the low/no-carb craze has caused some individuals to decrease their intake even further. In 2013–2016, only **15.8%** of total grain intake for adults on a given day came from whole grains. The contribution of whole grains to total grain intake increases with age and ranges from 12.9% among adults aged 20 to 39, to 19.7% for adults aged 60 and over (Ahluwalia et al., 2019). Whole grains contributed to a lower percentage of total grains intake among men (14.8%) compared with women (16.7%). Similarly, among adults aged 20 to 39, the percentage of total grains consumed as whole grains was lower among men (11.1%) than among women (14.7%).

In spite of the strong consensus and messaging on transitioning grain intake to more whole grains, Americans are not in alignment with dietary recommendations. Intake of refined grains is much higher than recommended and intake of whole grains is much lower than recommended..

Figure 3: Average Whole and Refined Grain Intake

LOW/NO-CARB SAFETY

Fad diets continue to influence population food habits, and in recent years all grains, including whole grains, have been pushed aside in the move to follow a low-carbohydrate diet. As noted earlier in the chapter, grains are significant sources of healthful fats, fiber, and other micronutrients. **When grains are totally removed from daily consumption, there is no another food group that can adequately replace these same nutrients**. In addition, when one macronutrient group is excluded from the diet, the consumption of the other two increases. Lowering carbohydrate intake usually translates particularly into a higher intake of fat, and to a lesser extent an increase in protein consumption, which Americans and Canadians already get enough of.

Whole grains continue to be recommended by many professional organizations and federal agencies despite the current popularity of low-carbohydrate diets. For example, the American Heart Association recommends eating three or more servings of fiber-rich whole grains every day. The United States Department of Agriculture makes this statement about the intake of grains: "Most Americans consume enough grains, but few are whole grains. At least half of all the grains eaten should be whole grains." The Centers for Disease Control also supports whole grain intake and notes that over the last decade, whole grain intake has increased for both men and women, but this trend seems to be most apparent in families with higher income levels (Ahluwalia et al., 2019). The USDA Food and Nutrition Service (FNS) requires that **80% of all grains/breads** offered in the National School Lunch and Breakfast programs be whole grain (Academy of Nutrition and Dietetics, 2022). One serving per day of grains in the Child and Adult Care Food Program (CACFP) must be whole grain-rich or at least 50% whole grain.

Americans should be encouraged to trade in some of the highly processed, refined grain items for more nutrient-dense whole grains. Similarly, in Canada, the 2020 Canada's Food Guide recommends that one-quarter of the plate should come from grains, namely whole grains. In this most recent version of Canada's Food Guide, serving sizes and number of servings per day for grains (and other food groups) are no longer specified, but rather a general recommendation is given to choose whole grains over refined grains and to choose grain foods prepared with little or no added sugar, salt, or saturated fat.

Benefit Versus Risk of Low-Carb/No-Carb Diets

There is a fair amount of evidence that following any kind of significantly restricted diet whether low or high in carbohydrates (and even if it is in line with national food guides) can result in a significant decrease in micronutrient intake (Gardner et al., 2010; Meckling et al., 2004; Noakes et al., 2005; Tay et al., 2015; Truby et al., 2008; Wyka et al., 2015). Among studies reviewed by Dietitians of Canada, reducing calories by 500 to 900 Kcal per day (the amount recommended for a weight loss of 1 to 2 pounds per week) using either high or low-carbohydrate diets **increased the risk of micronutrient inadequacy**. More restrictive lower carbohydrate diets (12% to 17% carbohydrate, 26% to 49% protein, 35% to 57% fat) such as Atkins® tended to have lower intakes of fiber and micronutrients such as non-heme iron, folic acid, thiamin, magnesium, calcium, potassium, vitamin D, vitamin B_6 and vitamin C (Gardner et al., 2010; Meckling et al., 2004; Truby et al., 2008). The low levels of iron, folic acid, and thiamin were thought to be due to the low intake of fortified cereals and grains. On the other hand, low-carb/higher protein diets may be associated with improvements in vitamin B_{12} and iron intake (Noakes et al., 2005).

The review by Dietitians of Canada also found that there is fair evidence that the lower the carbohydrate intake of a diet, the lower the fiber intake, on average (Gardner et al., 2010; Meckling et al., 2004; Truby et al., 2008). People following low carbohydrate diets should ideally be counseled to increase the nutrient density of their eating pattern, and a dietitian should evaluate if a multivitamin/multimineral supplement and fiber supplement may be beneficial for certain individuals.

Short-term studies (four to eight weeks) of low carbohydrate diets (5% to 35% energy from carbohydrate, 30% to 35% energy from protein) have shown **adverse changes in fecal metabolites and biomarkers that are associated with colonic health** (Aune, Chan, Greenwood, et al., 2012; Brinkworth et al., 2009; Duncan et al., 2007; Nilsson et al., 2013; Russell et al., 2011; Sieri et al., 2015). While there have not been studies to date showing an increased risk of colon cancer resulting from low carbohydrate intake, the low fiber consumption in these diets and often higher red meat and processed meat consumption has the potential to negatively impact intestinal health.

On the other hand, some research shows that there may be benefits to lower carbohydrate diets. Several meta-analyses and systematic reviews have shown that there is fair evidence that lower carbohydrate diets (<120 g per day) that last up to two years were associated with **weight loss and improved HDL cholesterol and triglyceride levels**. However, **the very low-carbohydrate diets sometimes resulted in increased LDL cholesterol**. Overall, the low-carbohydrate diets were associated with lower 10-year predicted risk of atherosclerotic cardiovascular disease than low-fat diets. This score is a better predictor of heart disease risk than LDL alone (Atallah et al., 2014; Clifton et al., 2014; T. Hu et al., 2012; Mansoor et al., 2016; Sackner-Bernstein et al., 2015; Santesso et al., 2012).

There is fair evidence from meta-analyses that among adults with type 2 diabetes, following a low carbohydrate diet (<130g per day) over the course of up to one year improves hemoglobin A1c, a marker of blood glucose management (Ajala et al., 2013; Kirk et al., 2008; Kodama et al., 2009). Short-term studies (six to 24 months) examining weight loss induced by following a low-carbohydrate diet have found no difference in the amount of weight lost on low-carbohydrate diets compared to other types of restrictive diets (Guldbrand et al., 2012, 2014; Jonasson et al., 2014; Rock et al., 2014; Saslow et al., 2014; Tay et al., 2014). Furthermore, longer-term studies show that restrictive eating patterns for the purpose of weight loss actually predict weight gain over time due to detrimental effects on metabolism among other factors (Schwartz et al., 2017). For more information on this topic, see the chapter on Obesity and Overweight.

In summary, those following low-carbohydrate diets are at risk for inadequate intakes of fiber and some important micronutrients. Low-carbohydrate diets **may** be beneficial for weight loss, reducing the risk of heart disease, and management of type 2 diabetes, but the research remains very mixed and definitive conclusions cannot yet be drawn.

LIFE STAGE AND GENDER INFLUENCES ON GRAIN INTAKE

As noted previously in Figure 3, neither males nor females of any age group meet the recommendations for whole grain intake. Women overall tend to do a little bit better (16.7%

whole grains to total grains) than men (14.8% whole grains to total grains). It does appear, however, that the intake of refined grains does decrease and whole grains increases as one ages — from 12.9% for those aged 20 to 39 to 19.7% for those 60 years and older, but still several servings short of the daily recommendations made by the United States Department of Agriculture (Ahluwalia et al., 2019).

Grain intake starts as an infant with most babies introduced to cereal around six months of age. Infant cereals include oats, barley, rice and multigrain blends. As chewing ability and swallowing safety matures, toddlers are transitioned to teething crackers, toast, and unsweetened breakfast cereals that may be made from corn, wheat, oats, or rice. Cereal and grain items such as bagels and muffins remain widely accepted breakfast items throughout the life span. Many ready-to-eat cereals have been created and marketed to children and adolescents. In fact, ready-to-eat cereals are one of the most common sources of whole grains in the American diet (Albertson et al., 2016). In the 2020–2025 Dietary Guidelines, it is recommended that toddlers age 12 to 23 months make upward of two-thirds of their grain intake whole grains to ensure that fiber and micronutrient needs are being met (Dietary Guidelines for Americans, 2020-2025).

In the middle-aged to older adult age range, the shift to less refined grains and more whole grains may be due to health reasons. Whole grains are recommended as prevention and treatment for a number of health conditions.

SECTION 3:

WHY ARE GRAINS SO HEALTHFUL?

In general, whole grains are excellent sources of manganese and fiber. Manganese is an essential micronutrient involved in several biochemical reactions such as lowering blood glucose, a coenzyme in the metabolism of vitamins including vitamin C and vitamin E, and it contains antioxidant properties that protect against free radicals.

Whole grains are a healthful source of nutrients, such as dietary fiber, iron, zinc, manganese, folate, magnesium, copper, thiamin, niacin, vitamin B_6, phosphorus, selenium, riboflavin, and vitamin E. **Whole grain foods contribute about 15% of the total dietary fiber in the American diet**, according to the What We Eat In America survey data (Kranz et al., 2017). Also, while one thinks of grains as a source of carbohydrates, whole grains also contain protein and small amounts of healthful fats. The protein content of different whole grains varies widely, and some whole grains with the **highest protein content include amaranth, KAMUT®, buckwheat, quinoa, spelt and wild rice** at around 6 g protein per serving (in 45 g uncooked grain). This is about the same amount as is present in an egg. However, except for **quinoa, buckwheat, and amaranth**, most whole grain protein is not a complete protein but is low in one or more essential amino acids. By enjoying a variety of plant proteins (such as legumes, nuts, seeds, etc.) throughout the week, the complementary proteins combine to create enough building blocks for the body's needs (Whole Grain Protein Power! | The Whole Grains Council). For more information on complementary proteins, see the Vegetarian Diet chapter. Additionally, a 45 g uncooked serving of whole grains has about 30 g of carbohydrates (including 3 to 7 g of fiber, which represents indigestible carbohydrates) and 1 to 3 g of lipid (Whole Grains Council). Whole grains also contain a variety of phytochemicals, and they support a healthful microbiome, as discussed below.

There is an abundance of grains to choose from, all with slightly different nutrient profiles. In 2012, the Grains and Legumes Nutrition Council developed a chart with comparative nutrient values for many grains. Values for macronutrients vary widely between the different grains, making a strong case for a varied diet. **Neither refined grains nor enriched grains can ever replace the total amount of nutrients lost in the processing of whole grains**, as shown in Table 4. Additionally, none of the phytonutrients that are lost during processing can be returned with enrichment.

Table 4: Comparing Nutrients in Whole Wheat to Refined Grains and Enriched Grains*

Nutrient	Refined Grain (% compared to whole wheat)	Enriched Grain (% compared to whole wheat)
B1 (thiamin)	24%	156%
B2 (riboflavin)	24%	299%
B3 (niacin)	25%	119%
B6	11%	
Folate	59%	661%
Vitamin E	8%	
Iron	33%	129%
Potassium	29%	
Magnesium	16%	
Protein	78%	

*Data in table recreated from
https://wholegrainscouncil.org/whole grains-101/whats-whole grain-refined-grain.
The amount of nutrients in whole wheat was set at 100% for comparison.

FIBER

Fiber is mainly found in the bran or the outer layer of a grain, which is removed in the processing of refined grains. Fiber includes carbohydrates known as polysaccharides and resistant oligosaccharides. Whole grains are one of the largest contributors to dietary fiber, and are particularly high in **insoluble fiber** (Anderson et al., 2009; Dhingra et al., 2012; Padayachee et al., 2017). Dietary fiber is an **essential nutrient** even though it is not digested by the body. Consumption of dietary fiber has been shown to be associated with a decreased risk of the following – cardiovascular disease, cardiovascular disease mortality, coronary artery disease, pancreatic cancer, gastric cancer and all-cause mortality (Veronese et al., 2018).

Fiber can be categorized by its physical characteristics, solubility, viscosity, and fermentability. It leads to satiety and satiation by adding bulk and slowing the digestion of foods found in a fiber-rich meal (Soluble and Insoluble Fiber). The various forms of fiber are discussed below:

- **Soluble fiber** — including pectins, beta-glucan, psyllium, and raw guar gum — is found in grains such as oats and barley, as well as apples, pears, flax seeds, nuts, legumes, and much more. In the digestive tract, soluble fibers combine with water and form a gel-like substance, which is mucilaginous. It is this gel-like, viscous mass that slows down the absorption of glucose across the intestinal wall (McRorie & McKeown, 2017). Bacteria in the colon digest some of this mass to produce gas and short-chain fatty acids. Soluble fiber has many beneficial health effects through its ability to decrease both cholesterol and fat absorption, as well as stabilizing blood sugar levels by slowing the digestion of carbohydrates. These benefits can lead to the following:
  - Reducing the risk of cardiovascular disease by lowering LDL and total cholesterol levels by 5% to 10% without changing HDL levels and reducing lipid levels (Surampudi et al., 2016)
  - Help with weight management by decreasing BMI, body weight, insulin resistance, and fasting blood glucose levels (Thompson et al., 2017)
  - Creating a healthful gut by providing gut bacteria the substrates they need to feed upon, which strengthens the gut barrier. Soluble fiber is fermented into short-chain fatty acids — mostly butyrate, acetate, and propionate — by the intestinal microbiota.
- **Insoluble fiber** includes cellulose and is found in foods such as wheat bran. Insoluble fiber — inulin, fructooligosaccharides, and wheat dextrin — is not digested in the intestines due to a lack of enzymes to break down the fibers found in the outer covering of the grain. Insoluble fiber helps move food along through the digestive tract and reduces the amount of time that harmful bacteria and toxins spend in the digestive tract, thereby reducing the risk of constipation, diverticulitis, diverticulosis and colorectal cancer. Undigested fibers also provide a food source for helpful bacteria in the gut.

- **Resistant starch** is a soluble fiber that is highly fermentable in the gut. It gets broken down by helpful bacteria to create short-chain fatty acids (which is discussed in further detail in the section on grains and the microbiome). Resistant starch is naturally found in grains as well as some fruits, vegetables, and legumes. Resistant starch is considered a prebiotic, which is a type of carbohydrate that gut bacteria feed upon; they are found in foods such as wheat, oats, onions and garlic (Slavin, 2013). Once fiber is broken down in the large intestine, it can feed the helpful bacteria in the gut. Eating a variety of fiber sources can improve the diversity of the microbiota, improve constipation and lactose intolerance, enhance immunity and reduce gut inflammation (British Dietetic Association, 2021).

Because whole grains are high in fiber, they improve satiety due to increased food volume and delayed gastric emptying in the case of soluble fiber. Whole grains also tend to have low glycemic indexes. The slow release of glucose into the bloodstream, along with the bulk created by high-fiber foods, helps to increase the sensation of fullness and reduce overeating. (Hartley et al., 2016; Tosh, 2013). Dietary fiber also helps in regulating blood glucose levels by slowing digestion and thus the release of glucose into the bloodstream. Despite the multitude of health benefits attributed to fiber, more **than 90% of women and 97% of men do not meet the daily requirement for fiber** (DGA 2020-2025). Table 5 lists the recommendation for fiber intake and Table 6 lists 'high' and 'good' sources of fiber.

Table 5: Fiber Recommendations by Life Stage

Age	Acceptable Intake of Fiber (g)
Infants	
0-12 months	Not determined
Young Children	
1-3 years	19
4-8 years	25
Males	
9-13 years	31
14-50 years	38
51+ years	30
Females	
9-18 years	26
19-50 years	25
51+ years	21

Source: Dietary Reference Intakes, Government of Canada and U.S. Food and Drug Administration

Table 6: Sources of Fiber from Grains

High Source (20% or more of the RDI/DRV, or more than 5.6 g per serving)	Good Source (10% to 19% of the RDI/DRV, or 2.8 to 5.5 g per serving)
1/3 cup bran (oat bran, wheat bran)	1 slice 100% whole-wheat bread
¼ cup All bran cereal	1 slice rye bread
1 cup cooked whole wheat pasta	1 cup cooked wild rice
1 cup cooked quinoa	1 cup cooked long-grain brown rice
1 cup cooked pearl barley	1 corn tortilla
1 cup cooked bulgur	3 cups popped popcorn
Fiber One granola bar	1 cup cooked oatmeal
30 grams rye wafer crackers	30 grams whole wheat crackers

PHYTOCHEMICALS

Epidemiological evidence consistently shows that higher whole grain intake reduces the risk of several chronic diseases such as type 2 diabetes, cardiovascular disease, and some types of cancer. The fiber content of whole grains is usually cited as the reason for these health benefits, however, increasing evidence from in vitro and in vivo studies shows that in addition to the fiber content of whole grains, the phytochemicals present in this food group likely also play an important role in disease prevention (Koistinen & Hanhineva, 2017; Van Hung, 2016; Zhu & Sang, 2017).

Phytochemicals are non-nutritive dietary bioactive compounds and secondary metabolites that are made by plants to protect themselves against environmental stressors and threats. Whole grains contain several phytochemicals, including:
1. Phenolic compounds such as phenolic acids, anthocyanins, tocols (tocotrienols and tocopherols), lignans, alkylresorcinols, and carotenoids (lutein, zeaxanthin, etc.)
2. Other phytochemicals such as phytic acid, phytosterols, γ-oryzanol, avenanthramides, and benzoxazinoids.

Phytochemicals in grains are mainly concentrated in the outer layers in the germ and bran portions, therefore whole grains contain higher levels of phytochemicals than refined grains (Koistinen & Hanhineva, 2017; Özer & Yazici, 2019; Van Hung, 2016).

Oats contain two unique phytochemicals, avenanthramides, and avenacosides A and B, which have strong antioxidant and anti-inflammatory effects and contribute to the ability of oats to reduce cardiovascular disease risk (Sang & Chu, 2017). Sorghum contains phytochemicals that help with glucose metabolism, are cholesterol-lowering and have anti-inflammatory and anti-cancer properties. The phytochemicals in sorghum include phenolic acids, flavonoids, condensed tannins, policosanols, phytosterols, stilbenes, and phenolamides. Most of these phytochemicals are concentrated in the bran portion (Dykes, 2019).

A study by Sytar et al. (2018) found that the color of grains and sprouts correlates with the antioxidant activity and contents of bioactive phytochemicals (Sytar et al., 2018). For example, anthocyanin, quercetin, and pelargonidin are higher in purple wheat sprouts than in blue or yellow wheat. Phenolic compounds from purple corn have anti-inflammatory and anti-cancer properties (Lao et al., 2017; Lao & Giusti, 2016; Yu & Beta, 2015). Natural anthocyanins have strong antioxidant capacities and help decrease the risk of diabetes, hypertension, and cardiovascular disease (Jing & Giusti, 2011; Putta et al., 2018). Yellow grains have yellow endosperms which are characterized by high carotenoid but lower anthocyanin levels (Seeram & Stoner, 2011). Pelargonidin chloride is found in higher amounts in the sprouts than in the grains of colored wheat and has been found to have anti-inflammatory and anti-diabetic properties (Amini et al., 2017; Cherian et al., 1992). Similarly, sprouts tend to be higher in flavonoids, total phenolic content, and total antioxidant activity than grains (Sytar et al., 2018). Consuming sprouted grain foods may be helpful in reducing the risk of chronic diseases for this reason.

Whole grains have a predominance of bound phytophenols (compared to fruits and vegetables which have largely free polyphenols) (Neacsu et al., 2013). Whole grains can also contribute vitamin E and phytosterols that have been linked to lowering markers of metabolic syndrome (Fardet, 2010). Higher total phenolic compound content is linked with higher antioxidant activity (Farasat et al., 2014). Wheat sprouts have a high antioxidant capacity and could play a role as a functional food supplement to help reduce the risk of diseases where free radicals play a role (Ravikumar et al., 2015).

GRAIN AND THE MICROBIOME

Some of the metabolic benefits of grains may be attributable to their effect on the gut microbiome (Korpela et al., 2014; Vanegas et al., 2017). When dietary fiber in whole grains is fermented in the gut by resident bacteria, short-chain fatty acids are produced, which improve gut health locally as well as overall health (Sekirov et al., 2010). For example, these short-chain fatty acids help maintain the gut barrier function by producing mucin, inhibiting growth of pathogens, and increasing nutrient absorption (Ríos-Covián et al., 2016). Short-chain fatty acids also act as signaling molecules for carbohydrate and lipid metabolism, and higher levels of these acids are associated with lower body weights and decreased risk of some cancers (Brahe et al., 2013; Ríos-Covián et al., 2016). Both gut microbiota and short-chain fatty acids are important for immune function and gut health (Bengmark, 2013; Benus et al., 2010).

A study by Matinez et al. (2013) found that groups randomized to consume whole grain barley and/or brown rice had more microbial diversity, a better Firmicutes/Bacteroidetes ratio, and more beneficial bacteria in fecal samples (Martínez et al., 2013). The changes in gut bacteria after consuming 60 g of these whole grains for four weeks were also associated with improvements in metabolic parameters such as better glucose and insulin levels.

A recent randomized controlled trial by Kopf et al. (2018) found that among people living in larger bodies, those randomized to consume a diet higher in whole grains (three servings per day of whole grains, compared to refined grains) had improvements in inflammatory markers (tumor necrosis factor-α and lipopolysaccharide-binding protein), which was linked to improvements in gut barrier function and modest changes in gut microbiota (Kopf et al., 2018). Several other studies have similarly found that increasing whole grains improves inflammatory markers and gut microbiota (Kristensen et al., 2012; Martínez et al., 2013; Tighe et al., 2010; Vitaglione et al., 2015). A study by Vanegas et al. (2017) found that consuming more whole grains (compared to refined grains) increased stool weight and frequency and had positive effects on gut microbiota, short-chain fatty acids, effector memory T cells and immune response (Vanegas et al., 2017).

While most studies examining the effect of whole grains on gut microbiota have found modest changes (Ampatzoglou et al., 2016; Cooper et al., 2017; Lappi et al., 2013; Roager et al., 2017; Vanegas et al., 2017; Vitaglione et al., 2015), other studies have reported more substantial changes in the gut microbiota, such as increases in beneficial bacteria and phylum-level changes (Costabile et al., 2008; Martinez et al., 2020). These differences may be due to the different types and quantities of whole grains used in each study.

SECTION 4:
TRADITIONAL STAPLE GRAIN SUBTYPES

CEREAL GRAINS

Rice, wheat, and maize comprise the common cereal grains. These grains, over millennia, have provided most of the daily calories and nutrients to populations. These grains went through natural genetic modification due to biological evolution, making them hardy, genetically diverse, and able to thrive in harsh climates.

Over time the grass family of cereal grains (wheat) diverged into several different subspecies which are the ancestors of modern wheat. Einkorn and emmer are two examples of ancient wheat families which were some of the first crops to be cultivated specifically for sustenance. About 12,000 years ago, einkorn and emmer wheat were being grown in the Near East (Boukid et al., 2018; Dinu et al., 2018).

Grain species grown today are a result of intentional crossbreeding coming from technological advancements in the 1930s–1960s which produced heartier and more resilient and pest-resistant plants. This gave rise to mono-cropping and decreased genetic diversity in the plants, leading to nutrient-depleted soils and the need for high chemical fertilizers and pesticides (A. Gupta et al., 2022).

Maize

Image: Maize

Maize, more commonly known in the United States as corn, is thought to have originated in southern Mexico 7,000 to 10,000 years ago from a wild grass. It was the Native Americans who first domesticated corn, making it into a food staple and one of the Three Sisters in their indigenous food legend. Today, maize is considered a dietary staple that looks far different than it did at its origin. Sub-Sahara Africa (SSA) considers maize a major staple crop, using it in wide-ranging food items from infant cereals to family main dishes (Ekpa et al., 2018).

Maize or corn is widely grown in the United States as well as in other countries, especially Brazil and China. While many may think of corn as only being yellow, other varieties like white, red, blue and black corn are also grown globally. While maize was widely used solely for human nourishment in the past, today in the United States over 40% of corn is diverted to the production of ethanol, and 36% is used for animal feed.

Nutritionally, corn is a source of many of the B vitamins, however, the B vitamin niacin exists in a bound form, so it cannot be absorbed without processing. Corn is also a source of minerals including potassium, copper, iron, zinc and manganese and is a good source of antioxidants such as carotenoids, lutein, and zeaxanthin which are involved in eye health.

Native Americans were some of the first food scientists. They instinctively soaked corn in a calcium hydroxide solution and then ground the product, creating the masa flour used for tortillas. This early process of soaking maize in a high pH (alkaline) solution and then grinding released the niacin from its bound state, making it available for intestinal absorption. This process protected the Native Americans from pellagra, the vitamin deficiency related to poor intakes of niacin.

As seen in other grains, processing methods have been used to make maize more palatable and adaptable, greatly increasing the number of ways it can be used in food preparation. Milling is still the most common method used to create ground maize products. Corn flour, cornmeal, corn starch, dry masa and hominy flour are used to make corn muffins, grits, polenta, tortillas, dry cereals, snack foods, breading for meats or vegetables and as a thickener. Corn flour has a fine texture and is light in color, while cornmeal is more coarsely ground. Cornmeal has a more distinctive yellow color (if made from yellow corn) than corn flour, and cornstarch is powdery and made only from the starchy endosperm of the plant.

The corn grown across the U.S. is predominately genetically modified to be herbicide-resistant. This is also seen in Sub-Saharan Africa, where corn has been modified to fit the climate and is hoped to be the answer to looming food insecurity due to population growth (Ekpa et al., 2018).

Rice

Image: Rice

Rice is one of the three main food crops globally, and over 40,000 varieties can be found worldwide. It originated in its wild form in Asia in approximately 2500 B.C. and then through genetic evolution emerged in its cultivated form. This domestication of rice occurred over 9,000 years ago. Rice continues to be a staple in Asian diets, although a decrease in intake has been noted over the past few decades (Shi et al., 2017).

Rice arrived in the U.S. about 400 years ago (H. Wang et al., 2017). As genetic evolution occurred, a common variety of rice emerged referred to as "weedy rice." This strand of the rice plant is invasive and can decrease crop yields by 80% if not contained. Rice production in the U.S. has been augmented by nutrient adaptations of the soil.

Based on processing, rice can be categorized as white, brown, black, purple or red. Brown rice (as well as colored rice like red rice and black or purple rice) contains the intact kernel and the bran, making it a better choice nutritionally than white rice due to a higher micronutrient and fiber content. This simple food provides 88% of the Recommended Daily Intake (RDI) of manganese, and lower but still double-digit percentages of thiamin, niacin, pyridoxine, copper, magnesium and selenium.

Parboiled rice (also known as converted rice) is a medium glycemic index food (generally lower than brown rice and wild rice) and can be a good substitute for those with diabetes wishing to improve their blood glucose management. Parboiled rice has been partially boiled in the husk, which improves its nutrient profile and also makes it more resistant to weevils – a type of beetle. Parboiled rice is more nutritionally similar to brown rice as the processing drives the nutrients, particularly thiamin, from the bran to the endosperm (Kyritsi et al., 2011).

Wheat

Image: Wheat

Wheat is the most common and dominant cereal grain produced, and when eaten in its whole form can provide benefits far beyond caloric energy. The most concentrated area of fiber, micronutrients, and phenolic compounds are found in the germ and bran parts of the wheat. These essential parts of the grain must be included in products labeled as "whole grain." Through the retention of the germ, whole wheat is an important source of folate, thiamin, magnesium, pyridoxine, iron, selenium, vitamin E and zinc. The bran part of the cereal grain contains fiber, B vitamins, and iron.

Whole grain foods are a part of a healthful diet and have been found to be protective against cancer, diabetes, and cardiovascular disease (Călinoiu & Vodnar, 2018). The glycemic index (rise of postprandial blood sugar) of whole grains has been studied and found that the slowly digestible starch found in whole grains can be helpful in controlling spikes in blood sugar levels. Unfortunately, the processing involved in the production of white flour removes both the germ and bran resulting in the loss of up to 70% of essential nutrients and an increase in the glycemic index. The refining of grains results in significant losses of thiamine, biotin, vitamin B_6, folic acid, riboflavin, niacin, pantothenic acid, calcium, iron and magnesium (Oghbaei & Prakash, 2016).

While millions of people currently use cultivated wheat as a food staple (Dinu et al., 2018), rice and maize also provide a significant amount of energy and nutrients to populations across the globe. Other popular grains such as rye, oats, and barley display a botanical structure similar to wheat. They too have an outer shell which is high in fiber, the germ that is high in micronutrients, and the carbohydrate-rich endosperm.

Rye

Image: Rye

Rye is genetically similar to wheat and is classified as a cereal grain. Like barley and oats, rye survives and thrives in cold and rainy climates. Before technology and transportation made wheat available almost everywhere, rye was perhaps the most accessible option for bread baking in northern Europe, from Russia and the Baltic States, west through Poland, Hungary, Austria, Germany, and the Netherlands, and up into Scandinavia. It is commonly consumed in Northern and Eastern Europe and brought to the United States" (Moskin, 2017). Rye is easy to grow even in cold, harsh temperatures. In the United States, it is mainly grown as a cover crop.

Rye bread, usually made from a mix of rye and wheat flour, has a different flavor, density, and color than wheat products. It is described as bitter, nutty, and because of a different matrix of gluten-forming proteins, is denser than wheat breads. Nutritionally, this grain has a higher protein content than many of the cereal grains and has a higher amount of the amino acid lysine. Rye has more dietary fiber and a higher proportion of gel-like, water-soluble fibers than wheat (Suhr et al., 2017). Rye adds vitamin E, calcium, iron and potassium to the diet and these nutrients have been associated with a reduction in cardiovascular disease, colon cancer, breast cancer and diabetes. Rye is also a source of soluble fiber and has a low glycemic index, making it a good option for blood glucose control and satiety.

In Europe, one can find rye crackers, flatbreads, and traditional roggebrood (rye bread) in grocery stores and bakeries. Most of these products can also be found in the United States as imports, or made from heirloom recipes at ethnic bakeries. Rye's history would not be complete without the mention of distilleries that for centuries used rye to make whisky. In the U.S., whisky distillers using rye date back to the 1700s, it then disappeared after the prohibition and emerged again in the 21st century.

Oats

Image: Oats

Oats are classified as a cereal grain and are widely consumed as a breakfast food, appearing on supermarket shelves as whole oats, instant oats, or as ready-to-eat cereal. Oats are rated as an excellent source of manganese and molybdenum, a very good source of phosphorus, and a good source of copper, magnesium, chromium, zinc, biotin and thiamin.

The familiarity with this grain may be due to decades of research indicating that oats have many health benefits due to their content of soluble fiber (beta-glucan). Beta-glucans are soluble cereal fibers that are found naturally in the bran of certain cereal grasses and are known to decrease LDL cholesterol (Ho et al., 2016). The soluble fiber in oats is also helpful in relieving constipation (Thies et al., 2014), and whole rolled oats have a low glycemic index, making them a good option for blood glucose management.

However, beta-glucan is not the only health-inducing substance in oats. This grain is also a robust source of phenolic acids and avenanthramides, compounds that promote gut health. According to Kristek et al. (2018), "The promotion of the growth of specific beneficial gut microbiota is believed to have preventative effects on CVD due to the influence of these bacteria on human physiology/ metabolism, including the ability to reduce total serum cholesterol" (Kristek et al., 2018).

Despite the impressive nutrition profile of minerals, fiber, healthful fats, protein and antioxidants, land given to oat production has been shrinking worldwide. Oats are a low yield crop due in part to its heavy husk which must be stripped to make the grain digestible for humans. Oat groats still contain part of the husk, increasing the fiber content but also require overnight soaking before cooking. Genetically pure oats do not contain gluten, however, cross-contamination of oats with gluten is common.

Barley

Image: Barley

Barley has a long history as a food product and was thought to have been domesticated about 5000 B.C. in Egypt. Nowadays, it is grown in a variety of locations as this grain is highly adaptable to many different climates. The countries that produce the most barley include Russia, Germany, Canada, France, and Ukraine (Food and Agriculture Organization of the United Nations). Barley is a cereal grain and, for centuries, was the primary grain used for bread making. Today, as the fourth-largest cereal crop grown worldwide, it is still used in soups, porridges, puddings and stews, in brewing beer and distilling alcohol (single malt scotch).

Like most other grains, barley also has an inedible outer husk, which is removed during processing. Interestingly, there is also a hull-less barley variety. There are many different forms of barley, including:
- Scotch barley, also known as "pot" barley, contributes almost 3 grams of fiber per serving and like most of the cereal grains is a good source of manganese. Scotch barley is not as common in the U.S., but it might appear in old recipes from Europe or Australia. It is not considered a whole grain.
- Pearl barley is a more polished form of barley with all or most of its bran layer removed. Malt barley is a form of barley specifically used for making beer. In the U.S., about three-quarters of barley grown is used for malting (Agricultural Marketing Research Center, 2022)
- Hulled barley, like hull-less barley, is virtually always whole grain. In the case of hulled barley, only the inedible hull is removed, leaving the other grain components intact. (In the case of hull-less barley, described above, the grain is grown without a hull at all and does not get polished.)

Barley flakes and barley flour are considered whole grain if they are made from whole barley (Whole Grains Council). One can replace up to half of the wheat flour in yeast breads with barley flour or all of the wheat flour in cookies and quick breads. Barley is also available as a sprinkle that can be added to breakfast cereals, porridge, cereal bars and baking to add additional fiber and nutrients to meals and snacks.

Barley contains the soluble fiber beta-glucan, which can decrease LDL cholesterol and help maintain stable blood sugar levels. Soluble fiber accounts for about 4% to 6% of barley's weight (Oscarsson et al., 1998). In the U.S., barley products that contain at least 0.75 g of beta-glucans per serving can display a health claim, and in Canada, barley products with at least 1 g of beta-glucans can show health claims (Bureau of Nutritional Sciences, 2016; FDA, 2013).

Pearl barley contains 2 g of fiber per one-half cup cooked, and 40 g of barley flour contains 4 g fiber. Whole barley flour is a source of protein with 4 g of protein per 40 g, but barley is low in the essential amino acid lysine (Canadian Nutrient File, 2021). Barley has a low glycemic index and raises blood glucose slowly, with the glycemic index of pearl barley ranging from 22 to 29 (on a scale of 100) (The University of Sydney). Barley does contain gluten and is not recommended for those with celiac disease.

For more information on barley, visit: How Well Do You Know Your Barley by Oldways Whole Grains Council. https://wholegrainscouncil.org/blog/2020/05/how-well-do-you-know-your-barley

ANCIENT GRAINS

Beyond wheat, rice, and corn, other grains frequently called "forgotten grains" go back to 10,000 B.C. when the hardy proso millet was highly cultivated across Eurasia because of its drought tolerance and resistance to bird and insect attack (Cheng, 2018). Recently, consumers have expanded their interest in and demand for many of the ancient grains that date back to earlier cultures and societies that have not been bred and have been changed by humans over time. Ancient grains such as quinoa, millet, and buckwheat date back 7000 to 10,000 years and have not been commercially cultivated or domesticated.

While technological advances stimulated crop production and larger harvests, the focus has now shifted to the nutritional qualities of ancient grains compared to the modern, intentionally cross-bred varieties (Boukid et al., 2018). These "forgotten" grains appear to have a more healthful phytochemical profile than modern grains and higher amounts of proteins, trace elements, and antioxidants. For example, einkorn and emmer wheat have been found to have higher selenium, iron, zinc, and manganese levels than some of the modern wheat species (Dinu et al., 2018). However, the nutrient content of ancient grains is variable depending on climate conditions and agronomic practices (Boukid et al., 2018).

Amaranth

Image: Amaranth

Amaranth is a tall broad-leaf plant classified as a "pseudo grain", and it comes from the same family as quinoa (Tang & Tsao, 2017; Whole Grains Council). It is a complete protein and gluten-free. There are many alternative names for amaranth, including Achis, achita, African spinach, bush greens, Indian spinach, Joseph's-coat, kiwicha, love-lies-bleeding, pigweed, princess-feather, spinach-grass, Surinam spinach, wild beet, and wild blite. There are over 60 different varieties of amaranth, and some are used for ornamental gardens (Whole Grains Council). This grain was first domesticated in the 1300s and was used as a sacred grain by the Aztecs in Columbia. Upon the arrival of the Spaniards in the 1700s and the resulting food acculturation, the grain faded in dietary importance as it was replaced by wheat, rye, and barley. In the 1970s, this grain emerged and gained popularity due to its protein content and the high level of the amino acid lysine which is often low in grain products (Cheng, 2018). Today, amaranth is grown mainly in China, Eastern Europe, and South America (The Jefferson Institute, 2002).

The active biochemicals of the amaranth are found in the outer seed coat and the healthful lipids in the seeds themselves. However, "quinoa seed oil has better nutrition quality than that of amaranth seeds based on the omega-6/omega-3 ratio" (Tang & Tsao, 2017). The seeds can be prepared as a porridge, combined with other grains like brown rice as a side dish, and can be ground into flour and used in baking. Replacing up to one-quarter of wheat flour in a recipe with amaranth flour yields a baked product with a desirable consistency and texture. **Amaranth flour also makes an excellent thickener for sauces, gravies, and soups**. Amaranth leaves are also eaten as a vegetable in some areas.

Amaranth is a good source of fiber, its flour is particularly high in fiber compared to many other flour options, with 6 g of fiber per 40 g of flour. Amaranth also contains 5 g of **complete protein** per one-half cup of cooked grain (or per 40 g of flour), a higher protein content than its quinoa cousin. Amaranth is also a good source of magnesium and phosphorus and contains more calcium and iron than many other grains (with 60 mg calcium per one-half cup cooked grain or 40 g flour, and 3 g iron per one-half cup cooked grain or 40 g flour) (Canadian Nutrient File, 2021). Amaranth is also higher in phytosterols than nut or vegetable oils with 543 µg to 834 µg per 100 (Marcone et al., 2003). Amaranth has a high glycemic index, similar to white bread and so may not be the best option for managing blood glucose. Amaranth grain contains about 7% oil, much of which is unsaturated fatty acids (75%), including linoleic acid (47%). Amaranth is high in the unsaturated hydrocarbon squalene (2% to 8%), which is used in synthesizing sterols.

Buckwheat

Image: Buckwheat

Buckwheat is also classed as a "pseudo-cereal" grain that originated in Eastern Asia as far back as 6000 B.C., certainly qualifying it as an "ancient grain." By the 1400s, this grain had arrived in Europe and was brought to America in the 1600s. Buckwheat is related to the rhubarb and sorrel family and is a triangular-shaped seed (Whole Grains Council). The countries producing the highest amounts of buckwheat include Russia, China, Ukraine, Poland, and France (Food and Agriculture Organization of the United Nations)

Grown easily in most of the Northern Hemisphere, the most commonly consumed part of the buckwheat plant is the seed which is ground into flour and is similar to oat bran. Buckwheat groats have the hull removed and are either whole or cracked. Another popular form is Kasha which is roasted buckwheat. As with the other "ancient grains," there is high demand for buckwheat products in the functional food industry, a trend which is expected to continue.

Nutritionally, buckwheat is superior in protein when compared to grains such as corn, rice, and wheat (Cheng, 2018). It is also a **complete protein**. Buckwheat provides 2 g of fiber per one-half cup cooked groats. It also provides 3 g of protein per one-half cup (Canadian Nutrient File, 2021). Depending on the variety, buckwheat fiber may be anywhere from 2% to 22% soluble fiber, and resistant starch counts for 4% to 7%. Buckwheat is also high in several trace minerals including zinc, copper, magnesium and manganese which are concentrated in the bran. However, the phytic acid in buckwheat may limit the absorption of some of these minerals. Buckwheat is also very high in lignans. Buckwheat bread has a glycemic index of 67, noodles a glycemic index of 59, and buckwheat groats have a glycemic index of 49 to 51 (out of 100) (The University of Sydney).

Buckwheat is considered to be safe for those with celiac disease since it is naturally gluten free. Although its prolamin content is low, buckwheat allergies have been documented in about 1% of people with celiac disease (Krkoskova & Mrazova, 2005; Wijngaard & Arendt, 2006). Buckwheat is one of Japan's top allergens, but wild buckwheat is likely a safe alternative for those who are allergic (Akiyama et al., 2011; Nordlee et al., 2011).

Millet

Image: Millet

Millet has been grown for over 10,000 years and is known in some areas as broomcorn. There are several different varieties of millet and their unique characteristics influence the use and consumption of this grain from the grass family. Finger millet has been used in snack foods and vermicelli and has a favorable glycemic index when compared to other grains (Shobana et al., 2018). Pearl millet is a commonly used cereal product in Africa and Asia. Pearl millet has attractive health characteristics such as high antioxidant activity and a low score on the glycemic index due to the slow digestibility of its starch, although the dietary fiber content is lower than the 'finger' variety (Dias-Martins et al., 2018).

The protein content of pearl millet is a mixed bag; it has more protein per gram than finger millet but the lowest amount of methionine of all of the grains. The amino acids leucine and isoleucine are higher in pearl millet than in corn, wheat, or rice. Prolamin is part of the gluten complex, however in millet and several other grains discussed here, prolamin in millet is considered safe to those who follow a gluten-free regimen (Rai et al., 2018).

Today, pearl millet is used widely in Indian and African foods such as porridges, flatbreads, sweets and drinks (Dias-Martins et al., 2018). Food scientists continue to look for ways to bring millet into mainstream markets. Its positive nutrition profile can be further enhanced through manufacturing processes which increase the bioavailability of nutrients and protein absorption of this grain (Dias-Martins et al., 2018).

Quinoa

Image: Quinoa

Perhaps one of the best-known "ancient grains" or "pseudo cereals" is quinoa. This grain's early history associates it with the religious practices of the Inca in the mountains of Chile, Peru, and Bolivia. Like amaranth, the Spanish explorers attempted to rid the country of this crop, and it did not remerge into mainstream farming until the 1970s. Nowadays, the top producers of quinoa are Peru, Bolivia, and Ecuador (Food and Agriculture Organization of the United Nations). Quinoa grows in both humid and semi-arid areas with hot days and cool nights (Salt Spring Seeds).

Quinoa is a small sesame-sized grain that comes from the same botanical family as beets and spinach and has been shown to be a very tolerant and resistant plant. Plant research has identified about 250 different types of quinoa including colorful varieties that are black, purple, red, ivory, orange and yellow (Whole Grains Council).

Quinoa contains 2 g fiber and 3 g protein per one-half cup cooked. **Quinoa is a complete protein** as it contains all essential amino acids. It supplies more omega-3 fatty acids than most other grains, with 140 mg omega-3 per 40 g quinoa flour (Canadian Nutrient File, 2021). Quinoa is also gluten-free and has a low glycemic index of 53 (out of 100) (The University of Sydney).

Quinoa flour can be mixed with cornmeal or wheat flour and results in highly acceptable baked products. Tang et al. (2017) stated that "quinoa can be used at the rates of 10% to 13% in bread, 30% to 40% in noodles and pasta, and 60% in sweet biscuits" with high sensory scores (Tang & Tsao, 2017). The quality of the bread product does decrease with an increase in the percentage of quinoa flour, which was attributed to a bitter taste and a decrease in texture (Sezgin & Sanlier, 2019). Most quinoa on the market today has been rinsed to remove bitter saponins on the surface. Quinoa is rarely pearled, as that creates an uneven cook without fully removing the saponins. Alternatively, some producers polish the quinoa by removing the saponin but leaving the bran intact.

Sorghum

Image: Sorghum

Sorghum has been used as a food crop in Africa for at least 8,000 years. This ancient grain was traditionally used as a porridge (thick and thin) or as a beverage, however, as cuisines have transitioned to include more Western foods, the consumption of sorghum has declined (Cisse et al., 2018). This grain is drought tolerant and there has been some interest in reviving the use of this crop as a food staple for small farmers. Barriers to increasing consumption of this cereal grain include stigma (it's known as a poor man's crop), low production which limits food scientists' development of new products using sorghum, and bird damage in the field.

From a nutritional perspective, sorghum's bioactive compounds are similar to that of millet. It has an attractive glycemic index and a slower gastric emptying time than wheat, which increases satiety (Bahwere et al., 2017).

Teff

Image: Teff

Teff also earns the right to be referred to as an "ancient grain" with domesticated use starting somewhere between 4000 to 10,000 B.C. It has the distinction of being billed as the "world's smallest seed" as it takes over 2.50 million seeds to make a kilo of this grain.

Teff is closely related to the finger millet described earlier in this section. This iron-rich, gluten-free grain is considered a food staple in Ethiopia and Eritrea but is not widely used in other countries (Nascimento et al., 2018). In the United States and Australia, teff is often used as a forage crop instead of an intentional human food crop (Cheng, 2018). However, even in Ethiopia, the land allocated to the production of teff has decreased. Research demonstrated that because the price of harvested teff was low, fewer farmers were interested in growing it. Food developers have used teff in breads, cookies, fermented beverages, weaning beverages and pasta, demonstrating the versatility of this grain, especially when mixed or added to other flours (Nascimento et al., 2018).

Ancient grain seeds are widely available from seed distributors. Ancient grain flours are available through many commercial baking outlets. Current interest in these flour varieties can be attributed to several factors, including the increased awareness of the importance of fiber, lipids, micronutrients, gluten-free status and sustainability.

Table 7: "Good" Nutrient Sources in Ancient Grains

Grain	'Good' Source of...	Gluten-Free	Glycemic Index
Buckwheat	Complete protein, zinc, copper, manganese, and soluble fiber	Yes	55 (Low)
Amaranth	Protein, fiber, calcium	Yes	75 to 100 (High)
Millet	Fiber, zinc, iron, magnesium	Yes	70+ (High)
Quinoa	Complete protein, zinc, magnesium, omega-3 fatty acids	Yes	53 (Low)
Sorghum	Fiber, iron, antioxidants	Yes	62 to 70 (Moderate)
Teff	iron	Yes	36 (Low)

SECTION 5:
GRAIN INTAKE AND HEALTH OUTCOMES

Some of the most widely researched benefits of eating whole grains include lower blood cholesterol and a lower risk of heart disease, decreased obesity, lower incidence of type 2 diabetes (T2D) and decreased risk of colon cancer. Many of these benefits are tied to the fiber in the bran portion of the grain, which is the very same portion that is removed during refining. This section will look at several chronic health issues and how grains may play a role in both prevention and intervention.

CONSTIPATION AND BOWEL DISORDERS

Whole grains contain more fiber than refined grains because of the retention of the bran layer. The extra fiber coupled with adequate fluids adds bulk to the stool, making it easier to pass without additional straining (de Vries et al., 2015). Insoluble fiber, of which whole grains are a primary contributor, speeds gastrointestinal transit, thereby helping to alleviate constipation (Anderson et al., 2009). Soluble fiber, which is present in grains such as oats and barley, slows gastrointestinal transit and allows stool to absorb water and improve consistency, leading to a stool that is neither too hard nor too soft and can therefore help with both diarrhea and constipation (Paruzynski et al., 2020). Fiber from whole foods such as whole grains, fruits, vegetables, nuts, seeds and legumes is preferable over fiber supplements for preventing and treating mild constipation as high-dose fiber supplements can be associated with increased gas, abdominal discomfort, and possibly worsening constipation in some cases (Lambeau & McRorie, 2017; Watanabe et al., 2018; Yang et al., 2012).

A systematic review including 29 studies found that oats and oat bran can help improve bowel health. One intervention study included in the review showed that oat bran provided small improvements in people with ulcerative colitis. The 14 studies included in the review on people without bowel disease found that oats or oat bran significantly increased stool weight and decreased constipation (Thies et al., 2014).

A study by Holma et al. (2010) looking at adults with constipation found that rye bread relieves mild constipation and improves colonic metabolism compared with white wheat bread and commonly used laxatives without causing negative gastrointestinal effects (Holma et al., 2010). The study showed that in comparison to white bread, rye bread shortened total intestinal transit time by 23%, increased weekly defecation by 1.4, softened feces and eased defecation. Compared to laxatives, rye bread reduced total intestinal transit time by 41%. A study by Grasten et al. (2000) found similar results when comparing rye bread to wheat bread (Gråsten et al., 2000).

A randomized controlled study on women with functional constipation found that consuming a brown rice-based diet decreased total intestinal transit time and increased frequency of stools compared to consuming a white rice-based diet (Jung et al., 2020). In a study examining children with infrequent bowel movements, the addition of two servings of oatmeal daily was effective at reducing symptoms that accompany constipation such as gas, straining, and the feeling of incomplete evacuation (Paruzynski et al., 2020).

DIABETES

Whole grains are important in achieving control of blood sugar which is foundational to diabetes management. The availability of soluble fiber can have a positive impact on the stabilization of blood sugars by slowing glucose absorption in the small intestine. In a review of the literature, Della Pepa et al. concluded that whole grains are effective in **both the prevention and treatment of type 2 diabetes** (Della Pepa et al., 2018).

High fiber diets (>25 g/day in women and >38 g/day in men) lowered the risk of developing type 2 diabetes by 20% to 30% in large prospective cohort studies. The reduced risk of diabetes is mainly due to high insoluble fiber intake from cereals (rather than from soluble fiber intake from vegetables and fruits). A review of recent studies noted that high intake of fiber from grains in human trials helps lower insulin resistance (Weickert & Pfeiffer, 2018). Davison and Temple (2018) also noted in their review of recent trials that the protective effect of cereal fiber on the risk of developing type 2 diabetes is likely due to the effect on gut microbiota which improves glucose tolerance by changing energy metabolism pathways, reducing inflammation and changing the immune system's response (Davison & Temple, 2018).

Similarly, Venn and Mann found in their review that epidemiological studies strongly support that whole grains reduce the risk of type 2 diabetes (Venn & Mann, 2004). People who eat three servings per day of whole grain foods have a **20% to 30% lower risk of diabetes than people who consume fewer whole grains**. Additionally, the emphasis should be on **whole food sources**, as studies in the review by Venn and Mann suggest that the improved glucose metabolism is at least partially associated with intact food structure. Fine grinding of the grains disrupts cell structures and makes the starch easier to digest, which does not seem to lend the same health benefits in terms of diabetes prevention (Venn & Mann, 2004). Other studies (not a complete list) that support both a reduction in and treatment for type 2 diabetes are presented in Table 8.

Oats and barley: Studies have found that beta-glucans (soluble fibers) from barley and oats can help diminish the postprandial rise in blood glucose, which may play a role in preventing the development of type 2 diabetes and also help with diabetes self-management. A 2013 literature review of 34 clinical trials found that consuming barley and/or oats as part of a meal resulted in a reduced postprandial rise in blood glucose by -1.28 to -3.57 mmol/L. Additionally, consuming 3 grams of beta-glucans from intact barley foods or oats (fermented, pearled, whole grains baked into wheat breads) or 4 grams of beta-glucans from processed barley foods and oat foods (bread made with barley flour or oat flour, pasta, cereals, beverages) is effective at lowering the postprandial glycemic response of a meal (Tosh, 2013).

Table 8: Type of Whole Grain and Its Effect on Diabetes Prevention and Control

Type of Grain	Results	Reference
Whole grains and cereal fiber	Preventing T2D	Meyer et al., 2000
whole grain intake and cereal fiber intake	21% to 27% lower risk for those in the highest quintile of whole grain intake, and 30% to 36% lower risk for those in the highest quintile of cereal fiber intake for developing T2D. Also, better blood glucose control in both people with and without diabetes when they consumed more whole grains	Murtaugh et al., 2003
Whole grain breakfast cereal with lower glycemic index	Preventing T2D	Kochar et al., 2007
Brown rice	Preventing T2D	Sun et al., 2010
Higher intake of whole grains, bran and germ	Preventing T2D	de Munter et al., 2007
Less processed or less finely milled grains	Better blood glucose control	Åberg et al., 2020; Reynolds et al., 2020; Tosh & Chu, 2015
Oatmeal, brown rice, whole grain breakfast cereal, dark bread, added bran, and wheat germ	Reduction in T2D development with total whole grains and the individual elements/grains listed. Stronger association in lean versus overweight or obese individuals	Hu et al., 2020

Ancient grains may be particularly helpful in reducing the risk of type 2 diabetes and in managing blood glucose amongst those with the disease.

- **Sorghum**: A 2016 systematic review found that consuming sorghum resulted in a lower postprandial rise in blood glucose and insulin compared to consuming whole grain wheat (Simnadis et al., 2016). All of the studies in the review showed a decrease in blood glucose (up to 26%) and insulin response (up to 55%) after consuming a meal with sorghum. This effect was seen in people with and without type 2 diabetes.
- **Buckwheat**: A 2018 systematic review and meta-analysis found that consuming 40 grams to 300 grams of buckwheat daily for one to 24 weeks decreased fasting blood glucose (Li et al., 2018). Buckwheat is concentrated in polyphenols and resistant starch as well as soluble fiber, protein, and quercetin which may contribute to its blood glucose-lowering effect (Tomotake et al., 2002; Whole Grains Council).

WEIGHT REGULATION AND OBESITY

Weight regulation and body size are highly complex issues. Genetics, mental health, medications, socioeconomic and sociocultural factors, eating patterns and physical activity all play a role. Higher body weight has been associated with higher risk of chronic health conditions such as type 2 diabetes, cardiovascular disease, and some types of cancer, however, a large body of research has shown that diets aimed at weight loss are ineffective at producing sustained weight loss due to changes in metabolism at lower caloric intakes, among other reasons (Canadian Adult Obesity Clinical Practice Guidelines). Rather than focusing on achieving a particular weight, the emphasis should instead be on following an eating pattern and lifestyle that gives health benefits and is tailored to the tastes and preferences of the individual.

Whole-grain foods are high in fiber, which helps with satiety, particularly when coupled with adequate fluids. Consuming high-fiber grains as part of a balanced eating pattern based on whole foods, along with mindful eating and Intuitive Eating, can help with weight stability and the prevention of excess weight gain. For more information on mindful eating and Intuitive Eating, see the Mindful Eating chapter. For more information on weight and body size, see the Obesity and Overweight chapter.

Research in this area has produced mixed results, but whole grain intake does appear to have an inverse relationship to body weight (Ye et al., 2012). A review by Cho et al. (2013) found that consuming a diet rich in cereal fibers, whole grains, and bran is modestly associated with less weight gain over time in an adult population (Cho et al., 2013). Aberg et al. (2020) found in a short-term randomized crossover trial that people with type 2 diabetes consuming more finely milled or more processed whole grains were more likely to gain weight compared to those consuming less processed whole grain foods (Åberg et al., 2020).

Recent studies comparing whole grain intake to refined grain intake observed weight loss as an unintended by-product of the higher fiber intake in the whole grain groups (Cooper et al., 2015; Roager et al., 2017). Similarly, Serra-Majem and Bautista-Castaño et al. (2015) found that among those following a Mediterranean style of eating pattern, consuming more white bread was associated with weight gain, but consuming more whole grain bread was not associate with weight gain (Serra-Majem & Bautista-Castaño, 2015). A randomized controlled trial by Schlesinger et al. (2019) comparing refined grain intake to whole grain intake found that whole grains increased resting metabolic rate and stool energy excretion, which may help explain epidemiological associations between whole grain consumption and lower body weight and adiposity (Schlesinger et al., 2019).

Soluble, viscous fiber (like those found in barley and rye) prohibits the digestion and absorption of some of the fat and protein, and their respective caloric contribution (Hervik 2019).

COLON CANCER

Diets that are higher in fiber are generally associated with lower risk of colon cancer because dietary fiber promotes colonic mobility and improves bowel movements, reducing the time that carcinogens stay in the intestinal tract (Guérin et al., 2014). A dietary pattern that includes whole grains on a regular basis and replaces refined grain products with whole grains is protective against colorectal cancer. The 2018 World Cancer Research Foundation (WCRF)/American Institute for Cancer Research (AICR) Continuous Update Project found strong evidence from six prospective cohort studies that **with every additional 90 grams of whole grains eaten per day, there was a 17% decrease in the risk of colorectal cancer**, and that the evidence for whole grains is actually stronger than the evidence for fiber alone. The protective effect of whole grains was most clearly seen for colon cancer (rather than rectal cancer) (World Cancer Research Fund/American Institute for Cancer Research, 2018).

A 2019 systematic review and meta-analysis commissioned by the World Health Organization found that people who consume high amounts of whole grains had a 13% lower risk of colorectal cancer compared to those who consumed low amounts of whole grains (A. Reynolds et al., 2019). There was also a dose-response effect on cancer incidence and cancer mortality, similarly to the WCRF/AICR report. In the World Health Organization (WHO) report, every 15 grams per day of additional whole grains provided benefits. The recommendation is to emphasize minimally processed whole grains (rather than highly processed whole grain products such as breakfast cereals) and to use whole grain foods to replace refined grains for the most benefit. Similarly, a systematic review and meta-analysis of prospective cohort studies by Aune et al. (2012) found that higher intake of whole grains reduced the risk of colorectal cancer in a dose-response fashion (Aune, Chan, Lau, et al., 2012).

One of the possible mechanisms by which whole grains may be protective against colorectal cancer is by providing a source of fiber, which ferments in the gut to short-chain fatty acids, speeds intestinal transit time, binds carcinogens and regulates blood glucose response (World Cancer Research Fund/American Institute for Cancer Research, 2018). The 2018 WCRF/AICR Continuous Update Project found that **for every additional 10 grams per day of fiber, there was a 9% decrease in risk of colorectal cancer**. The WHO report similarly found that for every 8 grams of additional fiber per day, there was a 16% decrease in colorectal cancer and the protective effect was most pronounced for cereal fiber (A. Reynolds et al., 2019).

Consuming at least 25 grams of fiber per day is likely adequate, and fiber intakes >30 g per day likely have additional health benefits in terms of reducing risk of noncommunicable diseases such as colorectal cancer. Additionally, another possible mechanism is that whole grains contain bioactive compounds such as vitamins and minerals (vitamin E, selenium, copper and zinc) and phenolic compounds, which stimulate antioxidant activity and have anti-cancer effects.

Other Cancers

A 2016 systematic review including three high-quality case-control studies found variable results regarding sorghum consumption and risk of a variety of cancers (Simnadis et al., 2016). Two studies from China found that people who consumed the most sorghum had a 5% lower risk of esophageal cancer, a 1% higher risk of gastric cardia cancer, a 12% lower risk of gastric non-cardia cancer, and a 65% lower risk of oral cancer (Gao et al., 2011; Zheng et al., 1993). A study from South Africa found that people who consumed the most sorghum had a 54% lower risk of esophageal cancer (Sewram et al., 2014). One high-quality randomized controlled trial in the review found lower biomarkers of oxidative stress (plasma polyphenol, protein carbonyl) in people consuming red sorghum pasta compared to whole grain wheat pasta (Khan et al., 2015). One of the potential reasons that sorghum appears to have anti-cancer and anti-inflammatory properties is that it has a high concentration of proanthocyanidins, 3-deoxyanthocyanidins, and flavones, though these phytochemicals are only found in some varieties of sorghum.

Few studies have investigated the relationship between whole grain intake and the risk of esophageal cancer. A prospective cohort study examining this relationship among Scandinavian adults found that there was a 45% lower risk of esophageal cancer among those consuming the highest tertile of whole grains compared to the lowest tertile. The association was strongest for whole grain wheat products (Skeie et al., 2016). A meta-analysis of 19 studies examining the relationship between grain intake and risk of stomach cancer found that whole grains were protective against gastric cancer, while refined grains increased the risk of gastric cancer (T. Wang et al., 2020).

CHOLESTEROL LEVELS

Cholesterol is a fat-like, waxy substance that is produced by the liver. It is essential for health as it comprises cell membranes and is a building block for hormones, fat-soluble vitamins, and bile acids. In spite of the important functions of this substance, if circulating cholesterol is above recommended limits it deposits on the walls of the arteries, narrowing the blood flow and increasing the risk of heart disease. Cholesterol is found in all animal products but is absent in plant products, therefore, whole grains do not contain cholesterol. Research done in the 1990s first identified that soluble fiber, like that found in oats, could bind cholesterol and package it for excretion, taking it out of the blood circulation. Soluble fiber can form a gel that can reduce nutrient diffusion rate across the small intestine and trap cholesterol in feces, helping the body eliminate cholesterol rather than absorbing it (Navarro-Perez et al., 2017). Today, **oats and barley along with fruits and vegetables are go-to foods to help reduce blood cholestero**l.

Beta-glucans are soluble cereal fibers that are found naturally in oats and barley. Beta-glucans in oats are known to decrease LDL cholesterol (Ho et al., 2016). More recently, studies have found that barley beta-glucans can also help lower blood cholesterol. A 2016 systematic review and meta-analysis found that consuming >6.5 grams per day of barley beta-glucans for four weeks decreased LDL by 0.25 mmol/L and >6.9 grams per day of barley beta-glucans can decrease non-HDL cholesterol by 0.31 mmol/L (Ho et al., 2016). This amount of beta-glucans can be found in a one-half cup of dried pearled barley.

Ancient grains may help reduce blood cholesterol by other mechanisms as well: their high levels of phytochemicals. Studies on the phytochemicals (phenolic compounds, betalains, fatty acids, tocopherols, carotenoids, squalene, saponins and phytates) in amaranth, as well as human trials with amaranth oil, suggest that **amaranth may help lower cholesterol and blood pressure**. A 2009 systematic review, a 2012 narrative review, and a 2017 narrative review found fair evidence that amaranth oil along with a heart-healthful diet resulted in a lower LDL, total cholesterol, and blood pressure in people with ischemic heart disease, coronary heart disease plus hypertension or hyperlipoproteinemia compared to the heart-healthful diet alone (Caselato-Sousa & Amaya-Farfán, 2012; Tang & Tsao, 2017; Ulbricht et al., 2009). More studies are needed to better understand the effect of the whole amaranth grain on heart disease risk since most studies to date have been on amaranth oil.

Consuming whole grains may also help lower serum triglycerides. A 2018 systematic review found one double-blind randomized controlled trial that found that consuming 25 grams of quinoa flakes per day for four weeks improved triglycerides, LDL, and total cholesterol among women (De Carvalho et al., 2014; van den Driessche et al., 2018). Additionally, a 2017 randomized controlled trial found that consuming 50 grams of quinoa daily for 12 weeks resulted in lower triglycerides (Navarro-Perez et al., 2017).

CARDIOVASCULAR DISEASE

Cardiovascular disease (CVD) is the leading cause of death in the United States. Included in the broad heading of this disease are strokes, heart attacks, and heart failure. As mentioned earlier, high blood cholesterol can contribute to heart disease so we might expect that there is also a correlation of whole grains to CVD in general. Ye, et al. (2012) conducted a systematic review in looking at whole grain consumption and CVD by comparing those who rarely or never consumed whole grains, to those reporting an average of 48 to 80 g/day of whole grain (three to five servings /day) and noted a 21% reduction in CVD risk in the whole grain consuming group (Ye et al., 2012).

A review by Cho et al. (2013) found that consuming a diet rich in cereal fiber, whole grains, and bran is modestly associated with a lower risk of CVD (Cho et al., 2013). Similarly, Mellen et al. (2008) found that higher whole grain consumption is associated with lower risk of CVD (Mellen et al., 2008).

Including a wider variety of whole grain foods and replacing refined grains in the diet with whole grains and ancient grains that are nutritionally dense can help improve cardiovascular risk markers. For example, there is fair evidence from randomized controlled trials that replacing modern wheat with KAMUT® Khorasan wheat improves cardiovascular risk markers (total cholesterol, LDL, triglycerides), decreases fat mass, and improves liver function markers (AST, ALT, ALP) (Cicero et al., 2018; Dinu et al., 2018; Trozzi et al., 2019). There are many possible mechanisms for the cardiovascular and other health benefits of KAMUT®. For example, this ancient form of wheat is very high in selenium polyphenols (10 times higher than modern wheat). In the study by Trozzi et al. (2019), the KAMUT® group had high phenol compounds in the gut compared to the control group, suggesting a possible role of the gut microbiome in the beneficial effects seen among those consuming KAMUT®. In the study by Cicero et al. (2018), the protein-derived bioactive peptides of KAMUT® may have played a protective role against stressors to the cardiovascular system.

In summary, in an umbrella review of observational studies on the benefits of whole grain, the following was concluded by Tieri et al. (2020):
- **Convincing evidence** that whole grain consumption decreases the risk of diabetes and colorectal cancer
- **Possible evidence** of a decreased risk of colon cancer and cardiovascular mortality

SECTION 6:

WHEN TO LIMIT CERTAIN GRAINS

GLUTEN ALLERGY OR FOOD INTOLERANCE

Gluten is a combination of over 100 different proteins including a high quantity of glutenin and gliadin. Gluten has been an integral part of wheat since the domestication of the plant as a diet staple and provides over 75% of the protein found in wheat products. Together these two proteins (glutenin and gliadin) are referred to as prolamins (Biesiekierski, 2017). Gluten has received much attention in the food industry as more and more consumers transition to a gluten-free diet for a variety of reasons beyond a diagnosis of celiac disease.

In wheat products, gluten acts as a binding agent and gives the product texture, supporting the "rise" seen in breads. Certain types of wheat flour have more gluten than others. For example, bread flour contains more gluten than all-purpose flour, meaning that this flour is higher in protein and best able to support the structure expected in a bread product. On the other end of the gluten spectrum is cake flour, which has a lower amount of gluten, resulting in a softer-structured product.

Allergies and sensitivities to wheat also exist meaning that wheat can cause symptoms in consumers who do not have celiac disease. This is an area requiring further study (Biesiekierski, 2017). See the chapter on the Gluten-Free Diet for more information. It is important to note that gluten-free doesn't equal grain-free, and gluten-free grains are listed in Table 9.

Table 9: Gluten-Free Grains

Gluten-Free Grains
Quinoa
Amaranth
Rice and wild rice
Arrowroot
Buckwheat
Corn
Millet
Sorghum
Teff

KIDNEY DISEASE

In renal disease, calcium and phosphorus homeostasis is affected as the kidneys have increased difficulty excreting these minerals. In later stages of kidney disease, foods that are high in phosphorus may need to be limited for this reason. The outer coating of cereal grains is high in phosphorus. In the early stages of kidney disease, whole grains are encouraged for their nutritional benefit, but as the disease progresses, high-phosphorus foods such as bran may need to be limited to prevent hyperphosphatemia.

Sprouting grains helps to break down the phosphorus, and so choosing sprouted grain breads can be one way of continuing to include whole grain and higher-fiber foods in the diet as renal disease progresses. Phosphates are also included in some anticaking agents, emulsifiers, and other additives in flour and bakery products. Checking the ingredient lists on grain products to limit phosphorus intake is important in promoting health for patients with kidney disease.

LOW FODMAP DIET

FODMAPS are fermentable oligosaccharides, disaccharides, monosaccharides and polyols. Many people with irritable bowel syndrome absorb FODMAPs poorly, causing bloating, gas, and abdominal discomfort. Studies have shown that following a low FODMAP diet with the help of a registered dietitian can help relieve symptoms. In the first stage of the diet, high FODMAP foods are removed for three to eight weeks to see if symptoms improve. Then in the second stage, foods are added back one at a time to test for tolerance and symptoms. In the final and third stage, the goal is to add back as many foods as can be tolerated.

Wheat, rye, and barley contain fermentable oligosaccharides (fructans), and these can be triggers of irritable bowel symptoms. When these foods are initially eliminated in the low FODMAP diet, they can be replaced with other low FODMAP grains such as rice, corn, and quinoa. Later, wheat, rye, and barley can be reintroduced one at a time to test for tolerance (Dietitians of Canada, 2019).

DIVERTICULITIS

Diverticulosis means having diverticula or small pouches that form in the wall of the colon; most people who have diverticulosis are asymptomatic. Diverticulitis is when these pouches or sacs become inflamed or infected. Symptoms of diverticulitis include pain or tenderness in the lower left abdomen, constipation, diarrhea, nausea, vomiting and fever. During an episode of diverticulitis or a "flare-up," a person may be able to continue eating a regular diet or may need to temporarily follow a low-fiber diet or a liquid diet, depending on symptoms. Once symptoms resolve, a return to a high-fiber diet is recommended.

Following a higher-fiber diet can help prevent diverticular disease in the first place and can prevent future flare-ups for someone who already has diverticula. Contrary to popular belief, someone with diverticular disease does not need to avoid fibrous foods and small round foods such as popcorn, seeds, nuts and whole grains. It is a common misconception that these fibrous foods will become stuck in diverticula and cause a flare-up of diverticulitis, however, in reality, these fibrous foods help to improve gut motility, prevent constipation, and reduce the amount of time bacteria spend in the colon, thereby reducing the risk of infection and diverticulitis. So, while whole grain foods may need to be limited during acute diverticulitis, they should be encouraged to prevent future flare-ups (HealthLinkBC, 2011).

DIARRHEA

While soluble fiber slows gastric emptying and gastrointestinal transit time, insoluble fiber speeds gut transit time. During times of diarrhea, insoluble fiber can worsen loose stools. Instead, choosing soluble fiber foods can help bulk up and thicken stools by forming a gel-like consistency without worsening frequent and loose stools. Many whole grain foods contain both soluble and insoluble fiber. Foods high in bran such as wheat bran are particularly high in insoluble fiber and can worsen diarrhea, whereas grains such as **oats and barley are high in soluble fiber and can improve loose stools**. In some cases, choosing lower-fiber grain foods such as white bread, crackers, noodles and white rice may be needed to help improve diarrhea. Once stools return to normal, a return to a higher fiber diet can resume (Dietitians of Canada, 2009).

SECTION 7:
GRAINS AND SUSTAINABILITY

Risks in grain consumption relate to the soil contamination found in some of the fields. Crops grown in polluted soil can contain heavy metals such as mercury, mycotoxins, and acrylamide. Ironically, processing the flour (dehulling and de-branning) appears to mitigate some of the contaminants but removes over half of the phytonutrients (Thielecke & Nugent, 2018). The risk of arsenic in rice has also been noted due to polluted water in the rice paddies.

Arsenic

Arsenic is a naturally occurring element found in varying degrees in soil and water. The inorganic form of arsenic is much more toxic than organic arsenic and it is considered a first level carcinogen (Gundert-Remy et al., 2015). Most of the inorganic arsenic is found in the bran layer of rice (Hojsak et al., 2015; G.-X. Sun et al., 2008). Avoiding foods and beverages that have added rice bran will help to lower one's exposure significantly. A 2021 study found that parboiling brown rice can remove up to 54% of inorganic arsenic from brown rice and 73% from white rice (outperforming soaking or rinsing) and can also preserve important micronutrients such as zinc (Menon et al., 2021).

Organic rice draws arsenic up from the soil the same way conventionally grown rice does.

On average, Americans eat 12 grams of rice per day, but Asian Americans eat more than 115 grams of rice per day, and Hispanics and Black Americans eat somewhere in between these amounts on average. The United States Environmental Protection Agency, which classifies inorganic arsenic as a carcinogen, sets a daily limit on arsenic in drinking water at 10 μg/L. There is no American standard for arsenic in food, however, for people who consume more than 115 grams per day of high-arsenic rice, they could be surpassing the drinking water limit (Potera, 2007).

The lowest levels of inorganic arsenic in brown rice comes from California, India and Pakistan (Consumer Reports, 2014). In South Central American-grown rice, arsenic averages 0.30 μg/g (compared to an average of 0.17 μg/g in California-grown rice). White rice grown in Louisiana has the highest amount of arsenic (0.66 μg/g), and organic brown rice from California has the lowest amount of arsenic (0.10 μg/g) (Potera, 2007).

How much rice is safe to eat, and is brown rice better than white rice in terms of contamination? To avoid any risks from high arsenic intake, a safe amount of rice to eat in America is up to 100 grams per day on average. This is about ½ cup of uncooked rice per day or this could be 1 cup of uncooked rice three days per week. Opting for brown rice from California, Pakistan and India rather than white rice, and parboiling before consumption can help reduce arsenic intake while conserving the necessary fiber and nutrients found in the bran.

Genetically Modified Grains (https://www.fda.gov/food/agricultural-biotechnology/gmo-crops-animal-food-and-beyond)

Gene mapping of a large variety of these grain species has provided information on how specific genome sequences can be spliced and new genes inserted resulting in crops with higher yields, more resistance to pests, and more tolerance to changing weather patterns; these altered seeds are referred to as genetically modified organisms, or GMOs. Although scientists have experimented with genetically modified staple crops including the Golden Rice Project in 1999, biofortification of maize with beta-carotene, and fortification of the amino acid lysine in wheat (Hefferon, 2015), none of these crops have actually gone to market. Contrary to popular belief, all grain crops (except for corn) commercially available in the U.S. are grown without GMO technology. The only FDA-approved GMO plant crops are corn, soybean, canola, sugar beets, potatoes, papayas, apples, summer squash, cotton and alfalfa.

SECTION 8:

GRAIN-DRUG INTERACTIONS

Whole grains and their inherent fiber can reduce the absorption of some minerals. It has also been proposed that the fiber from whole grains may decrease the absorption of certain drugs, though the research in this is very inconclusive, and any interaction is much **more likely to occur with fiber supplements** than with fiber from whole grains themselves. Questions regarding the interaction between drugs and whole grains or fiber supplements should be directed to the physician or pharmacist. Some medication classes where an interaction is proposed include tricyclic antidepressants (amitriptyline, doxepin, imipramine) and sulfonylureas (glyburide) (Pronsky et al., 2015). Fiber may also impair the absorption of digoxin and levothyroxine (Synthroid) (Christianson & Salling, 2020).

Nutrient interactions include a decrease in non-heme iron absorption with diets high in whole grains due to the phytate content of grains, which inhibits iron absorption. A diet that is very high in grains can also reduce the absorption of calcium and zinc (Abbaspour et al., 2014; Hurrell & Egli, 2010; Zijp et al., 2000). However, regularly eating a diet high in phytates can limit the impact on nutrient absorption over time. A study in the Journal of Nutrition found that after consuming a high-phytate diet with lots of whole grains for eight weeks, there was a 41% increase in serum iron response, indicating that the women were better able to absorb iron over time (Armah et al., 2015).

SECTION 9:

CLINICAL & CULINARY RECOMMENDATIONS AND COMPETENCIES

Messaging from the Menus of Change
Make whole, intact grains the new norm

Clinical recommendations and competencies are the foundation from which culinary competencies were created. The goal of the culinary medicine practitioner/food coach is to help clients and patients develop the skills necessary to meet the clinical recommendations by teaching skill-based learning outlined in the culinary competencies.

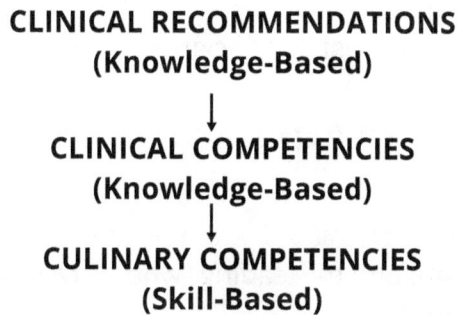

CLINICAL RECOMMENDATIONS
(Knowledge-Based)
↓
CLINICAL COMPETENCIES
(Knowledge-Based)
↓
CULINARY COMPETENCIES
(Skill-Based)

CLINICAL RECOMMENDATIONS

Grains are essential to a healthy diet. The most current USDA Dietary Guidelines 2020-2025 address optimal grain intake. They include:

1. The recommended amount of grains in the Healthy U.S.-Style Eating Pattern at the 2,000-calorie level is 6 ounce-equivalents per day
2. At least half of the grain recommendation should be whole grains
3. Limit refined grains to no more than half the daily requirement for whole grains; for a 2,000 calorie per day diet, that translates to less than 3 ounce-equivalents per day
4. If refined grains are consumed, they should be enriched
5. Replace refined grains with whole grains when possible
6. The American Heart Association recommends choosing minimally processed foods instead of ultra-processed foods (Lichtenstein et al., 2021)

CLINICAL COMPETENCIES

1. Compare and contrast whole grain, enriched grain, refined grain, and ancient grains, and list examples of each
2. Recall which nutrients for which grain supply a "good source"
3. Contrast soluble with insoluble fiber and list examples of each
4. Recall how many servings of whole grains are recommended per day
5. Identify which cohorts are most at risk of not meeting their daily whole-grain recommendation
6. Discuss the health benefits of consuming whole grains
7. Describe the unhealthful consequences of consuming refined or ultra-processed grains
8. Describe grains' influence on the microbiome
9. Identify health conditions that may require limiting whole grains
10. Discuss the benefits and risks of following a low-carbohydrate diet
11. Identify which grains interact with certain medications
12. Define and list gluten-free grains
13. Describe a low FODMAP diet and list specific grains to avoid

CULINARY COMPETENCIES FOR GRAINS
SHOPPING COMPETENCIES

1. Identify the fiber content in a serving of a grain product
2. Distinguish between accurate and misleading "whole grain" claims on a package
3. Purchase whole grain products
4. Determine if a refined grain product is enriched
5. Demonstrate how to purchase whole grain products within a budget
6. Select gluten-free grains and gluten-free products

COOKING/PREPARING COMPETENCIES
STOCKING THE KITCHEN COMPETENCIES

1. Stock a variety of whole grains
2. Quinoa, couscous, oats, barley, millet, etc....
3. Stock a variety of whole-grain products
   a. Bread, bagels, tortillas, pita, wraps
   b. Pasta
   c. Cereal
   d. Crackers
4. Stock grain flavor enhancers
   a. Various oils

b. Sources of acid – lemon, lime, flavored vinegars for example
c. Herbs and spices
d. Dried and fresh fruit

COOKING COMPETENCIES

1. Demonstrate cooking a variety of whole grains
2. Prepare and store grains in bulk
3. Demonstrate cooking whole grains when time is limited
4. Demonstrate parboiling grains
5. Demonstrate how to reduce arsenic in rice
6. Cook whole grains
7. Demonstrate substituting whole grains for refined grains in a recipe
8. Prepare a whole-grain salad
9. Prepare whole-grain pasta
10. Prepare a whole-grain bowl
11. Prepare/cook a whole grain-based breakfast cereal
12. Bake with whole grains

FLAVOR DEVELOPMENT COMPETENCIES

1. Salt grain dishes appropriately
2. Develop the flavor of whole grains using various ingredients
3. Develop the flavor of whole grains using culinary techniques

SERVING COMPETENCIES

1. Model eating whole grains
2. Serve the appropriate number of grain and whole grain servings a day
3. Utilize a variety of whole grains in meals and menu planning
4. Demonstrate introducing whole grains in a faded, stepwise fashion
5. Display proper serving sizes of grains
6. Prepare and serve a whole grain-based snack

SAFETY COMPETENCIES

1. Demonstrate the proper storage of grains
2. Identify grains that have an increased risk of developing foodborne illness
3. Demonstrate the prevention of cross-contamination when working with grains

4. Demonstrate culinary and safety techniques used when serving individuals with a grain or related allergy (e.g., gluten, wheat)

SECTION 10:
GRAINS AT THE STORE

In the International Food Information Council's (IFIC) 2018 Food and Health Survey, whole grains top the list of components considered to be healthful by consumers, following only vitamin D and fiber. Consumers are also able to differentiate between whole grains and enriched grains, as more than 80% recognize whole grains to be healthful — with less than 45% thinking that enriched grains are healthful. According to a food consumption analyst at NPD Group, 52% of shoppers intentionally seek out whole grains when they shop, and 51% are also interested in the fiber content of food products.

Defining Grain Products

Whole grain = berries = groats (whole grains separated from the hull)
Sprouted grain (the seeds are germinated and crack open)
Cracked grains = steel-cut oats = grits (whole grain cut into pieces)
Rolled grains = flakes (whole grains that are steamed and rolled)
Meal (whole grain ground to gritty consistency)
Polished grain = pearl grain (bran and germ are removed)
Flour (can be whole or refined grain that is ground into a powder)
Bran (the edible outer layer of the whole grain kernel)
Germ (the interior only, which is rich in vitamins and healthful oils)

ON THE LABEL

Image: The Whole Grain Stamp

Finding whole grain and ancient grain products in grocery stores and supermarkets is made easier with the Whole Grain Stamp on the front label. The Whole Grain Stamp, developed by the Oldways Whole Grains Council, is used to identify whole grains on thousands of products in 63 countries. These Stamps indicate if the product has 16 grams or more of whole grain (the equivalent of a whole serving of whole grains), or at least 8 grams of whole grains (equal to one half a serving of whole grains). The specific amount of whole grain per serving is listed on the Stamp as seen below in Figure 4.

Table 10: Whole Grain Stamps Defined*

100% Whole Grain Stamp	50% Whole Grain Stamp	Whole Grain Stamp
All the grain is whole-grain	At least half of the grain is whole-grain	Product primarily contains refined grains
Contains at least 16 grams of whole grain	Contains at least 8 grams of whole grain	Contains at least 8 grams of whole grain

*As defined by the Oldways Whole Grains Council

There are other front-of-package messaging about grains, but they may be misleading. For instance, the following claims do not mean that the product is a whole-grain product:
- "Multi-grains" and "Added fiber" does not mean the grains are made from whole grains.
- "Made with Whole Grains" does not mean the product has an appreciable amount of whole grain (one-half serving (8 grams) or more).

A Whole Grain claim on the front of the box doesn't tell the whole picture

A product can be made with whole grains, plus contain a lot of added sugar. This example of the Life Cereal has a front-of-the-box label that demonstrates this fact:

Image: Life Cereal Box

While it is great that there are 25 grams of whole grains in one cup of Chocolate Life cereal, the second ingredient is sugar. There are 9 grams (2 ¼ teaspoons) of sugar per serving.

The Ingredient List

The most important word to look for on the ingredient list is "whole" as the first word. This indicates that all of the first ingredient listed is whole grain, including the bran, germ, and endosperm of the grain. There are exceptions to this rule if multiple whole grains are used in the recipe.

Looking for Fiber

Whole grains vary in their dietary fiber content — see Appendix A. The amount of fiber in a product also depends on processing. A study by Heaton et al. (1988) showed that particle size affects the digestion rate and subsequent metabolic and health effects of wheat and maize (Heaton et al., 1988). For example, wheat flour or corn flour that is finely ground is absorbed more quickly than coarsely ground grains and causes a higher rise in blood sugar. The same is true for oats with the quick-cooking or instant varieties leading to a larger spike in blood glucose levels than the less processed varieties — steel cut, large flake, muesli and granola (Tosh & Chu, 2015). Therefore, choosing less processed forms of grains maintains more nutrients and is associated with more health benefits.

Tricks To Finding a Healthful Whole Grain Cereal:

1. Look for the Whole Grain Stamp, or look for 18 grams of whole grain per serving .
2. Look at the Nutrition Facts Panel to identify the amount of added sugar. You are looking for no more than 4 or 5 grams (4 grams = 1 teaspoon of sugar) of added sugar per serving.
3. Look for a 10:1 Ratio – there should be at least 1 gram of fiber for every 10 grams of carbohydrates.*
4. There should be at least 2 grams of fiber for every 100 calories.*

Enriched Grains

Image: Enriched on the Label

An enriched grain is not a whole grain, in fact, they are mostly refined grains. Enrichment is a process that adds iron and vitamins (thiamin, riboflavin, niacin and folic acid) back into grains. Note: Do not wash enriched grains as the vitamins and iron is added as a coating to the grain and washing will remove some of the nutrients. For example, rinsing white rice removes the majority of iron and B vitamins, whereas rinsing brown rice removes very little as the nutrients are within the grain of rice, not sprayed on top of it (Gray et al., 2016).

NUTRIENT CONTENT CLAIMS

For grains, fiber is looked upon as the health-promoting factor when it comes to nutrient and health claims.

- If a product has less than one gram of fiber, "not a significant source of dietary fiber" may be found on the label.
- The terms "more," "fortified," "enriched," "added," "extra" and "plus" can be used for dietary fiber if it is 10% or more of the Daily Value (DV) per serving.
- If a "fiber" claim is made and the food is not low in total fat, the label must state the level of total fat per serving.
- "High fiber" or "excellent source of fiber" means one serving contains 20% or more of the DV.
- "Good source of fiber" means one serving contains 10% to 19% of the DV.

QUALIFIED HEALTH CLAIMS

Health claims on food items need to be valid and approved by the Food and Drug Administration (FDA). There are two approved health claims in regard to whole grains. As long as the product contains a minimum of 51% whole grain and meets a specific fiber requirement, the following claims may be used: "Diets rich in whole grain foods and other plant foods and low in total fat, saturated fat, and cholesterol, may reduce the risk of heart disease and some cancers." The second is — "Diets rich in whole grain foods and other plant foods and low in total fat, saturated fat, and cholesterol, may help reduce the risk of heart disease." These are based on the following approved health claims (e-CFR; Nutrition, 2022).

- "Low fat diets rich in fiber-containing grain products, fruits, and vegetables may reduce the risk of some types of cancer, a disease associated with many factors."
- "Diets low in saturated fat and cholesterol and rich in fruits, vegetables, and grain products that contain some types of dietary fiber, particularly soluble fiber, may reduce the risk of heart disease, a disease associated with many factors."

SECTION 11:

GRAINS IN THE KITCHEN

ON THE TONGUE: THE TASTE OF GRAINS

There are subtle and not-so-subtle tastes and flavors from one whole grain to the next — see Table 11. While rye and certain types of wheat have very strong flavors, rice and sorghum have a mild flavor. The bitterness in whole wheat comes from the phenolic acid and tannins in the bran layer, as well as other molecules generated during heating, including pinellic acid (Borrell, 2009; Cong et al., 2021). A large contributor to the overall flavor experience is the texture of whole grain products compared to their processed counterparts. Refined grains have lost most of their texture as the endosperm is devoid of nearly all fiber. Getting used to the texture of various whole grain products can be difficult, and yet studies show time and time again that exposure helps drive acceptance and acceptability (De Leon et al., 2020; Haro-Vicente et al., 2017; Radford et al., 2014; Tritt et al., 2015).

One of the hardest changes to promote with food — besides eating more vegetables — is to switch from refined grains to whole grains in the diet. For certain, it is not a quick switch as it will take time for both an individual's taste buds and mechanoreceptors to learn to like the flavor and texture of whole grains, but it will also take time for the digestive tract to get used to an increase in fiber. Slow and easy wins this race.

Most Americans enjoy the taste of refined grains because the majority have added sugar, salt, and fat that can make those foods hyper-palatable (they are so tasty that it is hard to stop eating them once you start). This sets the bar for expecting and demanding that all food meets this hyper-palatable expectation.

Dr. Keith Williams of Penn State Hershey Medical Center talks about Transforming Your Tastebuds (https://www.youtube.com/watch?v=VfIerqR89dE) in regard to consuming whole grains in this video. Some tips from Dr. Williams' talk are listed below:
- **Fade** the amount of whole grains into a refined grain product over time. For example, mix a quarter cup of whole grain pasta into a cup of white pasta and change the ratio over time.
- **Repeated taste exposure** leads to a preference; the dose does not have to be large. In fact, in some studies, the dose of a new food was the size of a pea. Do not start with a serving.
- **The initial goal is cooperation, not nutrition.** Time will take care of the rest as the dose increases with repeat exposure.
- **Modeling** behavior that a significant other partakes in has been shown to be successful. For example, kids' peers, college boyfriends and girlfriends, or a parent and young child.

- Tasting is more likely to occur when a person is **hungry.** Present the novel food before a meal.
- **Positive reinforcement** like praise can encourage trying a new food. The repeated exposure will then lead to a preference.
- **Increasing availability** increases the likelihood a person will consume the food
- **Enhance the palatability** of the food through culinary techniques — using herbs and spices for example

Culinary Tip: Whole-grain pasta has a heavier and more gritty texture than white pasta. Serve with a robust, textured sauce like bolognese or mushroom ragu to disguise the "new" heartier texture of whole-grain pasta.

Table 11: Flavor and Texture of Various Grains

Grain	Flavor	Texture	Uses
Amaranth	Light, nutty, corn-like, and peppery taste	Slightly crunchy when cooked	Porridge, pop it like corn, sprinkle on salad
Freekeh	Earthy, nutty, and slightly smoky flavor	Firm, slightly chewy	Porridge, pilaf, use in soups and salads
KAMUT®	Rich, buttery taste	Like wheat	Mill into flour for bread, pasta
Millet	Mild flavor	Fluffy, sticky or creamy	Porridge, pilaf, add to bread, soup, stew, popped, milled into flour or prepared like polenta
Quinoa	Nutty flavor, mild, and grassy	Crunchy	Porridge, salads, added to granola
Sorghum	Neutral taste, absorbs the flavors it is cooked with	Chewy, similar to couscous	Porridge, pilaf, popped, milled into flour for baked goods
Teff	Mild, nutty, earthy, sweet, molasses-like flavor	Poppy seed texture	Porridge, add to stew, sprinkle on vegetables, milled into flour for baked goods

HOW TO INCREASE DIETARY FIBER INTAKE

Eating a higher-fiber diet improves the gut microbiome, enhances the immune system, improves bowel habits and reduces the risk of chronic diseases such as cardiovascular disease, diabetes, and bowel cancer (British Dietetic Association). It's important to increase dietary fiber gradually as increasing fiber intake too quickly may lead to gas, bloating, and could worsen bowel issues such as constipation or diarrhea. When increasing fiber intake, it's important to ensure adequate fluids as well, since soluble fiber absorbs water as it passes through the digestive tract to form a gel-like consistency and insoluble fiber traps water in the colon to keep stools soft and prevent constipation.

For example, you could start by increasing fiber at one meal per day (such as switching to whole grain oats at breakfast or 100% whole grain bread to your meal). Or you could start by switching one type of refined grain in your diet to a whole grain (such as switching from white bread to whole grain bread or from white rice to brown rice). Or you could start by adding legumes once or twice a week or adding nuts to a snack or trying a new type of vegetable every time you go to the supermarket. The possibilities are endless!

IN THE PANTRY

In stocking a pantry with whole grain products, many consumers start with whole grain pastas and brown rice as they are easy to cook and highly acceptable. Whole grain cereals are widely available, but it can be tricky to not be misled by the front of the package messaging (remember, the Whole Grain Stamp is a legitimate stamp). There are also a multitude of crackers, bread products, tortillas and snack foods that meet whole grain labeling requirements, making them strong pantry candidates.

If one is looking to make a switch to whole-wheat flour in baking, some modifications may be required such as titrating amounts of white flour to the whole wheat to ensure an acceptable product. For example, one cup of all-purpose flour can be replaced with up to ½ cup whole wheat flour plus ½ cup white flour with no noticeable change in texture and rise. See the chapter on Sugar for more healthful baking tips.

Specifically, pantries that reflect attention to whole grains frequently include grains from the following list. To take a deeper dive, click on each to be sent to the Whole Grain Council's summary sheet for each grain.
• Oats — whole oat groats, steel-cut oats (Irish or Scottish oats), rolled oats, quick-cook oats
• Barley
• Quinoa
• Popcorn
• Brown Rice, wild rice
• Whole wheat flour
• Whole grain crackers like Triscuits ™ and Wasa Crispbread ™
• Whole grain cereals like Kashi, Grape-Nuts, and many others
• Whole grain pasta

- Try adding a new grain each month like:
  - Buckwheat
  - KAMUT®
  - Amaranth
  - Millet
  - Teff
- Flavor enhancers
  - Herbs and spices: ginger, garlic, cumin, bay leaf, fresh herbs (cilantro and parsley), for example
  - Broth: vegetable, beef, or chicken
  - Flavored oils
  - Source of acid: lemon and lime juice and various vinegars (rice, white, flavored)
  - Dried fruit
  - Nuts

THE COST OF GRAINS

Grains are one of the least expensive staples in the diet. Many of these grains, even in whole form, take less than 30 minutes to cook and pair well with a lean or plant-based protein and a serving of vegetables. When stocking a low-cost pantry, focus on brown rice, whole oats, and millet.

Some cost-saving tips include:
- Shop at stores that sell grains in bulk bins as they are much cheaper that way.
- Shop at local ethnic markets.

STORING GRAINS

Part of the beauty of grains is their stability on the pantry shelf unless they are exposed to air, heat, or moisture. The Whole Grains Council recommends that partial packages of unused grain products be stored in airtight containers or zipped plastic storage bags. Grains that have been ground into flour have a shorter shelf life, and both intact grains and flours can be stored in the freezer for prolonged periods. Packaged grains do carry use-by dates, not necessarily for food safety but for optimal taste. See Appendix B for grains and storage times. You can also freeze raw grain to keep them from turning rancid. When freezing cooked grain, undercook them if you will be reheating them after thawing. When reheating grains, cook in a little bit of water, stock, or broth.

FLAVOR DEVELOPMENT

Image: Techniques to Add Flavor to Grains

Toasting — intensifies the flavor and adds depth and a nutty note
- Dry toast grains — wheat berries, quinoa, millet, freekeh, and farro — in a pan before cooking
- Toast grains in a bit of oil — best for rice
- Dry roast spices in the pan before adding the liquid — rosemary, thyme, cumin, coriander, and fennel, for example

Use flavorful liquid when cooking
- Use broth — vegetable, chicken, beef, mushroom – instead of water
- Adding a parmesan rind to the liquid adds flavor
- Saute onions, celery, carrots, garlic, or mushrooms before adding the liquid
- Add a bay leaf

Add flavorful ingredients after cooking
- When the grain is still warm, add:
- Acid — rice or other vinegar, lemon, lime or orange juice
- Oil — even flavored oils
- When the grain has cooled, add:
  - Nuts, dried fruit, chopped fresh herbs
  - Salt is necessary to enhance the flavor of grains. Add salt and pepper before and after cooking; taste after salting so that you don't overdo it.

PREPARING GRAINS

Grains are dry foods and need some type of processing before cooking in order to increase their digestibility and the availability of the nutrients. This usually is done by grinding, dehulling, or using heat. Since different grains have different properties, one is not necessarily a substitute for another without recipe modifications. The properties of the different grains discussed earlier in the chapter influence the end product of baked goods. The absence or presence of gluten in the flour is a major consideration when attempting to create a product that has the texture and rise of a traditional wheat product.

In cooking, whole grain products usually require a longer cooking time than processed grains due to the remaining fibrous portions of the plant. For example, brown rice may take double the amount of time to cook when compared to its processed white counterpart. Soaking whole grains in water (enough to cover them) overnight results in less cooking time the next day. In addition, many of the ancient grains cook in 30 minutes or less.

Grains should be rinsed and drained before cooking to remove any debris or excess starch on the surface, though **do not rinse bulgur wheat or enriched rice**.

COOKING WHOLE GRAINS

Cooking time: Depending on how much time is available, grains can cook up in as little as 10 minutes. You can also cook grains ahead of time (partially cook if you will reheat them later) in larger batches and refrigerate or freeze until ready to use. Grains will last three to four days in the refrigerator, and frozen, cooked whole grain can be used to create a quick hearty salad or stir-fry. The Oldways Whole Grain Council has a list of cooking time and liquids for various whole grains. Presoaking can also cut down on cooking time.

10 minutes	20 minutes	25 minutes	40+ minutes
Buckwheat	Amaranth	Millet	Whole rice
Bulgar	Teff		
Quinoa			

Amount of liquid: There are two ways to approach the amount of cooking liquid to use:
1. Measure the amount suggested in the instructions and cook until there is no remaining liquid.
2. Cook grains as you would pasta — in a lot of water — until they are tender, then drain.

With the first method, you can use a flavorful cooking liquid, as it will be absorbed by the grains. With the second method, water-soluble vitamins will be lost in the cooking water. This method is not generally recommended unless you are trying to remove toxins like arsenic.

Rinse grains to remove excess starch dirt and hidden debris. If the grains are enriched, do not rinse as that will cause some of the nutrients to be washed away.

Soaking grains is not necessary unless someone has an issue digesting whole grains or they are deficient (or at risk of becoming deficient) in iron, zinc, or calcium (Coulibaly et al., 2011; R. K. Gupta et al., 2015). Soaking can make them easier to digest while increasing the absorption of certain nutrients. This is because phytic acid in grains — known as an anti-nutrient due to its ability to bind to minerals (iron, zinc, and calcium) and prevent them from being absorbed — breaks down with soaking (Purdy et al., 2015). To soak, cover grains in warm water that has a source of acid (1 to 2 tablespoons lemon juice or vinegar) added to it. Soak at least 12 hours (Coulibaly et al., 2011). Rinse the soaked grains and cook as directed. Note: the cooking time will be shorter, and the amount of liquid will be less due to the soaking.

Amaranth — works well in soups, stews, and as a hot cereal
- To add flavor, toast first.
- Add grains to boiling water (use twice as much water as grain), which will prevent it from becoming sticky.
- Bring to a boil then simmer for 20 to 25 minutes with the lid on, remove from heat and let sit for 10 to 15 minutes to steam before serving.

Buckwheat — the groats work well as a porridge
- Wash well and remove any broken groats, then drain well.
- Bring two cups of water to a boil for every cup of groats. Add groats once the water is boiling, lower to a simmer and cook with the lid on for 10 minutes (or all the water is absorbed).
- Remove from heat, leave the lid on to steam for another 10 minutes.

Quinoa — comes in white, red, and black varieties
- To improve the taste, toast quinoa in a dry pan on medium-low for five to seven minutes before cooking in liquid to give it a nutty flavor. Rinsing after toasting will help to remove any saponins that can taste bitter.
- Rinse quinoa briefly while agitating to remove the outer layer that contains the bitter compound (saponin). Do not soak as this will cause the saponin to migrate inside the seed.
- Bring water or a flavored liquid (e.g., use broth, herbs, onions, etc....) to a boil (follow directions; if none, use 1.8 cups of liquid to 1 cup quinoa). Add quinoa, place lid on the pot, and simmer for 10 to 15 minutes until all the water is absorbed. Quinoa is fully cooked when the little tail sticks out of the seed.
- Take off the heat but leave the lid on to steam for 10 to 15 minutes. This will produce a light and fluffy grain.

Millet — comes in white, yellow, and red varieties. These tiny grains are popped or made into breads, porridge, malts and beers. They can be used to replace couscous or rice in a dish like risotto.
- To improve the taste, toast millet in a dry pan on low for four to five minutes (until they achieve a golden color) before cooking in liquid. There is no need to rinse after this step.
- Add twice as much liquid as millet to produce a nice pilaf and cook for 20 minutes. For porridge use three times more liquid than millet and stir often.

Sorghum — comes in light green, white, tan, bronze or red varieties. It is often used in porridges, flatbreads, and couscous.
- Sorghum (depending on the form — whole, pearled, or flake) can be boiled, popped, or baked.
- Do not sprout sorghum seeds as they can produce cyanide (McGee, 2004).

Teff — comes in brown (most flavorful), red, and ivory varieties and tastes like hazelnuts.
- Toast teff in hot oil (with onions or shallots if desired) while stirring constantly until they start to pop.
- Add liquid and cook until the liquid is absorbed.

Rice

Grain of rice with husk → Remove husk > brown rice → Remove bran > white rice

Rice comes in various forms, — brown, white, wild (a different species), and more. Rinse rice first to remove excess starch in order to create a fluffier end product and to reduce stickiness after cooking. The next steps involve removing arsenic from rice by parboiling and discarding the water.

Removing Arsenic from Rice

Rice absorbs more arsenic than wheat and barley (by 10 times) because of the amount of water that is used during growth (Williams et al., 2007). Arsenic sits in the outer bran layer so always rinse rice first before cooking and then parboil it – parboiling means to partially cook. The following parboiling method from Menton et al removes 50% of the arsenic in brown rice and 74% of the arsenic in white rice without removing micronutrients (Menon et al., 2021). Some chefs will cook the rice in step 2 with an excess of water – like pasta – and discard the leftover water after cooking. This will certainly remove more nutrients.

Image: Parboiling Rice to Remove Arsenic

Parboiled Rice

Parboiled rice sold in supermarkets are soaked, steamed, and dried with the husk on which causes nutrients to move from the bran layer to the inner endosperm (McGee, 2004). **This method does not remove arsenic.**

Rice is a potential source for food poisoning due to the microbe Bacillus cereus often found on the surface of raw grains. This bacterium can tolerate and survive high heat, so **always refrigerate cooked rice promptly**.

Wild Rice

Technically wild rice is not a rice but a wild grass. It has a distinctive, unique flavor that can be used in a dish by itself or mixed with other cooked grains to change the flavor profile. To prepare, use three to four times more water than wild rice. It doesn't absorb water very well so if necessary, drain any remaining liquid after it is cooked. Simmer for 35 to 60 minutes, until tender but not overcooked. Use wild rice in a stuffing, grain salad or as a side dish. It pairs well with dried fruit and nuts.

Rice Pilaf (Pilau)

A pilaf is traditionally a rice dish (although wheat and other grains can be used) that has added flavor, plus the grains of rice do not adhere to one another. Think light, fluffy, and separate grains of rice in a pilaf as opposed to the sticky rice you find in sushi. The rice is thoroughly rinsed to remove any extra starch, which lessens the chance for rice grains to stick together. Many ingredients can be added in the cooking process and after the rice is cooked — meat, vegetables, or herbs for example.

RECIPES & HOW TO

Chef Lyndon's Rice Pilaf

Yield 5 to 6 cups

Ingredients
- 2 tablespoons vegetable oil
- ½ cup minced onions
- 2 cups converted rice
- 3 ½ cups chicken or vegetable stock or water

Method
1. Heat oil in a saucepan; add onions and cook until softened (approximately 3 minutes)
2. Stir in the rice and coat the grains with the oil mixture (2 minutes)
3. Add the liquid (heated up)
4. Bring to a simmer, cover tightly, and cook 18 minutes or until rice is tender and the liquid is absorbed
5. Rest for 5 minutes, and fluff with a fork

Variations
- Brown Rice: increase liquid to 5 cups, and simmer 30 minutes or until tender.
- Curried rice: add ½ tablespoon of mild curry powder to onion mixture.
- Yellow Rice: add ½ teaspoon turmeric to onions.
- Roasted Pepper Rice: Fold in 1 each roasted red and green pepper (peeled, seeded, diced) to the fluffed rice.
- Lemon Rice: add juice and zest of one lemon to the liquid before cooking.
- Moroccan Rice: season to taste with cinnamon and cayenne, garnish with toasted almond and ½ cup currants or golden raisins. Place currants or raisins on top of rice when cooked, cover for 5 minutes. Add almonds just before serving.
- Herbed Rice: fold in 1 cup chopped fresh herbs of your choice just before serving.
- Scallion Rice: substitute ½ bunch of scallions for the onions. (Add scallion greens after cooking.)

Sticky Rice

Image: Sticky Rice

Sticky rice is a type of rice that has a large amount of the starch amylopectin. It requires the least amount of water to cook. Selecting a sticky rice — also referred to as sweet rice or glutinous rice (which does not have gluten) — can be tricky. You may need to try several brands in order to find the one you like best. Thai sticky rice has a longer grain and a more floral scent than Japanese sticky rice, which has a short grain (Guide to Sticky Rice).

Sticky rice can be cooked in two ways, but the steamed method is preferred:
1. Soak and steam method: Cover the rice with an extra 2 to 3 inches of water. Soak rice for 6 to 24 hours in room temperature water, or 2 to 4 hours in warm water. Drain and rinse in cold water. Place in a steamer (with a steamer liner or parchment paper), cover, and steam for 20 to 35 minutes (or as directed on the package) until it becomes tender and sticky.
2. Boil in a 1:1 rice-to-water ratio

Pasta

Whole Grain Pasta

Select a 100% whole grain pasta. Semolina flour is a type of flour made from Durum wheat, but it is not necessarily a whole grain unless it actually says 100% whole grain in the ingredient list.

Cooking tips for whole grain pasta include:
- Cook at a steady vigorous boil to evenly cook and prevent clumping
- Do not overcook but cook al dente
- Finish cooking in a sauce so that flavor can be absorbed more fully

Pasta Sauces

Image: Types of Pasta Sauce

There are many scrumptious pasta sauces that don't need to be made with saturated fat (cream and butter) but healthful fats (olive oil), nuts, and vegetables. Below is an outline of three base- sauces.

Tomato base with garlic, herbs and pureed vegetables	Olive oil base with fresh herbs and sauteed vegetables	Creamy base made with pureed vegetables, nuts or legumes

- To add nutrients to a tomato-based sauce, purée carrots, peppers, onions, zucchini and/or mushrooms. The vegetables add a complexity to the flavor and the sauce is a great way to get a nutrient-packed meal.
- One of the most delicious dishes is the simplest. Sautéing garlic and herbs in olive oil and adding al dente pasta, tossing and serving with fresh herbs and parmesan is as good as it gets.
- Instead of using heavy cream to make a creamy sauce, substitute plain Greek yogurt, skim milk, or coconut milk. Another option is to use non-dairy ingredients such as avocado, white beans, blended silken tofu, puréed cashews or cauliflower to make a creamy sauce.

To switch to a whole grain pasta, try any of the following methods:
- Start with one quarter whole grain pasta mixed with three-quarters refined pasta and slowly add more whole grain pasta over time. This will allow time for someone to get used to the heartier texture and different flavor profile.
- Serve whole grain pasta with a hearty sauce to cover some of the texture and taste differences.

You can also have fun cooking with pasta of varying colors. Make sure the colors come from natural ingredients like legumes, spinach, or other vegetables. There are a lot of pasta options made with legumes instead of grains. These include those made with red lentils, chickpeas, edamame and black beans. Most are high in fiber (look for 5 grams of fiber or more per serving) and have a good amount of protein.

Table 12: Chef's Advice for Saving Time

Chef	Grain Cooking Advice
Chef Scott	• Cooking with whole grains as they are whole, intact grains, takes longer to prepare so plan ahead. Try the use of Crock-Pots or Instant Pots to speed this up. • Cooking ahead of time and freezing is also an option if you are always on the go. • I do not soak them, but I do rinse them before cooking. • Ideally, I cook grains covered in the oven as they cook more evenly and are less likely to scorch. • Note, not all water to grain ratios are perfect, adjust as you need and like pastas, try to have your grains just al dente, not mushy. Mushy is bad for flavor and digests the sugars too quickly in your body.
Chef Kate	• Choose one new grain to try, and cook a larger quantity of it at the beginning of your week and store extras in the fridge safely for up to 7 days to add to meals as the week goes. This gives you a chance to try the grain in many different ways and when they are already cooked and good to go, it's a huge time saver.

Chef	Grain Cooking Advice
Chef Russell	• I recommend when trying a new grain, to purchase a small amount first to ensure you will like it. Enjoying a grain stems from the preparation of the grain and the ingredients that accompany it. Flavor is essential to the success of eating healthy cuisine. • When cooking dense grains such as: forbidden rice (black rice), arborio rice, farro, wild rice, sprouting red sienna rice, they take an extended period of time, usually 30 to 45 minutes. Parcooking the day before is helpful to save time when preparing for a meal. Parcook two-thirds of the way then finish when ready to eat. This will help with the timing. • Batch cook, cryovac and freeze whole grains. Pull what is needed at the time you need it. When cryovacing grains, be sure to cryovac flat to speed the thawing process.
Chef Cyndie	• Cook and chill in advance for stir-frying or flavored rice dishes, such as Spanish rice. The rice will absorb flavors better. • Soak grains such as bulgur in advance in desired flavor. For example, bulgur in water with lemon juice makes terrific tabbouleh.

Chef Cyndie's Easy Spanish Rice

Image: Spanish Rice

Ingredients
- 2 cups (cooked) brown rice, cooked, and chilled
- ½ cup onion, diced
- 1 tablespoon olive oil
- 1 cup salsa, prepared
- 2 tablespoons tomato paste

Method
1. Prepare rice at least a day in advance and keep it refrigerated
2. Sauté onions in olive oil until translucent

3. Add salsa and tomato paste and cook for 1 to 2 minutes until flavors bloom
4. Add rice and stir well to combine ingredients. Cook for 3 minutes. Heat to 165°F/74°C or above
5. Note: Save the remaining tomato paste in 2 tablespoon servings — wrap in plastic wrap and freeze for future use

BUILD A HEALTHFUL GRAIN-BASED BREAKFAST

Image: Build a Ready to Eat Breakfast Bowl

The first ready-to-eat cereals were very healthful — Shredded Wheat and Grape-Nuts to name a couple. Today, options with ready-to-eat breakfast cereals range from "candy in a box" (high added sugar and little to no fiber) to fiber-rich whole grains. While ready-to-eat cereals may be enriched and fortified with vitamins and minerals, it doesn't take away from the fact that they are refined grains containing a significant amount of added sugar. There are plenty of healthful options to choose from though.

Types of ready-to-eat cereal include muesli, granola, puffed rice, wheat and corn, baked (Grape-Nuts), and flakes.

Some tips that the cereal is not a healthful grain option are:
• It comes in a wide array of colors
• Candy or dessert-sounding names — Reese's Puffs and Cookie Crisp, for example
• You can see the sugar-coating
• Chocolate-based cereal

Steps to Identifying a Ready-to-Eat Breakfast Cereal
1. Look for the word "whole" in the first ingredient
2. Select options with no more than 4 grams (1 teaspoon) of added sugar per serving
3. Avoid cereals with added colors and flavors
4. Look for a short ingredient list

Build a Ready-to-Eat Breakfast Bowl

Once you have selected a healthful breakfast cereal, pair it with a whole fruit and milk serving (dairy or plant-based).

Build a Hot Cereal Bowl

Hot cereal, also referred to as porridge, gruel (not so appetizing sounding), and congee have been prepared since the beginning of civilization.

Step 1: Choose a grain or a combination of grains: steel-cut or rolled oats, brown rice, barley, quinoa, etc...

Step 2: Cook in water or milk (plant or dairy) with optional added flavor — cinnamon, nutmeg, and/or vanilla.

Step 3: Add flax or chia seeds, dried cereal, nuts, fruit (dried, fresh, or puréed).

Step 4: Optional: Top with a splash of maple syrup or honey.

Overnight Oats

Image: Overnight Oats

To a container, add:
- Rolled oats
- Milk (dairy or plant-based) in the same amount as rolled oats
- 1 teaspoon chia or flax seeds
- Stir and add cinnamon, nutmeg, and/or vanilla to taste
- Let rest overnight (or for a minimum of 5 hours).

Note: If substituting quick oats, soak for no longer than 30 minutes and consume within one hour or oats become gummy.

Add on any of the following to create a hot cereal bowl with your favorite ingredients:
- Fruit (fresh or dried)
- Nut butter
- Seeds or nuts
- Coconut flakes
- Granola

BUILD A SALAD-GRAIN BOWL/JAR

Image: Grain Jar

BUILD A GRAIN-BASED MEAL

To build a scrumptious grain bowl, think **grains** with **cooked vegetables** (roasted, caramelized, or grilled to add a depth of flavor) + **raw vegetables and greens** + **crunchy bits** (nuts, seeds, crisped chickpeas) + a bit of **protein** (plant or animal-based) + a delicious **dressing with acid** to bring it all together.

> Warm up cold, cooked grains in a little bit of water, stock or broth.

Lemon Vinaigrette by Chef Russell

Image: Lemon Vinaigrette

Ingredients
- 2 tablespoons dijon mustard
- 1 tablespoon honey

- ¼ teaspoon garlic, minced
- ½ cup extra virgin olive oil
- 3 tablespoons water
- 3 tablespoons lemon juice
- ½ cup apple cider vinegar
- ¼ teaspoon salt, sea or Himalayan
- ¼ teaspoon black pepper

Methods

1. Place the mustard, honey, garlic and shallots in a mixing bowl
2. Whisk the ingredients well
3. Slowly add the olive oil until fully incorporated
4. Add the water and lemon juice, mix well
5. Slowly add the vinegar until fully incorporated
6. Season with salt and pepper

BAKING WITH WHOLE GRAINS

(McGee, 2004; Oldways Whole Grains Council, 2017)

When switching to baking with whole grains, slow and easy is the way to go especially if an individual is not used to the stronger flavor and heartier texture of whole grains. The baking tips below list the end point so gradually work your way up to the full substitution. For example, if you intend to replace half of the flour in a recipe with whole wheat flour, start with replacing one-quarter of the flour and gradually increase. Taste buds will take time to adjust and chances are once someone is exposed to and used to whole grains, they will find the processed grains too bland and boring.

Table 13: Types of Whole Grain Flours and Their Uses in Baking

Traditional Whole Grains	Best Used For	Ancient Grain Flours	Best Used For
Whole wheat	Can be used in most recipes. It has an assertive flavor.	Amaranth Flour (gluten-free)	Pancakes, scones, and quick breads
White whole wheat	Can be used in most recipes. Has a milder taste than whole wheat.	Barley flour	Pancakes, muffins, and quick breads
Whole wheat pastry flour	Use for products that need a delicate flour — soft and tender.	Buckwheat flour (gluten-free)	Pancakes, scones, muffins and quick breads

Traditional Whole Grains	Best Used For	Ancient Grain Flours	Best Used For
Sprouted wheat flour	Use for products that result in a soft feel and a tender texture. Has a mild flavor.	KAMUT® flour	Scones, quick breads, and muffins
Irish-style wholemeal flour	Can be used in non-yeast recipes like pie crusts, biscuits, and Irish soda bread.	Millet flour (gluten-free)	Pancakes, scones, muffins and quick breads
Wheat berries	These are soaked and added to baked goods to add texture and a strong "wheat" flavor.	Quinoa flour (gluten-free)	Muffins and quick breads
Cracked wheat (berries)	Same as above but with smaller pieces. Can also be used to make a porridge-like oatmeal.	Spelt flour	Pancakes, muffins, and quick breads
Steel-cut oats (aka Irish or Scottish oats)	The pieces (groats) need to be soaked before adding to yeast bread and rolls.	Teff flour (gluten-free)	Pancakes, scones, quick breads and muffins
Rolled oats	Can be used in any baked treat — bread, muffins, cookies, granola scones and cake		
Oat flour	This is a fine powdered flour that can be used to make muffins, cakes, and cookies.		
Pumpernickel flour	This is a very dense and heavy flour, which can be mixed with other lighter flours to make bread.		

Whole Grain Baking Tips

- For yeast breads that need to rise, you can **replace half the all-purpose flour with whole-wheat flour**.
- For treats — cookies, scones, quick breads, muffins, pancakes and waffles — you can **replace all the flour with whole grain flour**. You will need to add an extra 2 teaspoons of liquid for every cup of whole-wheat flour used in the recipe.

- Weigh instead of measure flour as depending on how packed the measuring cup is, the amount can vary as much as 50%.

Whole Grain Baking Flavor Tips
- Replace 2 to 3 tablespoons of the liquid in a recipe with orange juice as it tempers the stronger whole grain flavors.
- For a sweet, mild flavor use white whole-wheat flour, freshly ground whole-wheat flour, or sprouted-wheat flour.
- There are several flavor sources in baked bread
  - The yeast product and fermentation products ("yeasty")
  - The flavor of different types of flour (from strong whole wheat to mild white flour)
  - Baking brings out "toast-like" flavors due to the browning reaction.

Baking with an eye on the sugar content and a thorough description of the "baker's percentage" is covered in the **Sugar** chapter.

Baking With Whole Grain Resources

Oldways Whole Grain Council has Expert Tips on baking with whole grains (https://wholegrainscouncil.org/blog/2015/04/expert-shares-tips-baking-whole grains) .

Baking with Ancient Grains (https://www.kingarthurbaking.com/learn/guides/baking-with-ancient-grains) and Baking with Whole Grains (https://www.kingarthurbaking.com/learn/guides/whole-grains) by King Arthur Baking Company is a great resource as is their cookbook Whole Grain Baking.

SECTION 12:

SERVING WHOLE GRAINS

Make sure when planning a menu that whole grains are served at breakfast, lunch, dinner and snack time. Table 14 lists the number of servings of grains recommended each day for various age and gender groups. Keep the total daily amount in mind when planning the menu and focus on whole grains.

Oldways Whole Grain Council has a resource for planning grain-based meals (recipes for up to 100 diners) throughout the week. The Plant Forward Plates Healthcare Toolkit has sample chapters. You can order it (at a cost) at https://oldwayspt.org/programs/plant-forward-plates.

Table 14: Grains Servings Per Day

Age of child (years)	Servings per day in ounce equivalents*	Serving size
2 to 3	3 total (at least 1 ½ whole grain)	½ ounce eq = ½ cup cereal; ½ slice bread; ¼ large muffin or ½ medium muffin
4 to 8	5 total (at least 2 ½ whole grain)	4 to 6 years: 1 ounce eq = 1 slice bread; 1 cup cold cereal; ½ cup oatmeal, rice, or pasta 7 to 8 years: 1 ½ ounce eq = 1 ½ slices bread; 1 ½ cup cold cereal; ¾ cup oatmeal, rice, or pasta
Boys 9 to 13	6 total (at least 3 whole grain)	2-ounce eq = 2 slices bread; 1 muffin; 1 cup oatmeal; rice or pasta
Boys 14 to 18	8 total (at least 4 whole grain)	
Girls 9 to 13	5 total (at least 3 whole grain)	
Girls 14 to 18	6 total (at least 3 whole grain)	
Women 19 to 30	6 total (at least 3 whole grain)	
Women 31 to 50	6 total (at least 3 whole grain)	
Women 51+	5 total (at least 3 whole grain)	
		2-ounce eq = 2 slices bread; 1 muffin; 1 cup oatmeal; rice or pasta
Men 19 to 30	8 total (at least 4 whole grain)	
Men 31 to 50	7 total (at least 3 ½ whole grain)	
Men 51+	6 total (at least 3 whole grain)	

*1-ounce equivalent = 1-inch mini bagel, 1 slice bread, ½ cup cooked grain, 5 whole wheat crackers, 7 round crackers, ½ English muffin, 1 small muffin (2 ½ inches), 1 pancake) 4 ½ inches), 3 cups popped popcorn, 1 cup ready-to-eat cold cereal, ½ cup cooked spaghetti or 1 ounce dry, 1 tortilla (6-inch).

EAT A VARIETY OF WHOLE GRAINS

Table 15 lists grain substitutions to broaden whole grain varieties in dishes. The larger grains — barley, farro, and wheat berries — hold up well in a grain salad, whereas the smaller, tiny grains — quinoa, amaranth, and millet — can be added to recipes (burgers, meatloaf) or as an accompaniment to dishes with sauces.

Whole grains can be added to:
- Stir-fries
- Soups
- Salads
- Meatloaf recipe
- Breakfast items — pancakes, waffles, and cooked hot cereal, for example

Table 15: Whole grain Substitutions for Standard-Grain Dishes

Instead of...	Use...
Rice as a side dish	Try bulgur wheat, millet, or teff
A pasta salad	A quinoa salad
White flour pancakes	Try a buckwheat blend (50%)
Oatmeal for breakfast	Try Fonio breakfast porridge (no gluten). Bump up your oatmeal by mixing in a variety of whole grains — quinoa, millet, and wheatberries make great additions — soak them overnight or use a slow cooker or Instant Pot
Risotto	Farrotto (Cooking farro the same way as risotto is delicious — so nutty and good!)
Pasta salad	Whole grain salad with bulgur, farro, wheat berries, etc. Can be served either warm or cold but it's always best to dress the grains while they are still warm so they absorb a little more flavor. Punchy dressings work best
Crepes	Try buckwheat galettes: 210 grams buckwheat flour, 2 cups water, 2 eggs, ½ teaspoon salt Mix well and let sit overnight for best results Cook in a cast iron pan if available Is great for both savory and sweet applications and is 100% gluten-free
Standard pancake batters	Buckwheat pancakes — buckwheat flour is high in protein, naturally gluten-free, and has a low glycemic index. Add sauteed apples to top the pancakes with a hint of maple syrup offers a more complex flavor profile with reduced sugars
Arborio rice risotto	Forbidden Rice (black rice) or Sprouting Red Sienna Rice (great source is Lundberg Family Farm Rice). Same cooking method as risotto
Croutons on salad	Toast dry, uncooked buckwheat groats until fragrant — they have the texture of an almond and provide a tasty crunch

ADDING WHOLE GRAINS TO THE MENU

The picture above focuses on how to use a whole grain as the star of the meal for breakfast, lunch, and dinner. Quinoa can be the main ingredient in a breakfast bowl or the main ingredient in salads for lunch or dinner.

ChooseMyplate recommends that 30% of the plate should contain grains and 20% protein. Since grains provide protein and grain-based dishes can have other plant-based sources of protein (nuts and seeds) added to it, 50% of the plate can be filled with grains, leaving the other 50% for fruits and vegetables for a vegetarian meal. Also, for those who are not ready to, or do not want to eat pure plant-based meals, the portion of grains can be increased, and the protein portion decreased (see the Protein Flip in the Protein chapter). Meat can be present, but in a much smaller portion, leaving more room for nutrient-dense plant-based products.

SECTION 13:

PRACTICAL TIPS TO INCREASE WHOLE GRAIN CONSUMPTION

1. Plan ahead; some grains should be soaked or washed before consumption. Grains are not ready-to-eat foods.
2. Introduce whole grains slowly; give your family and your digestive tract time to acclimate to a higher-fiber diet. Mix enriched and whole grains to ease the transition to eating more whole grains such as a 50/50 blend of all-purpose flour and whole grain flour.
3. Read labels to be sure that whole grains are the first item listed on an ingredient label.
4. Check front panels of food products for the Whole Grain Stamp.
5. Think about pulling out your Crock-Pot or upgrade to an Instant Pot to make quick work of cooking whole grains.
6. Use grains as the foundation of your next plant-forward meal. Rinse and repeat.
7. Stock your pantry with a variety of grains. Use blogs and recipe sites for inspiration.
8. Make large batches of grains so some can be frozen for a quick and easy meal later on.
9. If you have picky eaters remember it takes many encounters with a new food before it becomes a favorite. Don't give up.
10. Bask in the feeling of knowing that you took a major step to healthful eating with a transition to whole grains!

RESOURCES

* Whole Grains Council is (https://wholegrainscouncil.org/) an excellent resource for information, recipes, and research on whole grains. They have a long list of favorite whole grain cookbooks

- Oldways Whole Grain Council (https://oldwayspt.org/programs/whole-grains-council)
- Baking with Whole Grains King Arthur Baking Company (https://www.kingarthurbaking.com/learn/guides/whole-grains)
- Washington State University Bread Lab and recipes (https://breadlab.wsu.edu/

SUMMARY

Grains have been a dietary staple for thousands of years. Every culture includes some form of a staple grain in their diet which often represents unique climate attributes that made their native grains thrive. The messaging for grains is simple: increase whole grain intake and decrease/limit refined grains. In order for individuals to be able to follow this advice, culinary skills are essential. Individuals need to learn how to identify whole grain options, cook and prepare them, and introduce them into their and their family's diet in a stepwise manner in order to acclimate to the difference in texture and flavor.

Grains are an essential part of a healthful diet, and current dietary recommendations do not suggest a need to decrease grains, but rather to ensure that at least one-half of the grains consumed are "whole" grains meaning that the entire grain kernel was used in formulating the product. This will provide more dietary fiber and more nutrients such as vitamins, minerals, protein and healthful fats to the diet. There are many whole grain choices available to help consumers meet that mandate. This chapter provided culinary techniques to transform whole grains into delicious meals and side dishes, which will make it easier for individuals to reach their daily recommended intake.

APPENDIX A: Dietary Fiber: Food Sources Ranked by Amounts of Dietary Fiber and Energy per Standard Food Portions and per 100 Grams of Foods

Food	StandardPortion Size	Calories in Standard Portion[a]	Dietary Fiber in Standard Portion (grams)[a]	Calories per 100 grams[a]
High-fiber bran ready-to-eat cereal	⅓ – ¾ cup	60–81	9.1–14.3	200–260
Shredded Wheat ready-to-eat cereal (various)	1–1 ¼ cup	155–220	5.0–9.0	321–373
Wheat bran flakes ready-to-eat cereal (various)	¾ cup	90–98	4.9–5.5	310–328
Plain rye wafer crackers	2 wafers	73	5.0	334
Chia seeds, dried	1 tablespoon	58	4.1	486
Bulgur, cooked	½ cup	76	4.1	83
Popcorn, air-popped	3 cups	93	3.5	387
Whole-wheat spaghetti, cooked	½ cup	87	3.2	124
Oat bran muffin	1 small	178	3.0	270
Pearled barley, cooked	½ cup	97	3.0	123
Whole-wheat paratha bread	1 ounce	92	2.7	326
Quinoa, cooked	½ cup	111	2.6	120

Source: U.S Department of Agriculture, Agricultural Research Service, Nutrient Data Laboratory. 2014. USDA National Nutrient Database for Standard Reference, Release 27. Available at: http://www.ars.usda.gov/nutrientdata.

APPENDIX B: Storage Time for Grains

	Intact Grains	Ground Grains (Flour)
Amaranth	Pantry: 4 months Freezer: 8 months	Pantry: 2 months Freezer: 4 months
Barley	Pantry: 6 months Freezer: 1 year	Pantry: 3 months Freezer: 6 months
Brown/colored rice	Pantry: 6 months Freezer: 1 year	Pantry: 3 months Freezer: 6 months
Buckwheat	Pantry: 2 months Freezer: 4 months	Pantry: 1 month Freezer: 2 months
Corn/Popcorn	Pantry: 6 months Freezer: 1 year	Pantry: 3 months Freezer: 6 months
Farro	Pantry: 6 months Freezer: 1 year	Pantry: 3 months Freezer: 6 months
Millet	Pantry: 2 months Freezer: 4 months	Pantry: 1 month Freezer: 2 months
Oats	Pantry: 4 months Freezer: 8 months	Pantry: 2 months Freezer: 4 months
Quinoa	Pantry: 4 months Freezer: 8 months	Pantry: 2 months Freezer: 4 months
Rye	Pantry: 6 months Freezer: 1 year	Pantry: 3 months Freezer: 6 months
Sorghum	Pantry: 4 months Freezer: 8 months	Pantry: 2 months Freezer: 4 months
Spelt	Pantry: 6 months Freezer: 1 year	Pantry: 3 months Freezer: 6 months
Teff	Pantry: 4 months Freezer: 8 months	Pantry: 2 months Freezer: 4 months
Wheat	Pantry: 6 months Freezer: 1 year	Pantry: 3 months Freezer: 6 months
Wild Rice	Pantry: 4 months Freezer: 8 months	Pantry: 2 months Freezer: 4 months

Sourced from: Oldways Whole Grains Council

REFERENCES

Abbaspour, N., Hurrell, R., & Kelishadi, R. (2014). Review on iron and its importance for human health. Journal of Research in Medical Sciences : The Official Journal of Isfahan University of Medical Sciences, 19(2), 164–174.

Åberg, S., Mann, J., Neumann, S., Ross, A. B., & Reynolds, A. N. (2020). Whole grain Processing and Glycemic Control in Type 2 Diabetes: A Randomized Crossover Trial. Diabetes Care, 43(8), 1717–1723. https://doi.org/10.2337/dc20-0263

Academy of Nutrition and Dietetics. (2022). USDA Releases Transitional School Meal Standards to Strengthen Nutrition Quality. https://www.eatrightpro.org/news-center/on-the-pulse-of-public-policy/regulatory-comments/usda-releases-transitional-school-meal-standards-to-strengthen-nutrition-quality

Agricultural Marketing Research Center. (2022, February). Barley Profile. Agricultural Marketing Research Center. https://www.agmrc.org/commodities-products/grains-oilseeds/barley-profile

Ahluwalia, N., Herrick, K., Terry, A., & Hughes, J. (2019). Contribution of Whole Grains to Total Grains Intake Amomng Adults Aged 20 and Over: United States, 2013-2016 (No. 341). https://www.cdc.gov/nchs/products/databriefs/db341.htm

Ajala, O., English, P., & Pinkney, J. (2013). Systematic review and meta-analysis of different dietary approaches to the management of type 2 diabetes. The American Journal of Clinical Nutrition, 97(3), 505–516. https://doi.org/10.3945/ajcn.112.042457

Akiyama, H., Imai, T., & Ebisawa, M. (2011). Japan food allergen labeling regulation—History and evaluation. Advances in Food and Nutrition Research, 62, 139–171. https://doi.org/10.1016/B978-0-12-385989-1.00004-1

Albertson, A. M., Reicks, M., Joshi, N., & Gugger, C. K. (2016). Whole grain consumption trends and associations with body weight measures in the United States: Results from the cross sectional National Health and Nutrition Examination Survey 2001–2012. Nutrition Journal, 15(1), 8. https://doi.org/10.1186/s12937-016-0126-4

Amini, A. M., Muzs, K., Spencer, J. P., & Yaqoob, P. (2017). Pelargonidin-3-O-glucoside and its metabolites have modest anti-inflammatory effects in human whole blood cultures. Nutrition Research (New York, N.Y.), 46, 88–95. https://doi.org/10.1016/j.nutres.2017.09.006

Ampatzoglou, A., Williams, C. L., Atwal, K. K., Maidens, C. M., Ross, A. B., Thielecke, F., Jonnalagadda, S. S., Kennedy, O. B., & Yaqoob, P. (2016). Effects of increased wholegrain consumption on immune and inflammatory markers in healthy low habitual wholegrain consumers. European Journal of Nutrition, 55(1), 183–195. https://doi.org/10.1007/s00394-015-0836-y

Ancient Grains | The Whole Grains Council. Retrieved May 31, 2021, from https://wholegrainscouncil.org/whole grains-101/whats-whole grain/ancient-grains

Anderson, J. W., Baird, P., Davis, R. H., Ferreri, S., Knudtson, M., Koraym, A., Waters, V., & Williams, C. L. (2009). Health benefits of dietary fiber. Nutrition Reviews, 67(4), 188–205. https://doi.org/10.1111/j.1753-4887.2009.00189.x

Armah, S. M., Carriquiry, A. L., & Reddy, M. B. (2015). Total Iron Bioavailability from the US Diet Is Lower Than the Current Estimate. The Journal of Nutrition, 145(11), 2617–2621. https://doi.org/10.3945/jn.115.210484

Atallah, R., Filion, K. B., Wakil, S. M., Genest, J., Joseph, L., Poirier, P., Rinfret, S., Schiffrin, E. L., & Eisenberg, M. J. (2014). Long-term effects of 4 popular diets on weight loss and cardiovascular risk factors: A systematic review of randomized controlled trials. Circulation. Cardiovascular Quality and Outcomes, 7(6), 815–827. https://doi.org/10.1161/CIRCOUTCOMES.113.000723

Aune, D., Chan, D. S. M., Greenwood, D. C., Vieira, A. R., Rosenblatt, D. A. N., Vieira, R., & Norat, T. (2012). Dietary fiber and breast cancer risk: A systematic review and meta-analysis of prospective studies. Annals of Oncology: Official Journal of the European Society for Medical Oncology, 23(6), 1394–1402. https://doi.org/10.1093/annonc/mdr589

Aune, D., Chan, D. S. M., Lau, R., Vieira, R., Greenwood, D. C., Kampman, E., & Norat, T. (2012). Carbohydrates, glycemic index, glycemic load, and colorectal cancer risk: A systematic review and meta-analysis of cohort studies. Cancer Causes & Control: CCC, 23(4), 521–535. https://doi.org/10.1007/s10552-012-9918-9

Bahwere, P., Akomo, P., Mwale, M., Murakami, H., Banda, C., Kathumba, S., Banda, C., Jere, S., Sadler, K., & Collins, S. (2017). Soya, maize, and sorghum-based ready-to-use therapeutic food with amino acid is as efficacious as the standard milk and peanut paste-based formulation for the treatment of severe acute malnutrition in children: A noninferiority individually randomized controlled efficacy clinical trial in Malawi. The American Journal of Clinical Nutrition, 106(4), 1100–1112. https://doi.org/10.3945/ajcn.117.156653

Bengmark, S. (2013). Gut microbiota, immune development and function. Pharmacological Research, 69(1), 87–113. https://doi.org/10.1016/j.phrs.2012.09.002

Benus, R. F. J., van der Werf, T. S., Welling, G. W., Judd, P. A., Taylor, M. A., Harmsen, H. J. M., & Whelan, K. (2010). Association between Faecalibacterium prausnitzii and dietary fibre in colonic fermentation in healthy human subjects. The British Journal of Nutrition, 104(5), 693–700. https://doi.org/10.1017/S0007114510001030

Biesiekierski, J. R. (2017). What is gluten? Journal of Gastroenterology and Hepatology, 32 Suppl 1, 78–81. https://doi.org/10.1111/jgh.13703

Borrell, B. (2009). Fiddling with Flavors: Making Healthy Bread Taste Better. Scientific American. https://www.scientificamerican.com/article/why-bread-smells/

Boukid, F., Folloni, S., Sforza, S., Vittadini, E., & Prandi, B. (2018). Current Trends in Ancient Grains-Based Foodstuffs: Insights into Nutritional Aspects and Technological Applications. Comprehensive Reviews in Food Science and Food Safety, 17(1), 123–136. https://doi.org/10.1111/1541-4337.12315

Brahe, L. K., Astrup, A., & Larsen, L. H. (2013). Is butyrate the link between diet, intestinal microbiota and obesity-related metabolic diseases? Obesity Reviews, 14(12), 950–959. https://doi.org/10.1111/obr.12068

Brinkworth, G. D., Noakes, M., Clifton, P. M., & Bird, A. R. (2009). Comparative effects of very low-carbohydrate, high-fat and high-carbohydrate, low-fat weight-loss diets on bowel habit and faecal short-chain fatty acids and bacterial populations. The British Journal of Nutrition, 101(10), 1493–1502. https://doi.org/10.1017/S0007114508094658

British Dietetic Association. (2021, June 11). Fibre: Food Fact Sheet. https://www.bda.uk.com/resource/fibre.html

Bureau of Nutritional Sciences. (2016). Health Claims [Education and awareness]. https://www.canada.ca/en/health-canada/services/food-nutrition/food-labelling/health-claims.html

Călinoiu, L. F., & Vodnar, D. C. (2018). Whole Grains and Phenolic Acids: A Review on Bioactivity, Functionality, Health Benefits and Bioavailability. Nutrients, 10(11), 1615. https://doi.org/10.3390/nu10111615

Canadian Adult Obesity Clinical Practice Guidelines. Obesity Canada. Retrieved January 29, 2022, from https://obesitycanada.ca/guidelines/chapters/

Canadian Nutrient File. (2021, April 29). https://food-nutrition.canada.ca/cnf-fce/newSearch-nouvelleRecherche.do?action=new_nouveau

Carb Common Sense | The Whole Grains Council. Retrieved January 29, 2022, from https://wholegrainscouncil.org/blog/2015/06/carb-common-sense

Caselato-Sousa, V. M., & Amaya-Farfán, J. (2012). State of knowledge on amaranth grain: A comprehensive review. Journal of Food Science, 77(4), R93-104. https://doi.org/10.1111/j.1750-3841.2012.02645.x

Cheng, A. (2018). Review: Shaping a sustainable food future by rediscovering long-forgotten ancient grains. Plant Science: An International Journal of Experimental Plant Biology, 269, 136–142. https://doi.org/10.1016/j.plantsci.2018.01.018

Cherian, S., Kumar, R. V., Augusti, K. T., & Kidwai, J. R. (1992). Antidiabetic effect of a glycoside of pelargonidin isolated from the bark of Ficus bengalensis Linn. Indian Journal of Biochemistry & Biophysics, 29(4), 380–382.

Cho, S. S., Qi, L., Fahey, G. C., & Klurfeld, D. M. (2013). Consumption of cereal fiber, mixtures of whole grains and bran, and whole grains and risk reduction in type 2 diabetes, obesity, and cardiovascular disease. The American Journal of Clinical Nutrition, 98(2), 594–619. https://doi.org/10.3945/ajcn.113.067629

Christianson, E., & Salling, J. (2020). Meded101 Guide to Drug Food Interactions.

Cicero, A. F. G., Fogacci, F., Veronesi, M., Grandi, E., Dinelli, G., Hrelia, S., & Borghi, C. (2018). Short-Term Hemodynamic Effects of Modern Wheat Products Substitution in Diet with Ancient Wheat Products: A Cross-Over, Randomized Clinical Trial. Nutrients, 10(11), E1666. https://doi.org/10.3390/nu10111666

Cisse, F., Erickson, D. P., Hayes, A. M. R., Opekun, A. R., Nichols, B. L., & Hamaker, B. R. (2018). Traditional Malian Solid Foods Made from Sorghum and Millet Have Markedly Slower Gastric Emptying than Rice, Potato, or Pasta. Nutrients, 10(2), E124. https://doi.org/10.3390/nu10020124

Clifton, P. M., Condo, D., & Keogh, J. B. (2014). Long term weight maintenance after advice to consume low carbohydrate, higher protein diets—A systematic review and meta analysis. Nutrition, Metabolism, and Cardiovascular Diseases: NMCD, 24(3), 224–235. https://doi.org/10.1016/j.numecd.2013.11.006

Compare Nutrients in Various Grains | The Whole Grains Council. Retrieved January 29, 2022, from https://wholegrainscouncil.org/whole grains-101/health-studies-health-benefits/compare-nutrients-various-grains

Cong, W., Schwartz, E., & Peterson, D. G. (2021). Identification of inhibitors of pinellic acid generation in whole wheat bread. Food Chemistry, 351, 129291. https://doi.org/10.1016/j.foodchem.2021.129291

Consumer Reports. Which Rice Has the Least Arsenic? Retrieved April 16, 2022, from https://www.consumerreports.org/cro/magazine/2015/01/how-much-arsenic-is-in-your-rice/index.htm

Cooper, D. N., Kable, M. E., Marco, M. L., De Leon, A., Rust, B., Baker, J. E., Horn, W., Burnett, D., & Keim, N. L. (2017). The Effects of Moderate Whole Grain Consumption on Fasting Glucose and Lipids, Gastrointestinal Symptoms, and Microbiota. Nutrients, 9(2), 173. https://doi.org/10.3390/nu9020173

Cooper, D. N., Martin, R. J., & Keim, N. L. (2015). Does Whole Grain Consumption Alter Gut Microbiota and Satiety? Healthcare (Basel, Switzerland), 3(2), 364–392. https://doi.org/10.3390/healthcare3020364

Costabile, A., Klinder, A., Fava, F., Napolitano, A., Fogliano, V., Leonard, C., Gibson, G. R., & Tuohy, K. M. (2008). Whole grain wheat breakfast cereal has a prebiotic effect on the human gut microbiota: A double-blind, placebo-controlled, crossover study. British Journal of Nutrition, 99(1), 110–120. https://doi.org/10.1017/S0007114507793923

Coulibaly, A., Kouakou, B., & Chen, J. (2011). Phytic Acid in Cereal Grains: Structure, Healthy or Harmful Ways to Reduce Phytic Acid in Cereal Grains and Their Effects on Nutritional Quality. Science Alert. https://doi.org/10.3923/ajpnft.2011.1.22

Davison, K. M., & Temple, N. J. (2018). Cereal fiber, fruit fiber, and type 2 diabetes: Explaining the paradox. Journal of Diabetes and Its Complications, 32(2), 240–245. https://doi.org/10.1016/j.jdiacomp.2017.11.002

De Carvalho, F. G., Ovídio, P. P., Padovan, G. J., Jordão Junior, A. A., Marchini, J. S., & Navarro, A. M. (2014). Metabolic parameters of postmenopausal women after quinoa or corn flakes intake—A prospective and double-blind study. International Journal of Food Sciences and Nutrition, 65(3), 380–385. https://doi.org/10.3109/09637486.2013.866637

De Leon, A., Burnett, D. J., Rust, B. M., Casperson, S. L., Horn, W. F., & Keim, N. L. (2020). Liking and Acceptability of Whole Grains Increases with a 6-Week Exposure but Preferences for Foods Varying in Taste and Fat Content Are Not Altered: A Randomized Controlled Trial. Current Developments in Nutrition, 4(3), nzaa023. https://doi.org/10.1093/cdn/nzaa023

de Munter, J. S. L., Hu, F. B., Spiegelman, D., Franz, M., & van Dam, R. M. (2007). Whole grain, bran, and germ intake and risk of type 2 diabetes: A prospective cohort study and systematic review. PLoS Medicine, 4(8), e261. https://doi.org/10.1371/journal.pmed.0040261

de Vries, J., Miller, P. E., & Verbeke, K. (2015). Effects of cereal fiber on bowel function: A systematic review of intervention trials. World Journal of Gastroenterology, 21(29), 8952–8963. https://doi.org/10.3748/wjg.v21.i29.8952

Della Pepa, G., Vetrani, C., Vitale, M., & Riccardi, G. (2018). Wholegrain Intake and Risk of Type 2 Diabetes: Evidence from Epidemiological and Intervention Studies. Nutrients, 10(9), 1288. https://doi.org/10.3390/nu10091288

Dhingra, D., Michael, M., Rajput, H., & Patil, R. T. (2012). Dietary fibre in foods: A review. Journal of Food Science and Technology, 49(3), 255–266. https://doi.org/10.1007/s13197-011-0365-5

Dias-Martins, A. M., Pessanha, K. L. F., Pacheco, S., Rodrigues, J. A. S., & Carvalho, C. W. P. (2018). Potential use of pearl millet (Pennisetum glaucum (L.) R. Br.) in Brazil: Food security, processing, health benefits and nutritional products. Food Research International (Ottawa, Ont.), 109, 175–186. https://doi.org/10.1016/j.foodres.2018.04.023

Dietary Guidelines for Americans, 2020-2025. 164.

Dietitians of Canada. (2009). Managing Diarrhea. http://adultmetabolicdiseasesclinic.ca/resources/Managing-Diarrhea.pdf

Dietitians of Canada. (2019). Low FODMAP Diet.pdf. The Low FODMAP Diet: Healthy Eating Guidelines. https://www.scpcn.ca/wp-content/uploads/2020/03/Low-FODMAP-Diet.pdf

Dinu, M., Whittaker, A., Pagliai, G., Giangrandi, I., Colombini, B., Gori, A. M., Fiorillo, C., Becatti, M., Casini, A., Benedettelli, S., & Sofi, F. (2018). A Khorasan Wheat-Based Replacement Diet Improves Risk Profile of Patients With Nonalcoholic Fatty Liver Disease (NAFLD): A Randomized Clinical Trial. Journal of the American College of Nutrition, 37(6), 508–514. https://doi.org/10.1080/07315724.2018.1445047

Duncan, S. H., Belenguer, A., Holtrop, G., Johnstone, A. M., Flint, H. J., & Lobley, G. E. (2007). Reduced dietary intake of carbohydrates by obese subjects results in decreased concentrations of butyrate and butyrate-producing bacteria in feces. Applied and Environmental Microbiology, 73(4), 1073–1078. https://doi.org/10.1128/AEM.02340-06

Dykes, L. (2019). Sorghum Phytochemicals and Their Potential Impact on Human Health. Methods in Molecular Biology (Clifton, N.J.), 1931, 121–140. https://doi.org/10.1007/978-1-4939-9039-9_9

e-CFR. Electronic Code of Federal Regulations (eCFR). Subpart E: Specific Requirements for Health Claims [Text]. Electronic Code of Federal Regulations (ECFR). Retrieved May 31, 2021, from https://www.ecfr.gov/

Ekpa, O., Palacios-Rojas, N., Kruseman, G., Fogliano, V., & Linnemann, A. R. (2018). Sub-Saharan African maize-based foods: Technological perspectives to increase the food and nutrition security impacts of maize breeding programmes. Global Food Security, 17, 48–56. https://doi.org/10.1016/j.gfs.2018.03.007

Farasat, M., Khavari-Nejad, R.-A., Nabavi, S. M. B., & Namjooyan, F. (2014). Antioxidant Activity, Total Phenolics and Flavonoid Contents of some Edible Green Seaweeds from Northern Coasts of the Persian Gulf. Iranian Journal of Pharmaceutical Research: IJPR, 13(1), 163–170.

Fardet, A. (2010). New hypotheses for the health-protective mechanisms of whole grain cereals: What is beyond fibre? Nutrition Research Reviews, 23(1), 65–134. https://doi.org/10.1017/S0954422410000041

FDA. (2013). Guidance for Industry: Food Labeling Guide. U.S. Food and Drug Administration; FDA. http://www.fda.gov/regulatory-information/search-fda-guidance-documents/guidance-industry-food-labeling-guide

Food and Agriculture Organization of the United Nations. Retrieved April 5, 2022, from https://www.fao.org/home/en/

Gao, Y., Hu, N., Han, X. Y., Ding, T., Giffen, C., Goldstein, A. M., & Taylor, P. R. (2011). Risk factors for esophageal and gastric cancers in Shanxi Province, China: A case-control study. Cancer Epidemiology, 35(6), e91-99. https://doi.org/10.1016/j.canep.2011.06.006

Gardner, C. D., Kim, S., Bersamin, A., Dopler-Nelson, M., Otten, J., Oelrich, B., & Cherin, R. (2010). Micronutrient quality of weight-loss diets that focus on macronutrients: Results from the A TO Z study. The American Journal of Clinical Nutrition, 92(2), 304–312. https://doi.org/10.3945/ajcn.2010.29468

Gråsten, S. M., Juntunen, K. S., Poutanen, K. S., Gylling, H. K., Miettinen, T. A., & Mykkänen, H. M. (2000). Rye bread improves bowel function and decreases the concentrations of some compounds that are putative colon cancer risk markers in middle-aged women and men. The Journal of Nutrition, 130(9), 2215–2221. https://doi.org/10.1093/jn/130.9.2215

Gray, P. J., Conklin, S. D., Todorov, T. I., & Kasko, S. M. (2016). Cooking rice in excess water reduces both arsenic and enriched vitamins in the cooked grain. Food Additives & Contaminants. Part A, Chemistry, Analysis, Control, Exposure & Risk Assessment, 33(1), 78–85. https://doi.org/10.1080/19440049.2015.1103906

Guérin, A., Mody, R., Fok, B., Lasch, K. L., Zhou, Z., Wu, E. Q., Zhou, W., & Talley, N. J. (2014). Risk of developing colorectal cancer and benign colorectal neoplasm in patients with chronic constipation. Alimentary Pharmacology & Therapeutics, 40(1), 83–92. https://doi.org/10.1111/apt.12789

Guide to Sticky Rice: How to Make Glutinous Rice - 2022. MasterClass. Retrieved January 30, 2022, from https://www.masterclass.com/articles/how-to-make-sticky-rice

Guldbrand, H., Dizdar, B., Bunjaku, B., Lindström, T., Bachrach-Lindström, M., Fredrikson, M., Ostgren, C. J., & Nystrom, F. H. (2012). In type 2 diabetes, randomisation to advice to follow a low-carbohydrate diet transiently improves glycaemic control compared with advice to follow a low-fat diet producing a similar weight loss. Diabetologia, 55(8), 2118–2127. https://doi.org/10.1007/s00125-012-2567-4

Guldbrand, H., Lindström, T., Dizdar, B., Bunjaku, B., Östgren, C. J., Nystrom, F. H., & Bachrach-Lindström, M. (2014). Randomization to a low-carbohydrate diet advice improves health related quality of life compared with a low-fat diet at similar weight-loss in Type 2 diabetes mellitus. Diabetes Research and Clinical Practice, 106(2), 221–227. https://doi.org/10.1016/j.diabres.2014.08.032

Gundert-Remy, U., Damm, G., Foth, H., Freyberger, A., Gebel, T., Golka, K., Röhl, C., Schupp, T., Wollin, K.-M., & Hengstler, J. G. (2015). High exposure to inorganic arsenic by food: The need for risk reduction. Archives of Toxicology, 89(12), 2219–2227. https://doi.org/10.1007/s00204-015-1627-1

Gupta, A., Singh, U., Sahu, P., & Paul, S. (2022). Linking Soil Microbial Diversity to Modern Agriculture Practices: A Review. International Journal Environmental Research and Public Health, 19.

Gupta, R. K., Gangoliya, S. S., & Singh, N. K. (2015). Reduction of phytic acid and enhancement of bioavailable micronutrients in food grains. Journal of Food Science and Technology, 52(2), 676–684. https://doi.org/10.1007/s13197-013-0978-y

Haro-Vicente, J. F., Bernal-Cava, M. J., Lopez-Fernandez, A., Ros-Berruezo, G., Bodenstab, S., & Sanchez-Siles, L. M. (2017). Sensory Acceptability of Infant Cereals with Whole Grain in Infants and Young Children. Nutrients, 9(1), 65. https://doi.org/10.3390/nu9010065

Hartley, L., May, M. D., Loveman, E., Colquitt, J. L., & Rees, K. (2016). Dietary fibre for the primary prevention of cardiovascular disease. The Cochrane Database of Systematic Reviews, 1, CD011472. https://doi.org/10.1002/14651858.CD011472.pub2

Health Canada. (2021, January 14). Welcome to Canada's food guide. https://food-guide.canada.ca/en/

HealthLinkBC. (2011). Eating Guidelines for Diverticular Disease.

Heaton, K. W., Marcus, S. N., Emmett, P. M., & Bolton, C. H. (1988). Particle size of wheat, maize, and oat test meals: Effects on plasma glucose and insulin responses and on the rate of starch digestion in vitro. The American Journal of Clinical Nutrition, 47(4), 675–682. https://doi.org/10.1093/ajcn/47.4.675

Hefferon, K. L. (2015). Nutritionally enhanced food crops; progress and perspectives. International Journal of Molecular Sciences, 16(2), 3895–3914. https://doi.org/10.3390/ijms16023895

Ho, H. V. T., Sievenpiper, J. L., Zurbau, A., Mejia, S. B., Jovanovski, E., Au-Yeung, F., Jenkins, A. L., & Vuksan, V. (2016). The effect of oat β-glucan on LDL-cholesterol, non-HDL-cholesterol and apoB for CVD risk reduction: A systematic review and meta-analysis of randomised-controlled trials. British Journal of Nutrition, 116(8), 1369–1382. https://doi.org/10.1017/S000711451600341X

Hojsak, I., Braegger, C., Bronsky, J., Campoy, C., Colomb, V., Decsi, T., Domellöf, M., Fewtrell, M., Mis, N. F., Mihatsch, W., Molgaard, C., van Goudoever, J., & Nutrition, for the E. C. on. (2015). Arsenic in Rice: A Cause for Concern. Journal of Pediatric Gastroenterology and Nutrition, 60(1), 142–145. https://doi.org/10.1097/MPG.0000000000000502

Holma, R., Hongisto, S.-M., Saxelin, M., & Korpela, R. (2010). Constipation is relieved more by rye bread than wheat bread or laxatives without increased adverse gastrointestinal effects. The Journal of Nutrition, 140(3), 534–541. https://doi.org/10.3945/jn.109.118570

Hu, T., Mills, K. T., Yao, L., Demanelis, K., Eloustaz, M., Yancy, W. S., Kelly, T. N., He, J., & Bazzano, L. A. (2012). Effects of low-carbohydrate diets versus low-fat diets on metabolic risk factors: A meta-analysis of randomized controlled clinical trials. American Journal of Epidemiology, 176 Suppl 7, S44-54. https://doi.org/10.1093/aje/kws264

Hu, Y., Ding, M., Sampson, L., Willett, W. C., Manson, J. E., Wang, M., Rosner, B., Hu, F. B., & Sun, Q. (2020). Intake of whole grain foods and risk of type 2 diabetes: Results from three prospective cohort studies. BMJ, 370, m2206. https://doi.org/10.1136/bmj.m2206

Hurrell, R., & Egli, I. (2010). Iron bioavailability and dietary reference values. The American Journal of Clinical Nutrition, 91(5), 1461S-1467S. https://doi.org/10.3945/ajcn.2010.28674F

Jing, P., Bomser, J. A., Schwartz, S. J., He, J., Magnuson, B. A., & Giusti, M. M. (2008). Structure-function relationships of anthocyanins from various anthocyanin-rich extracts on the inhibition of colon cancer cell growth. Journal of Agricultural and Food Chemistry, 56(20), 9391–9398. https://doi.org/10.1021/jf8005917

Jing, P., & Giusti, M. M. (2011). Contribution of Berry Anthocyanins to Their Chemopreventive Properties. In N. P. Seeram & G. D. Stoner (Eds.), Berries and Cancer Prevention (pp. 3–40). Springer. https://doi.org/10.1007/978-1-4419-7554-6_1

Jonasson, L., Guldbrand, H., Lundberg, A. K., & Nystrom, F. H. (2014). Advice to follow a low-carbohydrate diet has a favourable impact on low-grade inflammation in type 2 diabetes compared with advice to follow a low-fat diet. Annals of Medicine, 46(3), 182–187. https://doi.org/10.3109/07853890.2014.894286

Jung, S.-J., Oh, M.-R., Park, S.-H., & Chae, S.-W. (2020). Effects of rice-based and wheat-based diets on bowel movements in young Korean women with functional constipation. European Journal of Clinical Nutrition, 74(11), 1565–1575. https://doi.org/10.1038/s41430-020-0636-1

Khan, I., Yousif, A. M., Johnson, S. K., & Gamlath, S. (2015). Acute effect of sorghum flour-containing pasta on plasma total polyphenols, antioxidant capacity and oxidative stress markers in healthy subjects: A randomised controlled trial. Clinical Nutrition (Edinburgh, Scotland), 34(3), 415–421. https://doi.org/10.1016/j.clnu.2014.08.005

Kirk, J. K., Graves, D. E., Craven, T. E., Lipkin, E. W., Austin, M., & Margolis, K. L. (2008). Restricted-carbohydrate diets in patients with type 2 diabetes: A meta-analysis. Journal of the American Dietetic Association, 108(1), 91–100. https://doi.org/10.1016/j.jada.2007.10.003

Kochar, J., Djoussé, L., & Gaziano, J. M. (2007). Breakfast cereals and risk of type 2 diabetes in the Physicians' Health Study I. Obesity (Silver Spring, Md.), 15(12), 3039–3044. https://doi.org/10.1038/oby.2007.362

Kodama, S., Saito, K., Tanaka, S., Maki, M., Yachi, Y., Sato, M., Sugawara, A., Totsuka, K., Shimano, H., Ohashi, Y., Yamada, N., & Sone, H. (2009). Influence of fat and carbohydrate proportions on the metabolic profile in patients with type 2 diabetes: A meta-analysis. Diabetes Care, 32(5), 959–965. https://doi.org/10.2337/dc08-1716

Koistinen, V. M., & Hanhineva, K. (2017). Mass spectrometry-based analysis of whole grain phytochemicals. Critical Reviews in Food Science and Nutrition, 57(8), 1688–1709. https://doi.org/10.1080/10408398.2015.1016477

Kopf, J. C., Suhr, M. J., Clarke, J., Eyun, S., Riethoven, J.-J. M., Ramer-Tait, A. E., & Rose, D. J. (2018). Role of whole grains versus fruits and vegetables in reducing subclinical inflammation and promoting gastrointestinal health in individuals affected by overweight and obesity: A randomized controlled trial. Nutrition Journal, 17(1), 72. https://doi.org/10.1186/s12937-018-0381-7

Korpela, K., Flint, H. J., Johnstone, A. M., Lappi, J., Poutanen, K., Dewulf, E., Delzenne, N., Vos, W. M. de, & Salonen, A. (2014). Gut Microbiota Signatures Predict Host and Microbiota Responses to Dietary Interventions in Obese Individuals. PLOS ONE, 9(3), e90702. https://doi.org/10.1371/journal.pone.0090702

Kranz, S., Dodd, K. W., Juan, W. Y., Johnson, L. K., & Jahns, L. (2017). Whole Grains Contribute Only a Small Proportion of Dietary Fiber to the U.S. Diet. Nutrients, 9(2), E153. https://doi.org/10.3390/nu9020153

Kristek, A., Schär, M. Y., Soycan, G., Alsharif, S., Kuhnle, G. G. C., Walton, G., & Spencer, J. P. E. (2018). The gut microbiota and cardiovascular health benefits: A focus on wholegrain oats. Nutrition Bulletin, 43(4), 358–373. https://doi.org/10.1111/nbu.12354

Kristensen, M., Toubro, S., Jensen, M., Ross, A., Riboldi, G., Pteronio, M., Bugel, S., Tenens, I., & Astrup, A. (2012). Whole Grain Compared with Refined Wheat Decreases the Percentage of Body Fat Following a 12-Week, Energy-Restricted Dietary Intervention in Postmenopausal Women. American Journal of Clinical Nutrition, 142(4), 710–716.

Krkoskova, B., & Mrazova. (2005). Prophylactic components of buckwheat—ScienceDirect. Food Research International, 38(5), 561–568.

Kyritsi, A., Tzia, C., & Karathanos, V. T. (2011). Vitamin fortified rice grain using spraying and soaking methods. LWT - Food Science and Technology, 44(1), 312–320. https://doi.org/10.1016/j.lwt.2010.06.001

Lambeau, K. V., & McRorie, J. W. (2017). Fiber supplements and clinically proven health benefits: How to recognize and recommend an effective fiber therapy. Journal of the American Association of Nurse Practitioners, 29(4), 216–223. https://doi.org/10.1002/2327-6924.12447

Lao, F., & Giusti, M. M. (2016). Quantification of Purple Corn (Zea mays L.) Anthocyanins Using Spectrophotometric and HPLC Approaches: Method Comparison and Correlation. Food Anal Methods, 9(5), 1367–1380.

Lao, F., Sigurdson, G. T., & Giusti, M. (2017). Health Benefits of Purple Corn (Zea mays L.) Phenolic Compounds. Comprehensive Reviews in Food Science and Food Safety. https://doi.org/10.1111/1541-4337.12249

Lappi, J., Salojarva, J., Kolehmainen, M., Mykkanen, H., & Poutanen, K. (2013). Intake of Whole grain and Fiber-Rich Rye Bread Versus Refined Wheat Bread Does Not Differentiate Intestinal Microbiota Composition in Finnish Adults with Metabolic Syndrome. The Journal of Nutrition, 143(5), 648–655.

Li, L., Lietz, G., & Seal, C. (2018). Buckwheat and CVD Risk Markers: A Systematic Review and Meta-Analysis. Nutrients, 10(5), E619. https://doi.org/10.3390/nu10050619

Lichtenstein, A. H., Appel, L. J., Vadiveloo, M., Hu, F. B., Kris-Etherton, P. M., Rebholz, C. M., Sacks, F. M., Thorndike, A. N., Van Horn, L., Wylie-Rosett, J., & on behalf of the American Heart Association Council on Lifestyle and Cardiometabolic Health; Council on Arteriosclerosis, Thrombosis and Vascular Biology; Council on Cardiovascular Radiology and Intervention; Council on Clinical Cardiology; and Stroke Council. (2021). 2021 Dietary Guidance to Improve Cardiovascular Health: A Scientific Statement From the American Heart Association. Circulation, CIR.0000000000001031. https://doi.org/10.1161/CIR.0000000000001031

Mansoor, N., Vinknes, K. J., Veierød, M. B., & Retterstøl, K. (2016). Effects of low-carbohydrate diets v. low-fat diets on body weight and cardiovascular risk factors: A meta-analysis of randomised controlled trials. British Journal of Nutrition, 115(3), 466–479. https://doi.org/10.1017/S0007114515004699

Marcone, M. F., Kakuda, Y., & Yada, R. Y. (2003). Amaranth as a rich dietary source of beta-sitosterol and other phytosterols. Plant Foods for Human Nutrition (Dordrecht, Netherlands), 58(3), 207–211. https://doi.org/10.1023/b:qual.0000040334.99070.3e

Martínez, I., Lattimer, J. M., Hubach, K. L., Case, J. A., Yang, J., Weber, C. G., Louk, J. A., Rose, D. J., Kyureghian, G., Peterson, D. A., Haub, M. D., & Walter, J. (2013). Gut microbiome composition is linked to whole grain-induced immunological improvements. The ISME Journal, 7(2), 269–280. https://doi.org/10.1038/ismej.2012.104

Martinez, I., Wallace, G., Zhang, C., Legge, R., & Benson, A. (2020). Diet-Induced Metabolic Improvements in a Hamster Model of Hypercholesterolemia Are Strongly Linked to Alterations of the Gut Microbiota | Applied and Environmental Microbiology. ASM Journals, 75(12). https://journals.asm.org/doi/10.1128/AEM.00380-09

McGee, H. (2004). On Food and Cooking: The Science and Lore of the Kitchen (1st edition). Scribner Books.

McRorie, J. W., & McKeown, N. M. (2017). Understanding the Physics of Functional Fibers in the Gastrointestinal Tract: An Evidence-Based Approach to Resolving Enduring Misconceptions about Insoluble and Soluble Fiber. Journal of the Academy of Nutrition and Dietetics, 117(2), 251–264. https://doi.org/10.1016/j.jand.2016.09.021

Meckling, K. A., O'Sullivan, C., & Saari, D. (2004). Comparison of a low-fat diet to a low-carbohydrate diet on weight loss, body composition, and risk factors for diabetes and cardiovascular disease in free-living, overweight men and women. The Journal of Clinical Endocrinology and Metabolism, 89(6), 2717–2723. https://doi.org/10.1210/jc.2003-031606

Mellen, P. B., Walsh, T. F., & Herrington, D. M. (2008). Whole grain intake and cardiovascular disease: A meta-analysis. Nutrition, Metabolism, and Cardiovascular Diseases: NMCD, 18(4), 283–290. https://doi.org/10.1016/j.numecd.2006.12.008

Menon, M., Dong, W., Chen, X., Hufton, J., & Rhodes, E. J. (2021). Improved rice cooking approach to maximise arsenic removal while preserving nutrient elements. Science of The Total Environment, 755, 143341. https://doi.org/10.1016/j.scitotenv.2020.143341

Meyer, K. A., Kushi, L. H., Jacobs, D. R., Slavin, J., Sellers, T. A., & Folsom, A. R. (2000). Carbohydrates, dietary fiber, and incident type 2 diabetes in older women. The American Journal of Clinical Nutrition, 71(4), 921–930. https://doi.org/10.1093/ajcn/71.4.921

Moskin, J. (2017, January 10). Rye, a Grain With Ancient Roots, Is Rising Again. The New York Times. https://www.nytimes.com/2017/01/10/dining/rye-grain-bread.html

Murtaugh, M. A., Jacobs, D. R., Jacob, B., Steffen, L. M., & Marquart, L. (2003). Epidemiological support for the protection of whole grains against diabetes. The Proceedings of the Nutrition Society, 62(1), 143–149. https://doi.org/10.1079/pns2002223

Nascimento, K., Paes, S., Oliveira, I., Reis, I., & Augusta, I. (2018). Teff: Suitability for Different Food Application and as a Raw Material of Gluten-free, a Literature Review. Journal of Food and Nutrition Research, 6.

Navarro-Perez, D., Radcliffe, J., Tierney, A., & Jois, M. (2017). Quinoa Seed Lowers Serum Triglycerides in Overweight and Obese Subjects: A Dose-Response Randomized Controlled Clinical Trial. Current Developments in Nutrition, 1(9), e001321. https://doi.org/10.3945/cdn.117.001321

Neacsu, M., McMonagle, J., Fletcher, R. J., Scobbie, L., Duncan, G. J., Cantlay, L., de Roos, B., Duthie, G. G., & Russell, W. R. (2013). Bound phytophenols from ready-to-eat cereals: Comparison with other plant-based foods. Food Chemistry, 141(3), 2880–2886. https://doi.org/10.1016/j.foodchem.2013.05.023

Nilsson, L. M., Winkvist, A., Johansson, I., Lindahl, B., Hallmans, G., Lenner, P., & Van Guelpen, B. (2013). Low-carbohydrate, high-protein diet score and risk of incident cancer; a prospective cohort study. Nutrition Journal, 12, 58. https://doi.org/10.1186/1475-2891-12-58

Noakes, M., Keogh, J. B., Foster, P. R., & Clifton, P. M. (2005). Effect of an energy-restricted, high-protein, low-fat diet relative to a conventional high-carbohydrate, low-fat diet on weight loss, body composition, nutritional status, and markers of cardiovascular health in obese women. The American Journal of Clinical Nutrition, 81(6), 1298–1306. https://doi.org/10.1093/ajcn/81.6.1298

Nordlee, J. A., Panda, R., Baumert, J. L., Goodman, R. E., & Taylor, S. L. (2011). Wild buckwheat is unlikely to pose a risk to buckwheat-allergic individuals. Journal of Food Science, 76(8), T189-191. https://doi.org/10.1111/j.1750-3841.2011.02372.x

Nutrition, C. for F. S. and A. (2022). Health Claim Notification for Whole Grain Foods. FDA. https://www.fda.gov/food/food-labeling-nutrition/health-claim-notification-whole grain-foods

Oghbaei, M., & Prakash, J. (2016). Effect of primary processing of cereals and legumes on its nutritional quality: A comprehensive review. Cogent Food & Agriculture, 2(1), 1136015. https://doi.org/10.1080/23311932.2015.1136015

Oldways Whole Grains Council. (2017, December 6). Expert Shares Tips for Baking with Whole Grains. Oldways Whole Grains Council. https://wholegrainscouncil.org/blog/2015/04/expert-shares-tips-baking-whole grains

Oli, P., Ward, R., Adhikari, B., & Torley, P. (2014). Parboiled rice: Understanding from a materials science approach. Journal of Food Engineering, 124, 173–183. https://doi.org/10.1016/j.jfoodeng.2013.09.010

Oscarsson, M., Andersson, R., Åman, P., Olofsson, S., & Jonsson, A. (1998). Effects of cultivar, nitrogen fertilization rate and environment on yield and grain quality of barley. Journal of the Science of Food and Agriculture, 78(3), 359–366. https://doi.org/10.1002/(SICI)1097-0010(199811)78:3<359::AID-JSFA126>3.0.CO;2-R

Özer, M. S., & Yazici, G. N. (2019). Phytochemicals of Whole Grains and Effects on Health. In A. Malik, Z. Erginkaya, & H. Erten (Eds.), Health and Safety Aspects of Food Processing Technologies (pp. 309–347). Springer International Publishing. https://doi.org/10.1007/978-3-030-24903-8_11

Padayachee, A., Day, L., Howell, K., & Gidley, M. J. (2017). Complexity and health functionality of plant cell wall fibers from fruits and vegetables. Critical Reviews in Food Science and Nutrition, 57(1), 59–81. https://doi.org/10.1080/10408398.2013.850652

Paruzynski, H., Korczak, R., Wang, Q., & Slavin, J. (2020). A Pilot and Feasibility Study of Oatmeal Consumption in Children to Assess Markers of Bowel Function. Journal of Medicinal Food, 23(5), 554–559. https://doi.org/10.1089/jmf.2019.0158

Potera, C. (2007). Food Safety: U.S. Rice Serves Up Arsenic. Environmental Health Perspectives, 115(6), A296–A296. https://doi.org/10.1289/ehp.115-a296

Pronsky, Z., Elbe, D., Ayoob, K., Crowe, J., Epstein, S., & RobertsW, W. H. R. M. (2015). Food Medication Interactions 18th Edition (Eighteenth edition). Food Medication Interactions.

Purdy, M., MS, & RDN. (2015). The Case for Soaking Your Grains—Food & Nutrition Magazine. https://foodandnutrition.org/blogs/stone-soup/case-soaking-grains/

Putta, S., Yarla, N. S., Kumar K, E., Lakkappa, D. B., Kamal, M. A., Scotti, L., Scotti, M. T., Ashraf, G. M., Rao, B. S. B., D, S. K., Reddy, G. V., Tarasov, V. V., Imandi, S. B., & Aliev, G. (2018). Preventive and Therapeutic Potentials of Anthocyanins in Diabetes and Associated Complications. Current Medicinal Chemistry, 25(39), 5347–5371. https://doi.org/10.2174/0929867325666171206101945

Radford, A., Langkamp-Henken, B., Hughes, C., Christman, M. C., Jonnalagadda, S., Boileau, T. W., Thielecke, F., & Dahl, W. J. (2014). Whole grain intake in middle school students achieves dietary guidelines for Americans and MyPlate recommendations when provided as commercially available foods: A randomized trial. Journal of the Academy of Nutrition and Dietetics, 114(9), 1417–1423. https://doi.org/10.1016/j.jand.2014.04.020

Rai, S., Kaur, A., & Chopra, C. (2018). Gluten-Free Products for Celiac Susceptible People. Front Nutr, 5, 116.

Ravikumar, P., Shalini, G., & Jeyam, M. (2015). Wheat Seedlings as Food Supplement to Combat Free Radicals: An In Vitro Approach. Indian Journal of Pharmaceutical Sciences, 77(5), 592–598.

Reynolds, A., Mann, J., Cummings, J., Winter, N., Mete, E., & Te Morenga, L. (2019). Carbohydrate quality and human health: A series of systematic reviews and meta-analyses. Lancet (London, England), 393(10170), 434–445. https://doi.org/10.1016/S0140-6736(18)31809-9

Reynolds, A. N., Akerman, A. P., & Mann, J. (2020). Dietary fibre and whole grains in diabetes management: Systematic review and meta-analyses. PLoS Medicine, 17(3), e1003053. https://doi.org/10.1371/journal.pmed.1003053

Ríos-Covián, D., Ruas-Madiedo, P., Margolles, A., Gueimonde, M., de Los Reyes-Gavilán, C. G., & Salazar, N. (2016). Intestinal Short Chain Fatty Acids and their Link with Diet and Human Health. Frontiers in Microbiology, 7, 185. https://doi.org/10.3389/fmicb.2016.00185

Roager, H., Vogt, J., Kristensen, M., Hansen, L., & Ibrugger, S. (2017). Whole grain-rich diet reduces body weight and systemic low-grade inflammation without inducing major changes of the gut microbiome: A randomised cross-over trial | Gut. Gut Microbiota. https://gut.bmj.com/content/68/1/83

Rock, C. L., Flatt, S. W., Pakiz, B., Taylor, K. S., Leone, A. F., Brelje, K., Heath, D. D., Quintana, E. L., & Sherwood, N. E. (2014). Weight loss, glycemic control, and cardiovascular disease risk factors in response to differential diet composition in a weight loss program in type 2 diabetes: A randomized controlled trial. Diabetes Care, 37(6), 1573–1580. https://doi.org/10.2337/dc13-2900

Russell, W. R., Gratz, S. W., Duncan, S. H., Holtrop, G., Ince, J., Scobbie, L., Duncan, G., Johnstone, A. M., Lobley, G. E., Wallace, R. J., Duthie, G. G., & Flint, H. J. (2011). High-protein, reduced-carbohydrate weight-loss diets promote metabolite profiles likely to be detrimental to colonic health. The American Journal of Clinical Nutrition, 93(5), 1062–1072. https://doi.org/10.3945/ajcn.110.002188

Sackner-Bernstein, J., Kanter, D., & Kaul, S. (2015). Dietary Intervention for Overweight and Obese Adults: Comparison of Low-Carbohydrate and Low-Fat Diets. A Meta-Analysis. PloS One, 10(10), e0139817. https://doi.org/10.1371/journal.pone.0139817

Salt Spring Seeds. Growing Amaranth & Quinoa Organically. Salt Spring Seeds. Retrieved April 5, 2022, from https://www.saltspringseeds.com/pages/growing-amaranth-and-quinoa

Sang, S., & Chu, Y. (2017). Whole grain oats, more than just a fiber: Role of unique phytochemicals. Molecular Nutrition & Food Research, 61(7). https://doi.org/10.1002/mnfr.201600715

Santesso, N., Akl, E. A., Bianchi, M., Mente, A., Mustafa, R., Heels-Ansdell, D., & Schünemann, H. J. (2012). Effects of higher- versus lower-protein diets on health outcomes: A systematic review and meta-analysis. European Journal of Clinical Nutrition, 66(7), 780–788. https://doi.org/10.1038/ejcn.2012.37

Saslow, L. R., Kim, S., Daubenmier, J. J., Moskowitz, J. T., Phinney, S. D., Goldman, V., Murphy, E. J., Cox, R. M., Moran, P., & Hecht, F. M. (2014). A randomized pilot trial of a moderate carbohydrate diet compared to a very low carbohydrate diet in overweight or obese individuals with type 2 diabetes mellitus or prediabetes. PloS One, 9(4), e91027. https://doi.org/10.1371/journal.pone.0091027

Schlesinger, S., Neuenschwander, M., Schwedhelm, C., Hoffmann, G., Bechthold, A., Boeing, H., & Schwingshackl, L. (2019). Food Groups and Risk of Overweight, Obesity, and Weight Gain: A Systematic Review and Dose-Response Meta-Analysis of Prospective Studies. Advances in Nutrition (Bethesda, Md.), 10(2), 205–218. https://doi.org/10.1093/advances/nmy092

Schwartz, M. W., Seeley, R. J., Zeltser, L. M., Drewnowski, A., Ravussin, E., Redman, L. M., & Leibel, R. L. (2017). Obesity Pathogenesis: An Endocrine Society Scientific Statement. Endocrine Reviews, 38(4), 267–296. https://doi.org/10.1210/er.2017-00111

Seeram, N. P., & Stoner, G. D. (Eds.). (2011). Contribution of berry anthocyanins to their chemopreventive properties. In Berries and Cancer Prevention (pp. 3–40). Springer New York. https://doi.org/10.1007/978-1-4419-7554-6

Sekirov, I., Russell, S. L., Antunes, L. C. M., & Finlay, B. B. (2010). Gut microbiota in health and disease. Physiological Reviews, 90(3), 859–904. https://doi.org/10.1152/physrev.00045.2009

Serra-Majem, L., & Bautista-Castaño, I. (2015). Relationship between bread and obesity. The British Journal of Nutrition, 113 Suppl 2, S29-35. https://doi.org/10.1017/S0007114514003249

Sewram, V., Sitas, F., O'Connell, D., & Myers, J. (2014). Diet and esophageal cancer risk in the Eastern Cape Province of South Africa. Nutrition and Cancer, 66(5), 791–799. https://doi.org/10.1080/01635581.2014.916321

Sezgin, S., & Sanlier, N. (2019). A New Generation Plant for the Conventional Cuisine: Quinoa. Trends in Food Science & Technology, 86(1).

Shi, L., Mu, K., Arntfield, S. D., & Nickerson, M. T. (2017). Changes in levels of enzyme inhibitors during soaking and cooking for pulses available in Canada. Journal of Food Science and Technology, 54(4), 1014–1022. https://doi.org/10.1007/s13197-017-2519-6

Shobana, S., Selvi, R. P., Kavitha, V., Gayathri, N., Geetha, G., Gayathri, R., Vijayalakshmi, P., Balasubramaniam, K. K. G., Ruchi, V., Sudha, V., Anjana, R. M., Unnikrishnan, R., Malleshi, N. G., Henry, C. J., Krishnaswamy, K., & Mohan, V. (2018). Development and evaluation of nutritional, sensory and glycemic properties of finger millet (Eleusine coracana L.) based food products. Asia Pacific Journal of Clinical Nutrition, 27(1), 84–91. https://doi.org/10.6133/apjcn.032017.18

Sieri, S., Krogh, V., Agnoli, C., Ricceri, F., Palli, D., Masala, G., Panico, S., Mattiello, A., Tumino, R., Giurdanella, M. C., Brighenti, F., Scazzina, F., Vineis, P., & Sacerdote, C. (2015). Dietary glycemic index and glycemic load and risk of colorectal cancer: Results from the EPIC-Italy study. International Journal of Cancer, 136(12), 2923–2931. https://doi.org/10.1002/ijc.29341

Simnadis, T. G., Tapsell, L. C., & Beck, E. J. (2016). Effect of sorghum consumption on health outcomes: A systematic review. Nutrition Reviews, 74(11), 690–707. https://doi.org/10.1093/nutrit/nuw036

Skeie, G., Braaten, T., Olsen, A., Kyrø, C., Tjønneland, A., Landberg, R., Nilsson, L. M., Wennberg, M., Overvad, K., Åsli, L. A., Weiderpass, E., & Lund, E. (2016). Intake of whole grains and incidence of oesophageal cancer in the HELGA Cohort. European Journal of Epidemiology, 31(4), 405–414. https://doi.org/10.1007/s10654-015-0057-y

Slavin, J. (2013). Fiber and Prebiotics: Mechanisms and Health Benefits. Nutrients, 5(4), 1417–1435. https://doi.org/10.3390/nu5041417

Soluble and insoluble fiber: MedlinePlus Medical Encyclopedia Image. Retrieved October 31, 2021, from https://medlineplus.gov/ency/imagepages/19531.htm

Springmann, M. (2019). Chapter 11 - Can diets be both healthy and sustainable? Solving the dilemma between healthy diets versus sustainable diets. In J. Sabaté (Ed.), Environmental Nutrition (pp. 197–227). Academic Press. https://doi.org/10.1016/B978-0-12-811660-9.00013-8

Suhr, J., Vuholm, S., Iversen, K. N., Landberg, R., & Kristensen, M. (2017). Wholegrain rye, but not wholegrain wheat, lowers body weight and fat mass compared with refined wheat: A 6-week randomized study. European Journal of Clinical Nutrition, 71(8), 959–967. https://doi.org/10.1038/ejcn.2017.12

Sun, G.-X., Williams, P. N., Carey, A.-M., Zhu, Y.-G., Deacon, C., Raab, A., Feldmann, J., Islam, R. M., & Meharg, A. A. (2008). Inorganic arsenic in rice bran and its products are an order of magnitude higher than in bulk grain. Environmental Science & Technology, 42(19), 7542–7546. https://doi.org/10.1021/es801238p

Sun, Q., Spiegelman, D., van Dam, R. M., Holmes, M. D., Malik, V. S., Willett, W. C., & Hu, F. B. (2010). White rice, brown rice, and risk of type 2 diabetes in US men and women. Archives of Internal Medicine, 170(11), 961–969. https://doi.org/10.1001/archinternmed.2010.109

Surampudi, P., Enkhmaa, B., Anuurad, E., & Berglund, L. (2016). Lipid Lowering with Soluble Dietary Fiber. Current Atherosclerosis Reports, 18(12), 75. https://doi.org/10.1007/s11883-016-0624-z

Sytar, O., Bośko, P., Živčák, M., Brestic, M., & Smetanska, I. (2018). Bioactive Phytochemicals and Antioxidant Properties of the Grains and Sprouts of Colored Wheat Genotypes. Molecules (Basel, Switzerland), 23(9), E2282. https://doi.org/10.3390/molecules23092282

Tang, Y., & Tsao, R. (2017). Phytochemicals in quinoa and amaranth grains and their antioxidant, anti-inflammatory, and potential health beneficial effects: A review. Molecular Nutrition & Food Research, 61(7). https://doi.org/10.1002/mnfr.201600767

Tay, J., Luscombe-Marsh, N. D., Thompson, C. H., Noakes, M., Buckley, J. D., Wittert, G. A., Yancy, W. S., & Brinkworth, G. D. (2014). A very low-carbohydrate, low-saturated fat diet for type 2 diabetes management: A randomized trial. Diabetes Care, 37(11), 2909–2918. https://doi.org/10.2337/dc14-0845

Tay, J., Luscombe-Marsh, N. D., Thompson, C. H., Noakes, M., Buckley, J. D., Wittert, G. A., Yancy, W. S., & Brinkworth, G. D. (2015). Comparison of low- and high-carbohydrate diets for type 2 diabetes management: A randomized trial. The American Journal of Clinical Nutrition, 102(4), 780–790. https://doi.org/10.3945/ajcn.115.112581

The Jefferson Institute. (2002). Grain Amaranth: A Lost Crop of the Americas. https://www.doc-developpement-durable.org/file/Culture/Culture-plantes-alimentaires/FICHES_PLANTES/amarante/amaranth_guide.pdf

The University of Sydney. Glycemic Index. Glycemic Index Research and GI News. Retrieved April 5, 2022, from https://glycemicindex.com/

Thielecke, F., & Nugent, A. P. (2018). Contaminants in Grain-A Major Risk for Whole Grain Safety? Nutrients, 10(9), E1213. https://doi.org/10.3390/nu10091213

Thies, F., Masson, L. F., Boffetta, P., & Kris-Etherton, P. (2014). Oats and CVD risk markers: A systematic literature review. The British Journal of Nutrition, 112 Suppl 2, S19-30. https://doi.org/10.1017/S0007114514002281

Thompson, S. V., Hannon, B. A., An, R., & Holscher, H. D. (2017). Effects of isolated soluble fiber supplementation on body weight, glycemia, and insulinemia in adults with overweight and obesity: A systematic review and meta-analysis of randomized controlled trials. The American Journal of Clinical Nutrition, 106(6), 1514–1528. https://doi.org/10.3945/ajcn.117.163246

Tieri, M., Ghelfi, F., Vitale, M., Vetrani, C., Marventano, S., Lafranconi, A., Godos, J., Titta, L., Gambera, A., Alonzo, E., Sciacca, S., Riccardi, G., Buscemi, S., Del Rio, D., Ray, S., Galvano, F., Beck, E., & Grosso, G. (2020). Whole grain consumption and human health: An umbrella review of observational studies. International Journal of Food Sciences and Nutrition, 71(6), 668–677. https://doi.org/10.1080/09637486.2020.1715354

Tighe, P., Duthie, G., Vaughan, N., Brittenden, J., Simpson, W. G., Duthie, S., Mutch, W., Wahle, K., Horgan, G., & Thies, F. (2010). Effect of increased consumption of whole grain foods on blood pressure and other cardiovascular risk markers in healthy middle-aged persons: A randomized controlled trial. The American Journal of Clinical Nutrition, 92(4), 733–740. https://doi.org/10.3945/ajcn.2010.29417

Tomotake, H., Shimaoka, I., Kayashita, J., Nakajoh, M., & Kato, N. (2002). Physicochemical and functional properties of buckwheat protein product. Journal of Agricultural and Food Chemistry, 50(7), 2125–2129. https://doi.org/10.1021/jf011248q

Tosh, S. M. (2013). Review of human studies investigating the post-prandial blood-glucose lowering ability of oat and barley food products. European Journal of Clinical Nutrition, 67(4), 310–317. https://doi.org/10.1038/ejcn.2013.25

Tosh, S. M., & Chu, Y. (2015). Systematic review of the effect of processing of whole grain oat cereals on glycaemic response. The British Journal of Nutrition, 114(8), 1256–1262. https://doi.org/10.1017/S0007114515002895

Tritt, A., Reicks, M., & Marquart, L. (2015). Reformulation of pizza crust in restaurants may increase whole grain intake among children. Public Health Nutrition, 18(8), 1407–1411. https://doi.org/10.1017/S1368980014001724

Trozzi, C., Raffaelli, F., Vignini, A., Nanetti, L., Gesuita, R., & Mazzanti, L. (2019). Evaluation of antioxidative and diabetes-preventive properties of an ancient grain, KAMUT® khorasan wheat, in healthy volunteers. European Journal of Nutrition, 58(1), 151–161. https://doi.org/10.1007/s00394-017-1579-8

Truby, H., Hiscutt, R., Herriot, A. M., Stanley, M., Delooy, A., Fox, K. R., Baic, S., Robson, P. J., Macdonald, I., Taylor, M. A., Ware, R., Logan, C., & Livingstone, M. (2008). Commercial weight loss diets meet nutrient requirements in free living adults over 8 weeks: A randomised controlled weight loss trial. Nutrition Journal, 7, 25. https://doi.org/10.1186/1475-2891-7-25

Ulbricht, C., Abrams, T., Conquer, J., Costa, D., Serrano, J. M. G., Taylor, S., & Varghese, M. (2009). An evidence-based systematic review of amaranth (Amaranthus spp.) by the Natural Standard Research Collaboration. Journal of Dietary Supplements, 6(4), 390–417. https://doi.org/10.3109/19390210903280348

van den Driessche, J. J., Plat, J., & Mensink, R. P. (2018). Effects of superfoods on risk factors of metabolic syndrome: A systematic review of human intervention trials. Food & Function, 9(4), 1944–1966. https://doi.org/10.1039/C7FO01792H

Van Hung, P. (2016). Phenolic Compounds of Cereals and Their Antioxidant Capacity. Critical Reviews in Food Science and Nutrition, 56(1), 25–35. https://doi.org/10.1080/10408398.2012.708909

Vanegas, S. M., Meydani, M., Barnett, J. B., Goldin, B., Kane, A., Rasmussen, H., Brown, C., Vangay, P., Knights, D., Jonnalagadda, S., Koecher, K., Karl, J. P., Thomas, M., Dolnikowski, G., Li, L., Saltzman, E., Wu, D., & Meydani, S. N. (2017). Substituting whole grains for refined grains in a 6-wk randomized trial has a modest effect on gut microbiota and immune and inflammatory markers of healthy adults. The American Journal of Clinical Nutrition, 105(3), 635–650. https://doi.org/10.3945/ajcn.116.146928

Venn, B. J., & Mann, J. I. (2004). Cereal grains, legumes and diabetes. European Journal of Clinical Nutrition, 58(11), 1443–1461. https://doi.org/10.1038/sj.ejcn.1601995

Veronese, N., Solmi, M., Caruso, M. G., Giannelli, G., Osella, A. R., Evangelou, E., Maggi, S., Fontana, L., Stubbs, B., & Tzoulaki, I. (2018). Dietary fiber and health outcomes: An umbrella review of systematic reviews and meta-analyses. The American Journal of Clinical Nutrition, 107(3), 436–444. https://doi.org/10.1093/ajcn/nqx082

Vitaglione, P., Mennella, I., Ferracane, R., Rivellese, A., Giacco, R., Ercolini, D., Gibbons, S., La Storia, A., Gilbert, J., & Jonnalagadda, S. (2015). Whole grain wheat consumption reduces inflammation in a randomized controlled trial on overweight and obese subjects with unhealthy dietary and lifestyle behaviors: Role of polyphenols bound to cereal dietary fiber |. American Journal of Clinical Nutrition, 101(2), 251–261.

Wang, H., Vieira, F. G., Crawford, J. E., Chu, C., & Nielsen, R. (2017). Asian wild rice is a hybrid swarm with extensive gene flow and feralization from domesticated rice. Genome Research, 27(6), 1029–1038. https://doi.org/10.1101/gr.204800.116

Wang, T., Zhan, R., Lu, J., Zhong, L., Peng, X., Wang, M., & Tang, S. (2020). Grain consumption and risk of gastric cancer: A meta-analysis. International Journal of Food Sciences and Nutrition, 71(2), 164–175. https://doi.org/10.1080/09637486.2019.1631264

Watanabe, N., Suzuki, M., Yamaguchi, Y., & Egashira, Y. (2018). Effects of resistant maltodextrin on bowel movements: A systematic review and meta-analysis. Clin Exp Gastroenterol, 11, 85–96. https://doi.org/10.2147/CEG.S153924

Weickert, M. O., & Pfeiffer, A. F. H. (2018). Impact of Dietary Fiber Consumption on Insulin Resistance and the Prevention of Type 2 Diabetes. The Journal of Nutrition, 148(1), 7–12. https://doi.org/10.1093/jn/nxx008

Wessel, T. (1984). The agricultural foundations of civilization. Agriculture and Human Values, 1(2), 9–12.

Whole Grain Protein Power! | The Whole Grains Council. Retrieved January 29, 2022, from https://wholegrainscouncil.org/blog/2014/02/whole grain-protein-power

Whole Grains Council. Oldways. Retrieved March 14, 2022, from https://oldwayspt.org/programs/whole grains-council

Wijngaard, H., & Arendt, E. (2006). Buckwheat—Wijngaard—2006—Cereal Chemistry—Wiley Online Library. Cereal Chemistry, 83(4), 391–401.

Williams, P. N., Villada, A., Deacon, C., Raab, A., Figuerola, J., Green, A. J., Feldmann, J., & Meharg, A. A. (2007). Greatly Enhanced Arsenic Shoot Assimilation in Rice Leads to Elevated Grain Levels Compared to Wheat and Barley. Environmental Science & Technology, 41(19), 6854–6859. https://doi.org/10.1021/es070627i

World Cancer Research Fund/American Institute for Cancer Research. (2018). Diet, Nutrition, Physical Activity and Cancer: A Global Perspective. Continuous Update Project Expert Report 2018. dietandcancerreport.org

Wyka, J., Malczyk, E., Misiarz, M., Zołoteńka-Synowiec, M., Całyniuk, B., & Baczyńska, S. (2015). Assessment of food intakes for women adopting the high protein Dukan diet. Roczniki Panstwowego Zakladu Higieny, 66(2), 137–142.

Yang, J., Wang, H.-P., Zhou, L., & Xu, C.-F. (2012). Effect of dietary fiber on constipation: A meta analysis. World Journal of Gastroenterology, 18(48), 7378–7383. https://doi.org/10.3748/wjg.v18.i48.7378

Ye, E. Q., Chacko, S. A., Chou, E. L., Kugizaki, M., & Liu, S. (2012). Greater whole grain intake is associated with lower risk of type 2 diabetes, cardiovascular disease, and weight gain. The Journal of Nutrition, 142(7), 1304–1313. https://doi.org/10.3945/jn.111.155325

Yu, L., & Beta, T. (2015). Identification and Antioxidant Properties of Phenolic Compounds during Production of Bread from Purple Wheat Grains. Molecules (Basel, Switzerland), 20(9), 15525–15549. https://doi.org/10.3390/molecules200915525

Zheng, T., Boyle, P., Willett, W. C., Hu, H., Dan, J., Evstifeeva, T. V., Niu, S., & MacMahon, B. (1993). A case-control study of oral cancer in Beijing, People's Republic of China. Associations with nutrient intakes, foods and food groups. European Journal of Cancer. Part B, Oral Oncology, 29B(1), 45–55. https://doi.org/10.1016/0964-1955(93)90010-c

Zhu, Y., & Sang, S. (2017). Phytochemicals in whole grain wheat and their health-promoting effects. Molecular Nutrition & Food Research, 61(7). https://doi.org/10.1002/mnfr.201600852

Zijp, I. M., Korver, O., & Tijburg, L. B. (2000). Effect of tea and other dietary factors on iron absorption. Critical Reviews in Food Science and Nutrition, 40(5), 371–398. https://doi.org/10.1080/10408690091189194

PROTEIN

~

By Deborah Kennedy PhD,
and Julia Hilbrands MS, MPH, RD
with
The Expert Chef Panel

*"No single food will make or break good health.
But the kinds of food you choose
day in and day out have a major impact."*
Quote by Dr. Walter Willett

WHILE CARBOHYDRATES AND FAT seem to go in and out of dietary favor with every changing season, protein often remains the steady, constant macronutrient. There are some fad diets like the Paleo diet that are high in protein, but very rarely will you come across dietary advice to limit protein. Protein provides many vital functions within the body and it also appears in a wide range of foods, both of animal and plant origins. And as you'll see, the various protein sources are associated with a variety of both positive and negative health outcomes. It all has to do with what accompanies the protein — fats with animal sources, or fiber, phytonutrients, vitamins and minerals with plant-based protein.

SECTION 1:

WHAT IS PROTEIN?

Protein is one of the three macronutrients in the diet (along with carbohydrates and fat), but it is also considered its own food group — indeed, there is a completely separate space on the MyPlate food graphic for protein. Foods within the protein group include animal products, like meat, poultry, fish, eggs, and dairy and also plant-based foods like beans, nuts, seeds and grains. While protein plays a central role in the diet, it is also a very important nutrient in the body.

It is a common belief that the most important role of protein in the body is to build muscle. However, support for muscle is only the tip of the iceberg when it comes to the importance of protein in the body. Protein also supports bones and connective tissue and is responsible for transporting molecules throughout the body. For example, oxygen is carried from the lungs to the rest of the body by a protein called hemoglobin. Other proteins in the blood help the body maintain fluid balance by keeping blood in the blood vessels and not leaking out. Hormones, enzymes, and neurotransmitters are all made of protein. Many components of the immune system are proteins, and a weakened immune system is one result of poor protein intake. Protein can also be used as an energy source if needed.

AMINO ACIDS

Image: Amino Acids

On a molecular level, a protein molecule is a string of amino acids, which are considered the building blocks of proteins. Amino acids are joined together by peptide bonds, and a long string of amino acids folds together on itself to create a protein molecule. The number and order of amino acids on this string determines how the protein will fold up and ultimately the function of that protein. There are 20 amino acids in all, so there are endless combinations, especially considering that each protein contains tens of thousands of amino acids.

Table 1 lists the amino acids that are found in the body. There are two different groups of amino acids: nonessential and essential. The 11 nonessential amino acids are amino acids that the body is able to make itself. However, the other nine amino acids cannot be made by the body and thus have to come from the diet; these are deemed the essential amino acids.

Table 1: Nonessential & Essential Amino Acids

Nonessential	Essential
Alanine	Histidine
Arginine	Isoleucine
Asparagine	Leucine
Aspartic Acid	Lysine

Nonessential	Essential
Cysteine	Methionine
Glutamic Acid	Phenylalanine
Glutamine	Threonine
Glycine	Tryptophan
Proline	Valine
Serine	
Tyrosine	

Any food that contains protein will have some amino acids, but the amount and variety depend on the type of protein source. Animal-based proteins such as meat, poultry, fish, eggs and dairy products contain ample amounts of all nine essential amino acids. Because of this, they are considered **complete proteins**. On the other hand, most plant-based proteins such as beans, nuts, seeds, and grains are low or entirely lacking in at least one essential amino acid, and therefore these foods are considered **incomplete proteins**. For example, legumes are low in the amino acids methionine and tryptophan, while nuts, seeds, and grains are low in the amino acid lysine. Because plant-based proteins are lacking in at least one amino acid, it is important that individuals eating vegetarian or vegan diets have a variety of protein sources in their diet so that they are still consuming each essential amino acid on a daily or weekly basis. Interestingly, there are two plant-based foods that are complete proteins and provide all nine essential amino acids, and these are **soy and quinoa**.

SECTION 2:

ANIMAL-BASED PROTEIN

Animal-based proteins like red meat and poultry are the foods many people think of when thinking about protein, but this subgroup also includes fish, eggs, and dairy products. In this section, we will describe each of these groups by their nutritional and culinary properties, and we will explore their associations with health outcomes in a later section.

RED MEAT — a great source of protein, iron, zinc, vitamins B_6 and B_{12}

Meat is the edible flesh from mammals and includes beef, lamb, and all pork products as well as wild game such as venison, elk, or rabbit. Red meat provides a rich source of protein, as one standard 3-ounce serving provides around 20 grams of protein that is easily digestible and absorbable.

Red meat is also a great source of heme iron, zinc, and several of the B vitamins. Iron helps to transport oxygen from the lungs to the rest of the body, and heme iron from red meat and other animal sources is more absorbable than the non-heme iron found in plants. Zinc is required for DNA synthesis and also provides support to the immune system, and like iron, zinc is more readily absorbed from animal sources than from plant sources. Red meat also provides several B vitamins, among which are vitamins B_6 and B_{12}. Vitamin B_6 is another nutrient that supports the immune system, and vitamin B_{12} is necessary for the nervous system. Vitamin B_6 can also be found in plant sources like grains, but **vitamin B_{12} is only attainable from animal sources**.

The fat content of red meat varies widely according to the breed and feeding regimen of the animal, as well as the cut of meat and the season of butchering (Williams, 2007). Lean cuts with less fat usually contain the words "round," "loin," "sirloin," "choice" or "select" on the packaging, while a "prime" cut usually indicates a higher fat content. All trimmed, lean red meat typically contains less than 5% to 7% fat and has a moderate cholesterol content (Williams, 2007).

Interestingly, red meat produced today is leaner and lower in fat content than meat produced a few decades ago due to a combined effect of changes in breeding, feeding practices, and butchering techniques (Higgs, 2000). It is a common belief that most of the fat in red meat is saturated fat, which is thought to contribute to increased blood cholesterol levels and increased disease risk. However, approximately 50% of the fat of beef and lamb is made up of unsaturated fatty acids, and red meat can be a significant source of omega-3 fatty acids depending on the cow's diet (McAfee et al., 2010; Williams, 2007).

Within the last several years, there has been increased attention paid to differences in grain-fed versus grass-fed beef. In terms of nutrient profile, the largest difference between these two farming methods is in the fatty acid profile. Grass-fed beef tends to have a higher unsaturated fatty acid content than grain-fed beef, including a higher omega-3 fatty acid content (Daley et al., 2010). In fact, in Australia, where animals are grass-fed for almost the entire year, the concentration of polyunsaturated fatty acids in lean beef can be up to six times higher than that of fish (Howe et al., 2007). The amount of saturated fat does not differ much between grass-fed and grain-fed beef, but grass-fed beef appears to have more saturated fats that have a neutral effect on cholesterol levels and less saturated fats that raise cholesterol levels compared to their grain-fed counterparts (Daley et al., 2010). It's also important to note that organic does not necessarily mean grass-fed when it comes to beef as cows can also be fed organic grain.

The differences in fat content can give grass-fed beef a different flavor profile, and the fat on grass-fed beef may even have a yellow tint due to its higher carotenoid content (Daley et al., 2010). Trained taste panels have consistently found grass-fed beef less palatable than grain-fed beef in both flavor and tenderness (Killinger et al., 2004). Particular attention should be paid to flavor and texture when serving grass-fed beef.

POULTRY — a great source of protein, niacin, and selenium; a good source of phosphorous, vitamin B$_6$ and vitamin B$_{12}$

If meat is the edible flesh or muscle from mammals, poultry is the edible flesh from birds. Common sources of poultry in many diets around the world are chicken and turkey, but this group also includes goose, duck, pheasant and other game birds. Like red meat, poultry is a good source of easily digestible protein, B vitamins, minerals and unsaturated fat. In general, poultry does not have quite as much iron as red meat, though it is still considered a good source of iron. Poultry can also be a source of omega-3 fatty acids, though this is dependent on the feed the bird has been eating (Alagawany et al., 2019).

The fat content of poultry is primarily found in the skin of the bird, and eating the skin increases the caloric value of poultry by 25% to 30% (Marangoni et al., 2015). Once the skin is removed, poultry becomes a low-fat food. The skin can be the key nutritional difference between breasts, thighs, and wings, as breasts are often served with the skin removed while thighs and wings are oftentimes served with the skin on. The way a chicken is raised, either conventional or free-range, also impacts fat content, as free-range chickens typically have slightly less fat than conventional chickens, though this difference largely diminishes once the skin is removed (Lin et al., 2014).

There is a longstanding debate — especially around American Thanksgiving tables — about whether dark meat or light meat poultry is better. While the difference in taste is a personal preference, there are some key nutritional differences to point out. Dark meat on a bird comes from the muscles that the bird uses more, such as the thighs, while breast meat is lighter because those muscles aren't used as much. Because dark meat muscles are used more, they contain more vitamins and minerals, especially iron and zinc (Marangoni et al., 2015). Dark meat may also contain a bit more fat than light meat, but the difference is fairly negligible.

PROCESSED MEAT

A subcategory of red meat and poultry is processed meats, which is any meat or poultry product that is preserved by smoking, curing, fermenting, salting or by the addition of chemical preservatives. This includes ham, bacon, pepperoni, pastrami, sausages, hot dogs, salami, jerky, and luncheon meats. It's common to think of processed meats as only being red meats, but chicken or turkey deli meat and sausages also meet this definition.

Some common additives or preservatives in processed meats are nitrites and nitrates, either synthetic or natural, as well as salt. In fact, processed meat contains about 400% more sodium and 50% more nitrates per gram than unprocessed meat (Micha et al., 2012). Processed meats are a common source of protein in the Standard American Diet, and there has been a lot of research surrounding the relationship between processed meat consumption and health outcomes, and how the processing of meat and poultry can make them more harmful to human health.

FISH — a great source of protein, omega-3 fatty acids (depending on the type), niacin, vitamin B$_6$, vitamin B$_{12}$, phosphorus and potassium

Fish and seafood play a primary role in the Mediterranean diet, but consumption is often limited in the Standard American diet. This group includes fish like salmon, tilapia, tuna and pollock as well as a wide range of seafood like shrimp, crab, and lobster. Fish and seafood can be a rich source of omega-3 fatty acids, an essential fatty acid that is an important nutrient for heart health (USDA & HHS, 2015). And while much of the benefit of seafood comes from its fat profile, seafood is also a big contributor to the protein food category. Seafood is low in saturated fat and an important source of many micronutrients, such as selenium, zinc, iodine, iron, and many B vitamins. Shellfish especially, like mussels, oysters, and clams, are packed with minerals like iron, zinc, selenium and calcium.

One concern with fish intake is its potential to contain mercury, which is a heavy metal found in seafood at varying levels. Seafood choices that are lower in mercury should be encouraged, especially for women who are pregnant or breastfeeding. However, pregnant and breastfeeding women should not avoid seafood altogether as essential fatty acids such as omega-3s are critical for fetal brain and eye development (Coletta et al., 2010; USDA & HHS, 2015). A recent study found that higher maternal fish consumption during pregnancy resulted in higher scores in visual recognition and verbal intelligence in infants (Oken & Bellinger, 2008). Seafood that is lower in mercury includes salmon, anchovies, herring, sardines, trout and Atlantic and Pacific mackerel. Seafood that should be avoided due to the potential to have a higher mercury content includes swordfish, tilefish, orange roughy, marlin, and king mackerel.

EGGS — a great source of protein, choline, and selenium; a good source of riboflavin, vitamin D, and phosphorous

Eggs contain high-quality protein, and in fact, protein from eggs is the most easily digestible and readily absorbable protein one can eat. Eggs, and especially egg yolks, are a rich source of many nutrients, such as choline, folate, and lutein and zeaxanthin, two carotenoids essential to eye health. Eggs are also inexpensive, easily accessible, and palatable to most people, making them an easy, healthful way to add protein to almost any meal.

Historically, it was thought that the cholesterol in foods was responsible in part for raising blood cholesterol levels and increasing the risk of heart disease. However, studies over the past few decades have shown this is not always the case (Hu et al., 1999). Many of the early studies on cholesterol and heart disease did not take saturated fat into account, and many high-cholesterol foods are also high in saturated fat, like many red and processed meats. However eggs have only a small amount of saturated fat, and more recent studies show that eggs can be a regular part of a healthful diet for many individuals (Fuller et al., 2018). Recommendations from the American Heart Association and the Dietary Guidelines do not recommend limiting eggs in order to improve blood cholesterol levels (Carson Jo Ann S. et al., 2020; USDA & HHS, 2015).

DAIRY — a great source of protein, calcium, vitamin D (if fortified), riboflavin, phosphorus and vitamin B$_{12}$

Cow's milk and other dairy products can also be a significant source of high-quality protein. A one-cup (8-ounce) serving of cow's milk provides 8 grams of protein. One cup of plain yogurt provides 13 grams of protein, and one cup of Greek yogurt contains roughly 24 grams of protein (FoodData Central). Cheese also contains some protein as a 1-ounce serving provides around 6 grams.

Milk has two major proteins: casein and whey. Casein constitutes approximately 80% of the total protein content of cow's milk with whey accounting for the other 20% (Davoodi et al., 2016). Cow's milk and other dairy products also contain high levels of the branched-chain amino acids (BCAAs) leucine, isoleucine and valine. BCAAs have been shown to promote protein synthesis and prevent muscle wasting (Blomstrand et al., 2006; Negro et al., 2008). See the chapter on Dairy for more information.

In addition to providing high-quality protein, dairy products are an important source of calcium, vitamin D, vitamin B$_{12}$, vitamin A, riboflavin, potassium and phosphorus (Davoodi et al., 2016).

SECTION 3:
PLANT-BASED PROTEIN

If you were to ask a non-vegetarian what vegetarians or vegans eat for protein, a common response would likely be tofu. While this certainly isn't wrong as tofu does serve as a great source of protein, the group of plant-based proteins is much larger than just this soy product. Among plant foods, protein can be found in ample amounts in beans and legumes, nuts, seeds and some grains.

LEGUMES — a great source of plant protein, fiber, B-vitamins, iron, folate, calcium, potassium, phosphorus, and zinc

One of the largest sources of plant-based protein in numerous healthful dietary patterns is legumes, which are sometimes referred to as pulses. By definition, legumes are plants that bear fruit in pods, and beans are a type of legume. Other legumes include lentils, peas, and peanuts, though, from a culinary perspective, peas are considered vegetables and peanuts are considered nuts. There is a wide variety of foods that fall into this category, including kidney beans, cannellini beans, Great Northern beans, fava beans, black beans, pinto beans, black-eyed peas, chickpeas, and lentils. Soybeans are also a legume and will be covered separately in the next section.

One half-cup serving of legumes provides about 8 grams of protein, though they are incomplete proteins because they do not contain all nine essential amino acids. Beans and legumes are also an important source of fiber, complex carbohydrates, B vitamins, iron, copper, zinc and phosphorus (Polak et al., 2015).

Due in part to all of these factors, bean consumption has been shown to play an important role in the prevention and management of a number of chronic health conditions, including type 2 diabetes, high cholesterol, hypertension and weight management (Orlich & Fraser, 2014). A recent study of individuals with type 2 diabetes found that those who consumed one cup of legumes per day had improved A1c levels and decreases in total cholesterol and triglyceride levels compared to the control group who were instructed to focus on wheat fiber foods (Jenkins et al., 2012). Beans and legumes are also an integral component of many health-promoting eating patterns, such as the Mediterranean diet, the DASH diet, and vegetarian and vegan diets.

SOY — a rich source of complete protein, fiber, B vitamins, magnesium and potassium

Soy is another member of the legume family, but it is unique in that it is a complete protein and provides all nine essential amino acids in ample amounts. Soy also provides more protein per serving than most other beans and legumes as a one-half cup serving of cooked soybeans provides almost 15 grams of protein. In addition to protein, soy is packed with vitamins, minerals, fiber, and healthful fats (Jenkins et al., 2010). Soy is also naturally high in isoflavones, a group of phytochemicals that have been shown to have antioxidant, anti-inflammatory, anticancer, and antimicrobial properties (Yu et al., 2016). As such, isoflavone intake has been associated with lower blood cholesterol concentrations and a reduced risk of cardiovascular disease and certain cancers (Lichtenstein, 1998).

Soybeans and other soy products have been a staple in Asian cultures for centuries, and the consumption of soy products in the U.S. and other Western cultures has been increasing over the past several decades (Messina & Messina, 2010). Recent estimates show that vegans in the United States consume about 10 to 12 grams of soy protein per day — roughly the amount in one serving of a soy product and an intake similar to what is seen in many Asian countries. Non-vegan vegetarians consume about half that amount daily, and the average American consumes only 2.2 grams of soy protein per day, mostly in the form of soy as an additive to other food products (Messina & Messina, 2010). The intake of soy, which is rich in plant-based protein, healthful fats, and isoflavones, has been linked to a decreased risk of certain cancers and a decrease in mortality from gastric, colorectal, and lung cancer; a lower risk of coronary heart disease and osteoporosis (Koh et al., 2009; Messina & Lane, 2007; Nachvak et al., 2019; Wu et al., 2008).

Soy-based foods are sometimes controversial as some consumers have heard and believe that soy isoflavones are estrogenic and may have adverse effects on health and development. However, population studies out of Asia tell us the exact opposite. In Asia, many people consume much more soy on a daily basis than in most other regions of the world, and studies in Asia have shown a lower risk of breast cancer among women consuming a high amount of soy compared to those consuming little to no soy (Messina & Messina, 2010). Moderate amounts of soy have also been shown to have no adverse effects on childhood development, male or female fertility, male testosterone levels, or thyroid function (Dwyer et al., 2008; Hamilton-Reeves et al., 2010; Messina & Redmond, 2006; Mínguez-Alarcón et al., 2015). For reference, a moderate amount of soy is approximately one to two servings per day. Population-based studies suggest that the greatest health benefits are seen among individuals who consume two to four servings of soy per day (Messina, 2016). To note: The research is supporting soy food (edamame, soy milk, tofu) not soy supplements like soy isoflavone or textured vegetable protein and soy protein isolate.

NUTS & SEEDS — a great source of fiber, plant protein, polyunsaturated fats and magnesium, and depending on the kind of nut or seed, many other nutrients

Nuts and seeds are another significant source of plant-based protein. A 1-ounce serving of nuts provides between 3 to 7 grams of protein, depending on the nut, while the protein content of seeds ranges from 5 to 9 grams per 1 ounce serving. A 1-ounce serving of either nuts or seeds is equal to about one small handful.

Peanuts are by far the highest consumed nut in the United States and make up about two-thirds of all nut intake (Here's the Shocking Number of Peanuts You Eat Every Year | National Peanut Board, 2016). Peanuts actually have more protein than any other nut at up to 7 grams per 1-ounce serving (FoodData Central). Peanuts and tree nuts were shown to decrease the total risk of both cardiovascular disease (by 13%) and coronary heart disease (by 15%) when consumed at least twice weekly (Guasch-Ferre et al., 2017).

Other commonly consumed and well-researched nuts include almonds and walnuts. Walnuts are a significant source of alpha-linoleic acid, an essential fatty acid that is beneficial to cardiovascular health. Studies have shown that consuming walnuts can improve cardiovascular risk factors and is beneficial to gut microbiota (Holscher et al., 2018). In the study by Guasch-Ferre and colleagues mentioned previously, consuming walnuts at least once weekly resulted in a 19% lower risk of cardiovascular disease and a 23% lower risk of coronary heart disease (Guasch-Ferre et al., 2017). Almonds are a good source of vitamin E, riboflavin, and magnesium, and studies have observed that the addition of 1.5 ounces of almonds per day can reduce LDL cholesterol levels and maintain HDL cholesterol levels (Kalita et al., 2018). Other nuts include hazelnuts, pecans, and pistachios. Hazelnuts are a fantastic source of folate, vitamin E, and monounsaturated fatty acids (FoodData Central).

Moving onto seeds, chia seeds are an excellent source of omega-3 fatty acids as well as calcium and fiber (Onneken, 2018). Flaxseed is also known for its numerous health benefits, and regular consumption of flaxseed has been linked to a reduction in cardiovascular disease, diabetes, cancer, and even autoimmune and neurological disorders (Goyal et al., 2014). Some other seeds to explore include hemp seed, pumpkin seeds or pepitas, sunflower seeds and sesame seeds.

In addition to protein, nuts and seeds are also a good source of healthful unsaturated fats, vitamins, minerals and fiber. They also contain phytochemicals that have antioxidant and anti-inflammatory properties (Sugizaki & Naves, 2018). In fact, observational studies have shown that eating 1.5 servings of unsalted nuts and seeds each day can reduce the risk of cardiovascular disease by 30% to 50% (Fraser, 1992; Hu et al., 1998). Other studies have shown that a small handful of tree nuts can lower blood cholesterol levels when substituted for another high-calorie snack food (Rehm & Drewnowski, 2017).

Tree Nuts: Almonds, Brazil nuts, cashews, hazelnuts, macadamia nuts, pecans, pine nuts (pignolias), pistachio nuts, and walnuts

Many of these same nutritional properties and health benefits can be seen when consuming nut and seed butters rather than the whole form (van den Brandt & Schouten, 2015). However, nut and seed butters come with a caution as oftentimes additional sugar and salt are added during processing to enhance flavor and extend shelf life. When nut and seed butters contain significant amounts of additives, their health benefits diminish. Be sure to check nutrition labels and ingredient lists when purchasing nut and seed butters.

GRAINS

Grains are often thought of as being a significant source of carbohydrates, but there are several grains that have a high protein content as well. One of these grains is **quinoa**, and while quinoa is technically a seed, it is treated as a grain for culinary and nutritional purposes. Quinoa is unique among the grains and most plant-based foods in general as it is a complete protein, meaning it provides all nine essential amino acids in ample amounts. Incomplete protein grains with a higher protein content include spelt, KAMUT®, teff, whole wheat pasta, wild rice, millet, oatmeal, and buckwheat (Fraser, 1992; Hu et al., 1998).

Table 2: Protein Content of Grains (FoodData Central)

Grain	Protein (g) per ½ cup serving (cooked)
Spelt	5.4 g
Teff	4.9 g
KAMUT®	4.9 g
Whole wheat pasta	4.2 g
Quinoa	4.1 g
Wild rice	3.3 g
Millet	3.1 g
Buckwheat	2.8 g
Oatmeal (cooked w/ water)	2.7 g

COMPLEMENTARY PROTEINS

Image: Rice and Beans

While most plant-based foods are incomplete proteins, it is sometimes a practice to pair certain plant-based foods so that together they provide all nine essential amino acids. These pairs are called **complementary proteins**, and the two foods involved in the pair essentially make up for the limitations of the other in terms of essential amino acids. Nuts and legumes are limited in the amino acids methionine and tryptophan, whole grains are lacking in lysine. By serving a legume and a grain together as complementary proteins, these limitations are accounted for as the grain provides the methionine and tryptophan that are not present in the legume, and the legume makes up for the lack of lysine in the grain. Some common complementary protein pairings include rice and beans, hummus with whole grain pita, peanut butter on whole grain bread, bean and barley stew, or a bean burrito on a whole wheat tortilla.

While these dishes offer convenient pairings, it's important to note that complementary proteins don't always need to be served together at the same meal. For vegans and those eating primarily plant-based foods, it's important to eat a variety of protein sources throughout the day and week so that all amino acids are consumed, but they do not need to be consumed at the same time.

SECTION 4:

RECOMMENDATIONS FOR PROTEIN INTAKE

The Dietary Guidelines stress that healthful eating patterns should include a variety of protein foods in nutrient-dense forms, and this includes protein from both animal and plant-based sources. At a 2,000-calorie level diet, the recommendation is for 5 ½ ounce-equivalents of protein foods per day, with 8 ounces of seafood each week. Each ounce of meat, poultry, or fish counts as an ounce equivalent, and the standard serving size for these foods is 3 ounces, which is about the size of a deck of playing cards. One egg is also equal to a 1-ounce equivalent of protein. Other 1-ounce equivalents of protein include ½ ounce of nuts, 1 tablespoon of nut butter, or ¼ cup of beans. Protein needs are actually quite lower than most people think, and in developed countries, protein needs are easily met through typical diets, even in vegetarian and vegan diets.

The current recommended daily allowance for protein for adults is 0.8 grams of protein per kilogram body weight (USDA & HHS, 2015). However, it may be more useful to use the acceptable macronutrient distribution range (AMDR) of 10% to 35% of total calories when assessing protein intake as it allows for more flexibility to meet individual needs and preferences (Wolfe et al., 2017). Wolfe et al. calculated the amount of flexible caloric intake left over after the minimum recommended amounts of carbohydrate, fat, and protein were added together – greater than or equal to 60% of discretionary calories remained. His team concluded that instead of filling those calories with refined grains or saturated fat, that protein was a healthful option, and that one should not rely on prescribing the "minimal amount" of protein required, especially when protein requirement is influenced by physiological circumstances.

There are a few instances where protein needs may be increased, such as during recovery from illness or injury, for elite athletes, during the aging process or weight loss in order to preserve muscle mass. However, the average daily exerciser does not need large amounts of protein to support health; refer to the **Competitive Athlete** chapter for more information in this area. Table 3 outlines these and other recommendations for protein intake from various authoritative bodies.

Table 3: Recommended Vegetable Intake From Different Authoritative Bodies

Source	Recommended Servings
Recommended Dietary Allowance (RDA)	0.8 grams protein/kilogram body weight (0.35 grams/pound)
Acceptable Macronutrient Distribution Range	10% to 35% of total calories from protein
2015 -2020 Dietary Guidelines for Americans	5.5 oz-equivalents per day, including 8 oz seafood per week
DASH* Diet Plan	Lean meats, poultry, fish: 6 oz or less per day Nuts, seeds, and legumes: 4 to 5 servings/week
American Heart Association	Poultry, meat, eggs: 8 to 9 servings/week Fish, other seafood: 2 to 3 servings/week Nuts, seeds, beans, legumes: 5 servings/week

*DASH = Dietary Approaches to Stop Hypertension
Sources: (Institute of Medicine, 2006; NHLBI; USDA & HHS, 2015; Van Horn Linda et al., 2016)

SECTION 5:

PROTEIN INTAKE AMONG AMERICANS

An analysis of NHANES data from 2015–2016 found that for almost 60% of Americans, protein intakes meet the minimum population and individual requirements, while protein intake is below recommendations for a little over 40% of individuals (Pannucci). The cohorts with protein intake below recommendations are adolescent females (12 to 19 years) and older women (60-plus years).

Figure 1: Average Daily Protein Intake Compared to Recommended Intake

Even for those Americans whose intake of total protein meets requirements, the average intake of protein foods in various subgroups does not always meet recommendations (USDA & HHS, 2015). Figures 2 and 3 from the Dietary Guidelines 2015–2020 show that while Americans' intake of meat, poultry, and eggs tends to meet (for females) or exceed (for males) recommendations, average intake of seafood, nuts, seeds, soy products and legumes often falls below recommendations (2015-2020 Dietary Guidelines | Health.Gov). Average intake of meat, poultry, and eggs are especially high for teen boys and adult men.

Figure 2: Average Intake of Protein Subgroups Compared to Recommended Intake Ranges (U.S. Department of Agriculture and U.S. Department of Health and Human Services, 2020)

Figure 3: Recommended Versus Average Weekly Intake of Legumes

The most commonly consumed protein foods in the United States include beef, especially ground beef; chicken; pork; processed meats such as hot dogs, sausages, ham and luncheon meats; and eggs. The most common seafood choices are shrimp, tuna, and salmon. The most common nut choices are peanuts, peanut butter, almonds and nut mixes. About half of all protein in the United States is consumed as a separate food item, like a chicken breast, fish filet, or egg, while the other half is consumed as part of a mixed dish, such as on hamburgers, pizza, or tacos (U.S. Department of Agriculture and U.S. Department of Health and Human Services, 2020).

SECTION 6:

PROTEIN INTAKE AND HEALTH OUTCOMES

Protein is an essential component of many different structures and processes in the human body, and in previous sections, it was established that protein can come from many different sources. While the protein from all of these sources is metabolized and used the same way by the body, there is a wide range of other components that accompany the protein, depending on the source. When we eat what we would consider a protein food, we're not only consuming the protein but also everything else that comes with it, including fat, sodium, fiber, vitamins and minerals and potentially some preservatives or additives. Much of the difference in health outcomes between different sources of protein is not due to the protein itself but to the other elements that come along with it.

For example, let's compare four different protein-containing foods, outlined in Table 4. A 3-ounce sirloin steak provides a whopping 25 grams of protein, but it also comes with 5 grams of saturated fat. A 3-ounce piece of ham provides 19 grams of protein and less saturated fat than the steak, but it also comes with over 1,000 mg of sodium, close to half of the recommended daily limit in a single serving of food. Option number three is a 4-ounce piece of grilled salmon which provides 21 grams of protein, very little sodium, only 1 gram of saturated fat, and is an excellent source of omega-3 fatty acids. And finally, a cup of cooked black beans provides about 15 grams of protein but also provides 15 grams of fiber, which is roughly half of one's fiber needs for the day, along with practically no sodium or saturated fat.

Table 4: Protein Content of Four Foods (FoodData Central)

Protein Source	Protein	Saturated Fat	Sodium	Fiber
3oz sirloin steak	25 g	3.5 g	58 mg	0 g
3oz ham, roasted	19 g	2 g	1180 mg	0 g
3oz grilled salmon	21 g	1 g	77 mg	0 g
1 cup black beans	15 g	0 g	2 mg	15 g

As the example in Table 4 illustrates, these four different foods provide a good amount of protein, but the other nutrients that accompany that protein are vastly different. The preparation methods of different protein sources will also impact their health outcomes if additional fat or sodium is added during preparation or cooking.

Given these differences, what does the research say about protein sources and health outcomes? A lot of research has focused on the health impacts of red and processed meat, and many studies have shown that eating healthful protein sources like beans, nuts, fish or poultry in place of red and processed meat can lower the risk of several chronic diseases (Bernstein et al., 2010; Pan et al., 2012). However, keep in mind that there are a lot of nuances in this research, and broad classifications of animal and plant proteins as being healthful or not may be over simplistic (Richter et al., 2015).

PROTEIN & MUSCLE MASS

Research on the effects of plant-based protein on skeletal muscle mass is mixed. A review by van Vliet and colleagues concluded that soy protein does not induce muscle protein synthesis to the same extent as protein from animal sources (van Vliet et al., 2015). In contrast, a cross-sectional study by Miki and colleagues found that vegetable protein intake was associated with higher skeletal muscle mass in elderly patients (Miki et al., 2017). Research has consistently shown that branch chain amino acids (BCAAs), and leucine in particular, can stimulate muscle protein synthesis and decrease exercise-induced muscle damage (Blomstrand et al., 2006; Layman et al., 2015; Negro et al., 2008). BCAAs are found in particularly high amounts in whey protein from dairy products. Refer to the chapter on the *Competitive Athlete* for more information.

HEART DISEASE

In general, population studies point to an association between even small intakes of red meat and especially processed meat and an increased risk of heart disease and stroke (Preis et al., 2010). In an investigation of over 120,000 participants in the Nurses' Health Study and Health Professionals Follow-Up Study, each additional 3-ounce serving of unprocessed red meat per day increased the risk of dying from cardiovascular disease by 13% (Pan et al., 2012). The link between processed meats and cardiovascular disease death was even stronger, as each additional 1.5-ounce serving of processed meat each day was associated with a 20% increase in the risk of dying from cardiovascular disease. Another meta-analysis found that individuals with diets high in red meat had higher triglyceride levels — a risk factor for heart disease — than those with low red meat intake (Guasch-Ferre et al., 2019).

Replacing red and processed meat with more healthful protein sources like beans, soy, nuts, fish and poultry may very well reduce these risks. In the same meta-analysis that was mentioned above, it was found that when participants replaced red meat with plant-based protein in their diets, they experienced a reduction in cardiovascular disease risk factors (Guasch-Ferre et al., 2019). In another study of over 1,700 healthy middle-aged men, intake of plant-based protein was inversely related to both systolic and diastolic blood pressure, whereas intake of animal-based protein had a positive association with blood pressure (Stamler et al., 2002). Replacing one serving of red meat with a serving of a plant-based protein may reduce CHD risk by up to 30% (Bernstein et al., 2010; Pan et al., 2012). A large reason why plant-based protein sources as well as poultry and fish are associated with a lower risk of heart disease is because of differences in fat, both in amount and type. Red and processed meat have primarily saturated fat, which can raise LDL cholesterol, while fish, poultry, and nuts have mostly healthful unsaturated fats, and legumes have very little fat at all.

However, results from these types of studies are not always consistent. In the EPIC cohort, a positive association with CVD mortality was seen for processed meat consumption but not for the consumption of red meat or poultry (Rohrmann et al., 2013). A 2013 meta-analysis found similar results and concluded that only processed meat intake, not red meat intake, was associated with a greater risk of CHD (Micha et al., 2012). One confounding factor in this research is that individuals who eat more plant-based or vegetarian diets also tend to be non-smokers, consume less alcohol, have a lower body weight, and be more physically active, all of which are lifestyle factors that also lower the risk of CVD and other chronic diseases (Richter et al., 2015).

When considering protein intake and heart health, it's also important to consider the impact of fish intake, as fish can be an important source of omega-3 fatty acids. Omega-3 fatty acids can lower blood pressure and heart rate, improve the function of blood vessels, and recent evidence suggests it is anti-inflammatory (Souza et al., 2020). A meta-analysis of 19 separate studies found that each 100-gram serving of fish per week was associated with a 5% reduced risk of acute coronary syndrome (Leung Yinko et al., 2014). According to the American Heart Association, eating two servings of fatty fish per week has been linked to a lower risk of heart attack and other cardiac issues (Arnett Donna K. et al., 2019).

Eggs are another protein source that receive a lot of attention in discussions about heart health. Eggs are packed full of protein and beneficial nutrients, but they are also high in dietary cholesterol. More recent research has shown however that dietary cholesterol does not impact serum or blood cholesterol as much as was previously thought (Hu et al., 1999). Thus, the American Heart Association suggests that for people who have low risk factors for heart disease, one egg or two egg whites per day can still be a part of a healthful diet (Arnett Donna K. et al., 2019).

DIABETES

When considering the risk of type 2 diabetes, there are similar associations with red and processed meat and disease risk that are seen with heart disease. A study conducted in 2011 found that those who had diets high in red meat, and especially processed red meat, had a higher risk of type 2 diabetes than those with lower intakes (Pan et al., 2011). However, among this group of study participants, replacing a serving of red meat with a serving of nuts, low-fat dairy, or whole grains decreased the risk of type 2 diabetes by 16% to 35%. Another study found that people who increased their red meat intake increased their risk of type 2 diabetes by 50% over a four-year period (Pan et al., 2013).

CANCER

There have been many research studies focused on the association between red and processed meats and cancer. In fact, in October 2015, the World Health Organization's International Agency for Research on Cancer concluded that consumption of processed meat is carcinogenic to humans and that the consumption of red meat is probably carcinogenic as well (Bouvard et al., 2015). These conclusions were based primarily off of evidence that links processed meats to an increased risk of colorectal cancer (Norat et al., 2005), and there have also been some positive associations between processed meat and stomach cancer as well as between red meat and pancreatic and prostate cancer (Bouvard et al., 2015).

A study among over 89,000 women followed for over 20 years found that high consumption of red meat in adolescence may also be associated with premenopausal breast cancer

(Farvid et al., 2015). Researchers observed a 22% higher risk of breast cancer among women who ate 1.5 servings or more of red meat per day while in high school in comparison to women who only had one serving per week during the same time. In contrast, those with higher intakes of poultry, nuts, and legumes experienced a lower risk of breast cancer.

There remains some speculation about what makes processed meats so unhealthful. Is it the added preservatives, such as nitrates and nitrites? Is it the copious amounts of sodium? Or could it possibly be the additional saturated fat that is found in most processed meats? Additionally, many studies do not differentiate between processed red meats and processed poultry products. Research to date suggests that poultry is typically better for health than red meat, so is this same relationship observed among processed meats? More research is needed to answer that question.

With the increasing concern over processed meats and health, there has been a push in the market for processed meats made with "natural" preservatives such as celery juice or powder rather than synthetic preservatives. However, natural preservatives still contain nitrates and nitrites, and the impact on disease risk of these new products has yet to be studied (Karwowska & Kononiuk, 2020).

In general, it's best to limit processed meats and added preservatives whenever possible. The World Cancer Research Fund recommends limiting red meat to no more than three servings per week and to eat very little or completely avoid processed meats (World Cancer Research Fund/American Institute for Cancer Research, 2018).

For more information on dietary influences on the risk of cancer, see the chapter on **Cancer**.

PREPARATION METHODS

The way a protein food is prepared can also profoundly affect disease risk. For example, poultry and fish are not typically associated with an increased risk of chronic disease. However, this changes if poultry or fish is battered and deep-fried. The addition of batter and oil significantly alters the nutrient profile of the food, no longer making it a health-promoting protein source.

There is also evidence that how meat is cooked has implications for cancer risk. Grilling at very high temperatures can create compounds called polycyclic aromatic hydrocarbons and heterocyclic amines on the grilled or charred surface of the meat, and these compounds can be carcinogenic (Farvid et al., 2015). High-temperature grilling can also lead to the formation of advanced glycation end-products, compounds that can raise blood pressure and lead to oxidative stress (Tuttle et al., 2012). When grilling, be cautious that the meat doesn't get too charred. Using marinades before grilling can also reduce the production of these compounds (Salmon et al., 1997).

Some other preparation methods for meat and poultry that are not associated with an increased risk of disease include baking, broiling, braising, roasting and stir-frying. See the chapter on Cooking, Nutrition, and Bioavailability for more information on the benefits and risks of varying cooking methods for protein.

SECTION 7:
CLINICAL & CULINARY RECOMMENDATIONS AND COMPETENCIES

Messaging from the Menus of Change Annual Report 2020

SERVE LESS RED MEAT LESS OFTEN;
SERVE MORE KINDS OF SEAFOOD MORE OFTEN;
MOVE LEGUMES AND NUTS TO THE CENTER OF THE PLATE

Clinical recommendations and competencies are the foundation from which culinary competencies were created. The goal for the culinary medicine practitioner is to help clients and patients develop the skills necessary to meet the clinical recommendations by teaching skill-based learning outlined in the culinary competencies.

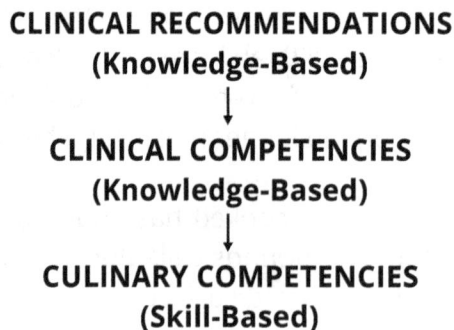

CLINICAL RECOMMENDATIONS
(Knowledge-Based)
↓
CLINICAL COMPETENCIES
(Knowledge-Based)
↓
CULINARY COMPETENCIES
(Skill-Based)

CLINICAL RECOMMENDATIONS

Protein Specific Recommendations:

1. Eat a variety of protein foods, including seafood, lean meats and poultry, eggs, legumes (beans, lentils, and peas), and nuts, seeds, and soy products (DGA 2015-2020, DGA 2020-2025)
2. Most intake of meats and poultry should be from fresh, frozen, or canned, and in lean forms (e.g., chicken breast or ground turkey) versus processed meats (e.g., hot dogs, sausages, ham, luncheon meats) (DGA 2020-2025)
3. Eat nuts but because they are calorically dense, replace them rather than add them to the diet (DGA 2015-2020)
4. Eat 8 ounces or more of a variety of seafood per week (DGA 2015-2020)
5. Seafood choices higher in EPA and DHA but lower in methyl mercury are encouraged (DGA 2015-2020, DGA 2020-2025)
6. Choose main dishes that combine meat and vegetables together, such as low-fat soups or a stir-fry that emphasizes veggies (AHA)
7. Watch portion size for meat: Aim for 2- to 3-ounce servings (AHA)
8. For poultry, meat, and eggs — lean and extra-lean; skin and visible fat removed (AHA)

Associated Clinical Recommendations:

1. Consume less than 10% of calories per day from saturated fats
2. Consume less than 2,300 milligrams (mg) per day of sodium

CLINICAL COMPETENCIES

1. Describe a complete protein and list animal and plant sources of complete protein
2. Compare and contrast the health benefits of consuming various sources of protein
3. Explain the unhealthful consequences of consuming processed meat and red meat
4. Recall how many servings of various sources of protein are recommended per day
5. Identify which cohorts are most at risk of not meeting their daily protein requirement
6. List sources of protein that supply a "good source" of nutrients found in the various sources of protein
7. Identify essential and nonessential amino acids

CULINARY COMPETENCIES FOR PROTEIN
SHOPPING COMPETENCIES

1. Demonstrate how to shop for healthful sources of protein within a budget
2. Purchase the most healthful cuts of meat and poultry

3. Define "plumping" and identify meat that has been plumped
4. Describe organic as it applies to meat and poultry items
5. Compare the various types of eggs available on the market
6. Purchase the most healthful type of fish
7. Purchase an assortment of dried and/or low-salt canned legumes
8. Purchase an assortment of nuts
9. Purchase healthful vegetarian options of traditional meat-based food — burgers, for example
10. Purchase nitrite/nitrate-free processed meat

COOKING/PREPARING COMPETENCIES

Stocking the Kitchen

1. Stock a variety of protein sources at home
   a. Legumes — an assortment of dried or canned soybeans, chickpeas, lentils, black beans, kidney beans, pinto beans, etc...
   b. Fish — canned, frozen, and/or fresh
   c. Chicken
   d. Eggs
   e. Lean cuts of meat for occasional use
   f. Nuts and seeds
   g. Grains (complete protein) – quinoa and amaranth

Knife/Instrument Skills

1. Select an appropriate knife or tool for the task
2. Slice meat to enhance tenderness
3. Remove visible fat from meat
4. Remove the skin from poultry
5. Tenderize meat
6. Cut through meat, cartilage, and bone (advanced)

FLAVOR DEVELOPMENT COMPETENCIES

1. Utilize non-meat savory (umami) ingredients
2. Utilize acid and salt to enhance the flavor profile
3. Select cooking methods to increase flavor and texture
4. Demonstrate how to build flavor by creating a marinade

COOKING COMPETENCIES

1. Prepare a more healthful dish by mixing animal and plant sources of protein together. For example:
   a. Blended burger
   b. Taco
2. Explain why it is important to remove visible fat before cooking meat and poultry
3. Demonstrate Healthful Dry Methods for Cooking Meat/Poultry/Fish
   a. Roast meat, poultry and fish
   b. Sauté meat, poultry, and fish
   c. Grill meat, poultry, and fish
   d. Pan-fry meat, poultry, and fish
   e. Stir-fry meat, poultry, and fish
4. Demonstrate Healthful Moist Methods for Cooking Meat/Poultry/Fish
   a. Stew meat, poultry, and fish
   b. Braise meat, poultry, and fish
   c. Steam meat, poultry, and fish
   d. Poach meat, poultry, and fish
5. Demonstrate Cooking Eggs Healthfully
   a. Poach eggs
   b. Bake eggs
   c. Pan cook eggs: scrambled eggs, frittata
   d. Boil eggs
6. Demonstrate Preparing and Cooking Legumes Healthfully
   a. Prepare/cook legumes (dried and canned)
   b. Cook with tofu
   c. Cook with tempeh
   d. Cook with seitan

SERVING COMPETENCIES

1. Model eating healthful sources and quantities of protein
2. List the amount of protein recommended in the *Eat Lancet Report*
3. Serve the appropriate number of protein servings per day
4. Utilize plant-based protein in meals and menu planning
5. Utilize the protein-flip (CIA, 2016)
6. Demonstrate the proper serving size of meat, poultry, and fish
7. Demonstrate the proper serving size of legumes
8. Explain the concept of complementary plant-based protein sources and give an example

SAFETY COMPETENCIES

1. Demonstrate proper storage of meat, poultry, and fish
2. Demonstrate the prevention of cross-contamination when working with raw and undercooked meat, poultry, and fish
3. Cook meat, poultry, and fish to the appropriate temperature
4. Wash hands often when working with raw meat, poultry, and fish
5. Explain how to use marinades and the role they play in the development of toxic compounds
6. Describe the culinary techniques that lead to the production of toxic compounds
7. Explain why it is important to remove charred, overcooked areas before serving meat, poultry, and fish

SECTION 8:

PROTEIN AT THE STORE

As discussed earlier, protein is found in both plant and animal products and table 5 lists the amount of protein found in various sources. When deciding on which types of protein to buy, the **decision shouldn't be based on the amount of protein as most people consume enough, but rather what else accompanies the protein, or the "package" it comes in.** Do the ingredients promote health or not? Following a plant-forward diet is the foundation of this work but it doesn't mean that animal sources of protein are off the table. In fact, by following the culinary tips listed in the next section, there are healthful ways to enjoy both sources of protein.

Table 5: Amount of Protein in Various Food Sources

Food	Grams of Protein
¼ cup raw peanuts	9
¼ cup dry roasted almonds	8
¼ cup walnuts	4
¼ cup sunflower seeds	8
1 cup whole wheat pasta	8
2 oz chicken breast	16
2 oz ground beef 90%	15
1 cup whole milk	9
1 boiled egg	6

Food	Grams of Protein
1 cup chickpeas	15
1 cup black beans	15
1 cup lentils	18

Source: (FoodData Central)

PROTEIN ON THE LABEL

Image: Nutrition Facts Panel

You can determine how much protein a product has by the grams of protein listed on the Nutrition Facts Label. There is no % Daily Value listed for protein because unlike other nutrients, the amount of protein needed is based on a person's weight (usually 0.8 grams per kilogram body weight) and not the amount of calories that they take in. That translates into about 7 grams of protein per day for every 20 pounds of body weight.

You will also find other labels and symbols on protein products. Below is a list of some of them.

Natural: The FDA has not defined the word "natural," so it doesn't really mean much of anything on a product. The current guideline is that the term natural is to be used on food products as long as it "is truthful and not misleading" and the product does not contain artificial colors or flavors or "synthetic substances."

For meat and poultry products, the term "natural" may be used when products contain no artificial ingredients or preservatives and are no more than minimally processed. Beyond that, the USDA does not have oversight into the treatment of the animals as it does when the "organic" seal is used.

Organic: This term can be used on meat, poultry, eggs, and dairy products that come from animals that:
• Are given no antibiotics or growth hormones
• Are raised in living conditions that accommodate their natural behaviors (grazing, for example)

• Are fed 100% organic feed and forage

For a list of livestock and poultry standards, visit https://www.ams.usda.gov/grades-standards/organic-standards

Sustainable: This term applies to locally grown food and meat that utilize sustainable agricultural practices that conserve natural resources. These include growing food using techniques that do not harm the environment, thus preserving the land, and are seasonal. Organic and sustainable do not mean the same thing. Sustainable practices also protect and support the local farmer by making sure they are paid fairly and help with the distribution of their food. However, this term is not regulated or legally defined for use on food labels.

EGGS

Buying eggs can be very confusing as there are many different terms you can find on a carton of eggs: cage-free, free-range, organic, high in omega-3s and vegetarian-fed. What should you pay more for and what is just a gimmick? It really depends on what is important to you: how they treat the chickens, what they feed the chickens, taste or added ingredients, for example. Decide for yourself by learning what each term means.

Cage-free: This label is used for poultry and eggs and merely means the bird was not housed in a cage. It doesn't mean that they had access to the outdoors or were humanely treated. There is no oversight for this labeling so assess with caution.

Free-range: Free-range is a term used for poultry and egg products and is defined by the USDA as "the bird having access to open air for five minutes per bird each day", which really doesn't make a difference in the long run for the bird or their health. There are no regulations on what they are fed, and beak cutting and forced molting through starvation are permitted under this term. While there is a federal definition of "free-range", there is no oversight for this label.

Pasture-raised: These are eggs from birds raised outdoors or with access to the outdoors.

Vegetarian-fed: These birds eat feed that does not contain animal byproducts. There are no regulations pertaining to the chicken's living conditions with this label.

Organic: Chickens that lay organic eggs are fed an organic, all-vegetarian diet free of antibiotics and pesticides. They are cage-free inside barns or warehouses and have access to the outdoors. That doesn't mean that they go outside often, if at all, but they aren't packed in as tightly as standard chickens. A third party oversees that the standards are followed.

High in omega-3s: Most individuals do not consume enough of the anti-inflammatory fatty acids known as omega-3s. Chickens that lay eggs high in omega-3s are fed a diet that is high in omega-3 fatty acids (polyunsaturated fats and kelp meal) which are passed into the egg and onto the consumer. There are no regulations pertaining to the chicken's welfare or living conditions with this label.

Natural: Natural means nothing with regard to how chickens are treated and, in the end, it doesn't mean a whole lot for eggs. Natural just means that nothing was added to the egg.

Fertile: These eggs are gathered from chickens that lived with roosters so most likely they are not caged and can roam around.

Bottom line for eggs: Most labels on eggs do not mean much when it comes to how the egg-laying chickens are treated. In terms of nutrition, paying more for eggs high in omega-3 fatty acids may be worth it if you do not get this essential fatty acid from other sources (fatty fish for example). For a unique experience and fabulous taste, try finding a local egg farm in your neighborhood – you may never go back to conventional store-bought eggs!

Eggs should be kept in the refrigerator and preferably not in the door where the jarring motion from opening and closing can disturb and thin the egg whites (McGee, 2004).

For more information, visit USDA Definitions of labels on eggs. (https://www.usda.gov/media/blog/2012/04/06/eggstra-eggstra-learn-all-about-them)

FISH

Selecting the most healthful fish has become a complicated task, partly because some varieties of fish are high in mercury. Fatty fish provides essential omega-3 fatty acids that most individuals' diets are lacking, but you do not want to trade a good (omega-3 fatty acid) for a bad (mercury). The most common source of mercury for Americans is tuna fish because we eat so much of it. Mercury poses a health threat to the brain and nervous system, especially in growing children and pregnant women.

For tuna: Limit children's consumption of canned chunk light tuna to less than one ounce per week for every 12 pounds of body weight to stay below the level of mercury the Environmental Protection Agency considers safe. That means that a child who weighs 36 pounds should not eat more than 3 ounces (half a standard-sized can of chunk light tuna) per week. Children should also avoid albacore or white tuna because the levels of mercury are higher.

The Smart Seafood Buying Guide (https://www.nrdc.org/stories/smart-seafood-buying-guide) has a list of seafood from highest to lowest amount of mercury. Below are the highest and lowest categories of mercury in seafood.

Fish with the least amount of mercury: Anchovies, butterfish, catfish, clam, domestic crab, crawfish, Atlantic croaker, flounder, Atlantic haddock, hake, herring, jacksmelt, mackerel (North Atlantic or chub), mullet, oyster, plaice, pollock, canned and fresh salmon, sardine, scallop, shrimp, sole, squid, tilapia, freshwater trout, whitefish and whiting.

Fish with the highest amount of mercury: Bluefish, grouper, king mackerel, marlin, orange roughy, shark, swordfish and tuna (bigeye or ahi).

Go to the Seafood Watch (https://www.seafoodwatch.org/) to find Best Choice, Certified, Good Alternative, and Avoid options for seafood.

LEGUMES

Vegetable sources of protein are very healthful as they are low in calories, high in fiber and other healthful nutrients. Serve edamame (soybeans), chickpeas, hummus, split peas, black-eyed peas, lentils, and beans (kidney, lima, pinto, white, navy and black) as they are all inexpensive powerhouses of nutrients.

If consuming non-genetically modified (GMO) soybeans is a priority for you, look for non-GMO varieties. In the United States, labels do not need to say GMO, although many consumer groups are fighting to have this done. If you'd like more information on GMOs, the website Signal to Noise Special Edition: GMOs and Our Food ("Signal to Noise Special Edition") explores many different topics related to GMOs.

To save money, buy dried peas, beans, or lentils, but know they do take some time to prepare. If you decide to trade some convenience for cost, select canned varieties without added salt. Another issue to consider when purchasing canned goods is the fact that today most aluminum cans contain BPA, a chemical that lines the can and has been linked to having possible negative health effects on the brain. It won't be easy, but you may be able to find BPA-free cans (Eden

Foods switched to BPA-free cans in 1999). This may be a good enough reason to cook your own beans if you have trouble finding BPA-free cans.

Did you know? Peanuts are a legume.

NUTS AND SEEDS

Nuts and seeds are a healthful source of protein as long as they have little to no salt added. It is important though to be aware of serving sizes as they tend to be high in calories too – a little bit goes a long way with nuts and seeds. They are not only filling but some have been found to be heart-healthy as well. There are technically 18 tree nuts: almonds, Brazil nuts, cashews, chestnuts, hazelnuts (filberts), macadamia nuts, pecans, pistachios and walnuts are the most common.

Pumpkin, sesame, and sunflower seeds also make great additions to the diet. For individuals with a nut allergy, the following can be substitutions: sunflower seeds and sunflower seed butter or soybeans and soy butter.

POULTRY

Like labels on eggs, labels on other poultry products can be confusing as well. Don't pay extra for "free-range" or "natural" unless the label explicitly states "free of antibiotics", but it may be worth spending more for "organic". The USDA bans the use of hormones in all chickens so that isn't something to look for when buying chicken. You can save money when purchasing cut-up poultry (breast, thighs) by removing the skin yourself before cooking as you pay more for the bone and skin to be removed.

Plumping

It is hard to find cooked poultry that has not been injected with a saltwater solution — even in "all-natural" and organic birds. The reason for this is that breeders want to provide a juicier, better textured, more flavorful experience to make up for the flavor lost with breeding leaner animals. "Natural flavoring," processed ingredients, chicken broth, carrageenan (a seaweed extract), sugar, gums, modified food starch and more are also added. Look for "self-basting" as a clue, but more importantly, look on the Nutrition Label to see how much sodium is in a standard serving size (3 ounces). The Consumer Reports looked at the nutrition information for 16 rotisserie chickens on the company's website and the results are listed in Table 6 (Santanachote, 2021). As you can see, there are some that provide about eight times more sodium than what is present in **plain (no salt added) roasted chicken (70 milligrams)**.

Table 6: Amount of Sodium in a 3-ounce Serving of Rotisserie Chicken

Brand	Amount of Sodium in a 3-ounce Serving
Sam's Club	550 mg
Costco	460 mg
BJ's, Boston Market, Publix, Safeway, Stop & Shop, Walmart and Wegmans (nonorganic)	170 to 368 mg
Kroger (Simple Truth)	40 mg
Wegmans (organic chicken)	95 mg

(Santanachote, 2021)

MEAT

Beef/Pork/Lamb/Veal/Ham

Choose the leanest cuts of beef and avoid prime cuts as they have the most fat. Also avoid beef with marbling, which are streaks of fat. Table 7 lists cuts of beef that are lower in fat and make tasty choices.

The leanest pork choices include pork loin, tenderloin, center loin and ham.

Table 7: Lean Cuts of Beef

Lean Cuts of Beef	Extra Lean Cuts of Beef
Round steak	Eye of round roast
95% lean ground beef	Top round steak
Chuck shoulder roast	Mock tender steak
Arm pot roast	Bottom round roast
Shoulder steak	
Strip steak	
Tenderloin steak	
T-bone steak	

Get to know the butcher at your grocery store. They can advise on lower-fat cuts of meat and how best to prepare them. They can also — when asked — cut and prepare meat that requires advanced knife skills. For example, butterfly or spatchcock a chicken; fillet and remove the bones from fish; remove the skin from poultry and much more.

Processed Meats

Processed meats are not a healthful selection but for those occasional times, look for cold cuts, hot dogs, sausages and bacon that are nitrite- and nitrate-free (uncured). When selecting processed meat choose those made from turkey, soy, or chicken as they are lower in fat and pay particular attention to the salt content.

If you want to read more about the scientific data around healthful protein sources, go to Harvard's Nutrition Source for Protein. (https://nutritionsource.hsph.harvard.edu/what-should-you-eat/protein/)

SECTION 9:
PROTEIN & SUSTAINABILITY

The Food Planet Health Summary Report does not mince words. It starts with "Food is the single strongest lever to optimize human health and environmental sustainability on Earth. However, food is currently threatening both people and the planet." What do people need to eat so that by 2050 people's health and the planet's health are in line? The EAT-Lancet report, created by 37 leading international scientists, looked into just that question. They set "universal scientific targets for the food system" in order to protect both people and the planet in the future. **Fruit, vegetable, legume, whole grain and nut consumption needs to double, and the amount of meats and treats needs to be cut in half** in order to reach the 2050 goal (The EAT-Lancet Commission on Food, Planet, Health). Graph 1 outlines the daily sources of protein needed to achieve this goal.

The amount of animal-based protein listed in the *Eat Lancet Report* for planetary and personal health, depicted on Graph 1, translates into:

Total of beef, pork, and lamb: 0.49 ounces per day or 3.4 ounces per week
Total poultry: 1 ounce per day or 7 ounces per week
Total fish: 1 ounce per day or 7 ounces per week
Total eggs: 0.5 ounces per day or 3.2 ounces per week
Serving fish 2/week, poultry 2/week, eggs 2 to 3/week, and beef 1/week (using standard serving sizes)

Graph 1: Eat Lancet Recommendation of Daily Protein Sources

Consumption of animal sources of protein needs to be drastically reduced because they require the most resources, as seen in Figure 4.

Figure 4: Amount of Resources Needed for Plant Versus Animal Foods

SECTION 10:
PROTEIN IN THE KITCHEN

ON THE TONGUE — THE TASTE OF PROTEIN

The taste of protein is high in umami (savory), which carries with it a tactile sensation of "fullness" (Beauchamp, 2009; Ninomiya, 2015). Pure umami compounds are unpalatable alone but they are quite delicious when mixed with other ingredients. An umami taste sensation occurs when L-glutamate (mostly) and other amino acids including L-aspartate activate an umami receptor. L-glutamate and thus the taste of umami is not just present in protein from animal sources, it is also present in mushrooms, tomatoes, green peas and wine for example. In many plant-based protein dishes – like tofu and tempeh– monosodium glutamate is added, which adds an umami element to the dish.

Babies are exposed to umami tastes in utero and through breast milk (which is high in free glutamate) but it is unclear whether or not a preference for umami is innate or learned. There is individual variability in the ability to taste umami, which is thought to occur from variations in the TAS1R3 gene as well as one's exposure to the taste of umami (Chen et al., 2009; Raliou et al., 2009; Shigemura et al., 2009). Some individuals cannot taste umami (but for some, with repeat exposure they can become tasters), some are hypo-tasters, while in the taster group, some are very sensitive to the taste of umami.

PREPARING ANIMAL-BASED PROTEIN

Image: Tenderizing Protein

Tenderizing

Pounding chicken, turkey, beef, pork, lamb and other meats with a tenderizer helps to create a more tender end product. The muscles of these animals can be tight (various cuts have differing levels of toughness) and hitting them with a hammer-like instrument helps to break up the fiber creating a more tender piece of meat. There is a flat side for creating thin cutlets and a jagged side that breaks up the muscle. The increased surface area will allow for an increase in absorption of marinades as well.

Image: Removing Excess Fat

Removing Excess Fat

With a sharp knife cut off any visible fat on red meat and the skin off of poultry. If you do not have the proper knife or skill (yet) ask the butcher to do this at the store.

Marinating

Marinating meat in an acidic solution (vinegar, wine, buttermilk, citrus) helps to make a juicier, more flavorful, and more tender product by breaking down and weakening the muscle tissue. It works best with thin cuts of meat as the flavor does not penetrate much beyond the surface. Select ingredients from the four boxes below.

Ingredients for a Marinade

Image: Build a Marinade

Flavor Enhancers	Salt–To Draw Water Soluble Flavors Into The Meat	Oil–To Transfer Fat Soluble Flavors To The Meat's Surface	Acid–To Change The Texture And Add Flavor
Herbs and spices	Soy or tamari sauce	Olive oil	Wine
Mustards	Salt	Flavored oils	Vinegars
Worcestershire sauce		Toasted sesame seed oil	Tomatoes
Ketchup			Buttermilk
Honey			Citrus juice

- The rule of thumb is a half-cup of marinade is needed for every pound of meat
- Marinating for too long with an acidic or salty solution can create a mushy end product.
- Marinate in the refrigerator — up to two hours if citrus juice is used; up to four hours if salt, alcohol, or other acidic ingredients are used; overnight is fine as long as no alcohol, salt, or acid is being used (Stradley, 2015)
- Do not marinate in a cast iron, aluminum or metal pan or foil; glass containers are preferred. A plastic bag also works as it provides for easy cleanup and it helps make sure all parts of the meat are exposed to the marinade.

COOKING ANIMAL-BASED PROTEIN

Eggs

Eggs

The Oven	The Stove Top
Frittata	Boiled
Baked eggs	Scrambled
Quiche	Omelet
Shakshuka	Poached
	Fried

Table 8: The Nutrient Composition of Egg Whites Versus Egg Yolks

Nutrient	Egg White	Egg Yolk
Water	88%	55%
Protein	11%	16%
Carbohydrate	1%	1%
Fat	<1%	27%
Vitamins	Lower amounts of B vitamins, and less than half the amount of vitamin A, vitamin E, and vitamin D than found in yolks	All vitamins except vitamin C. Fun fact: chickens can make their own vitamin C
Minerals — rich in calcium, phosphorous, and potassium, plus all the trace elements	More potassium and magnesium than found in yolks	More iron and zinc than found in whites
Other nutrients		Choline

(Réhault-Godbert et al., 2019)

Poaching	Simmering	Boiling
180°F/ 82°C	185°F to 200°F 85°C to 93°C	212°F/ 100°C

Boiled

The simplest way to prepare an egg is to boil them as nothing needs to be added (like fat). The trick is to cook them in bubble-less water (simmer at 180°F to 190°F / 80°C to 85°C), as the rolling boil may crack the shell.

• Soft-boiled (coddled) — three to five minutes (whites are not cooked through and liquid yolk)
• Medium (mollet eggs) — five to six minutes (the whites are cooked, and the yolk is semi-liquid)
• Hard — 10 minutes (firm throughout)

For a quick check on the freshness of an egg — place a raw egg in water, if it floats it is old and should be discarded.

Baked/Shirred, en Cocotte

Eggs can be baked in a separate dish in the oven, in a separate dish surrounded by water (en cocotte), in a pan surrounded by vegetables (e.g., shakshuka — tomatoes, peppers, onion and garlic), or actually baked in a vegetable (peppers, squash, tomatoes, avocado).

Bake at 375°F/190°C until they reach an internal temperature of 160°F/71°C (or a knife inserted in the center comes out clean).

Poached Eggs

- Add vinegar and a bit of salt (1 tablespoon vinegar and ½ teaspoon salt) to the water, which helps to coagulate the whites so they don't spread
- Crack an egg into an almost but not boiling water
- Remove with a slotted spoon to drain the water and serve

Image: Fried Eggs

Fried Eggs

- Use oil, not butter
- Heat oil in a pan (when a drop of water in the oil sputters, the oil is hot enough)
- Add the egg and cook until the desired outcome is reached:
  - Sunny-side up — the egg is not flipped
  - Over easy — flip but cook for just a short time (about 10 seconds, and the yolk will be runny)
  - Over medium — flip and cook until the yolk is only slightly runny
  - Over well — the yolk is firm and cooked through

Scrambled Eggs

- Whisk eggs together and add a bit of water (optional for fluffier eggs). Milk can also be used.
- Add some oil to the pan and when it sputters, add the egg mixture.
- Use low heat and stir depending on desired consistency — stir infrequently for large curds, whereas stirring a little more frequently will provide smaller curds. Do not stir constantly as this will produce watery eggs.

- Remove the pan from the heat before the eggs are completely cooked as they will continue to cook off of the heat.
- When liquid starts to leach out of the scrambled eggs, they have been overcooked.

Omelet — this is a great way to add vegetables to a breakfast dish although it can be served any time of day.
- Select the right number of eggs for the diameter of the pan. The word omelet means thin layer so don't add too many eggs (three eggs in a medium-size frying pan).
- Requires a hotter pan than for scrambled eggs. Use oil, not butter.
- Cook vegetables beforehand and make sure the water in vegetables like mushrooms and tomatoes evaporates before adding the eggs.
  - Cook using one of the various methods — waiting for the bottom to be cooked before folding in half, lifting up the omelet to let the uncooked egg run over the side to cook, or scramble the eggs quickly and push them into a circle before folding in half.

Table 9: Eggs: Cooking Methods and Nutrient Retention

Cooking Method	Positives	Negatives
Scrambling	Retains more vitamin D, vitamin K, and healthful fats compared to boiled eggs	Decreases vitamin B and selenium
Boiled	Greater retention of vitamin D than baking	Decrease in lutein and zeaxanthin (soft boiling will prevent some of the loss) and overall antioxidant capacity
Frying	Greater retention of vitamin D than baking	Cholesterol in eggs can become oxidized to oxysterols, which are harmful. Decrease in lutein and zeaxanthin and overall antioxidant capacity. Compared to poaching, frying lowers the amount of omega-3 fatty acids by 14% to 23%. The amount of the harmful advanced glycation end products (AGEs) is magnitudes higher than other cooking methods.
Poached		Reduction in omega-3 fatty acids but not as much as frying.
Baking		Larger loss of vitamin D than boiling or frying

Cooking Method	Positives	Negatives
Cooking eggs in general (compared to raw)	Improves the digestibility of the protein in eggs, increases the availability of protein from 51% to 91%, and decreases the risk of salmonella poisoning	

(Goh & Lim, 2004; Jakobsen & Knuthsen, 2014; Nimalaratne et al., 2016; Uribarri et al., 2010)

Summary: Eggs are full of nutrients. To improve the healthfulness of eggs and to limit the production of harmful byproducts — cook eggs in water or oil, not butter; cook on lower heat for shorter periods of time. The least healthful method is frying an egg and the most healthful methods are soft-boiled and poached whereby the egg white is fully cooked but the yolk remains relatively uncooked (Réhault-Godbert et al., 2019). Fully cook the yolk for individuals who are at risk of food poisoning — the elderly, young children, immune-compromised, and those pregnant and lactating. Other healthful methods include the addition of vegetables to the egg mixture without overcooking.

Fish

Focus on cooking fish that is low in mercury. For the times when you do serve fish that may be high in mercury, serve a side dish that supplies a good source of selenium (a large serving of shiitake mushrooms, or cooked spinach and couscous) or make a crust that has crushed brazil nuts (note: can be extremely high in selenium, so a little goes a long way) (Gribble et al., 2016; Khan & Wang, 2009). Selenium binds to mercury which neutralizes its harmful effects.

Method 1: Steam over boiling water

Step 1: Marinate the fish by choosing ingredients from Table 10, or make your own marinade

Table 10: Building a Fish Marinade

Sodium	Spices	Acid
Tamari or soy sauce,	Garlic, ginger, dill, chili	Vinegar, citrus juice and zest, Dijon mustard, capers
Example 1 Tamari sauce	Grated ginger and garlic	Lemon zest
Example 2 Soy sauce	Garlic	Balsamic vinegar, Dijon mustard

Step 2: Prepare steamer by boiling water. Add parchment paper to the top of the steamer to catch the juices from the marinade.

Step 3: Steam with the lid on for 5 to 20 minutes depending on the size of the piece of fish. If it is a thin filet, it will be quick so check at 5 minutes – when cooked through it should be firm to the touch but still have some bounce in it. Some people like their fish well done and others like it only just cooked, this takes a little bit of practice to cook it just right. A piece of salmon should only take about 7 to 10 minutes maximum (depending on the thickness). A whole sea bass (or other fish that is medium-sized) should take about 15 to 20 minutes.

Step 4: Serve with lemon slices, the cooked marinade, and/or fresh herbs

Method 2: Poisson en Papillote/ Fish Cooked in Parchment Paper

Image: Fish en Papillote

This is an impressive dish, and once you get the hang of folding the parchment paper, it is super easy to make. Cooking in parchment allows the fish to steam and cook in the aromas it is surrounded in, without the use of saturated fats. To create a delicious papillote, choose from the ingredients below or create your own.

Build a Papillote

1. **Acid and Liquid**
   a. The juice of a lemon, lime or orange
   b. The zest or slices of lemon, lime or orange
   c. Wine, broth, soy sauce, fish sauce
2. **Aromatics**
   a. Onion, shallot or scallion
   b. Garlic
   c. Ginger
3. **Herbs and Spices**
   a. Thyme,

    b. Basil

    c. Oregano

    d. Dill

4. **Vegetables *the fish will cook quickly so make sure the vegetables are cut small enough to steam in the same amount of time**

    a. Thinly sliced carrots, fennel, mushrooms, zucchini

    b. Peas, asparagus, peppers

    c. Olives, capers

Step 1: Prepare the parchment paper by folding a piece in half and cutting into a heart shape. (A folded piece of aluminum foil can also be used but the presentation is not as dramatic.)

Step 2: Add the fish (bloodline down, skin up) and other ingredients — lemon slices, capers, a sundried tomato, garlic, mushrooms and fresh chives are used in the picture above, but you can add whatever will cook quickly. Mushrooms work well because they pick up the juices and become very flavorful. Add just a splash of white wine, citrus juice, broth, or a combination of liquids.

Step 3: Assemble the papillote by securing the sides with an egg white that has been beaten into a froth. Brush the edges with the beaten egg white, fold the paper heart in half pressing the sides together to seal. Brush the edge of the paper heart with the egg white. Make a series of short folds along the edges. Brush it again with the egg white. With a pastry brush, gently oil the top of the papillote.

Step 4: Place the papillotes on a sheet pan and place in a 450°F/232°C preheated oven for about 8 to 10 minutes, depending on the thickness of the fish being used.

Step 5: Serve and open the papillote at the table, this allows the diner to experience the presentation and delicious aroma. Be careful as lots of steam will escape.

Method 3: Poaching

Image: Poached Fish in a Soup

Poaching is an underutilized tool for cooking fish but if you make a flavorful bouillon, it can be delicious and healthful.

Step 1: In a large pot, bring 8 cups water, ½ cup white wine, 1 teaspoon black peppercorns, 1 lemon that is halved and juiced into the pot, 1 bundle of thyme, 1 leek roughly chopped, and a pinch of salt to a gentle simmer. This is a good base recipe but feel free to add, remove, and alter as you see fit. Love ginger? Throw some chopped ginger in there.

Step 2: Gently lower your fish pieces into the simmering water and let it gently cook to your desired doneness.

Step 3: Remove carefully with a slotted spoon or fish spatula and enjoy with a fresh squeeze of lemon and some chopped herbs.

Another option is to poach your fish directly in a sauce you are going to serve it with. For example, poach the fish in a coconut curry broth or in a spicy tomato, caper, and bell pepper sauce as shown in the picture above.

Method 4: Roast

Image: Fish Roast

Step 1: Preheat the oven to 400°F/200°C.

Step 2: Prepare the fish and other vegetables (optional). This can be as simple as adding salt and pepper to the fish and adding sliced lemons. Toss vegetables in a bowl with a small amount of oil, salt and pepper, and dried spices of your choosing (rosemary, dill). The trick for adding other vegetables is that they have to be cut thin enough that they cook at the same time as the fish.

Step 3: Lay the fish and vegetables on a cookie sheet lined with parchment paper. Cook until done — it depends on the thickness of the fish — anywhere from 10 to 20 minutes.

Step 4: This is optional. Add capers and lemon juice to the cooked fish, serve and enjoy!

Method 5: Pan Frying

Image: Fish Pan Fry

Pan frying fish in a little bit of oil is a quick, easy and delicious way to serve fish. Marinating it first will allow for a flavorful bite. Pan frying however results in more of a loss of vitamin D than does steaming, baking, or microwaving (Ložnjak & Jakobsen, 2018).

Method 6: Grilling

Image: Fish Grilled

Grilling whole fish allows for the outside to take on the char, which is removed before eating. That way the potential carcinogens present in the blackened pieces are not ingested.

Step 1: Take the fish out of the refrigerator about a half hour before cooking for a more even cook. Prepare the grill — clean off the grates and heat to a fairly high temperature — about 400°F/204°C. If possible, leave one side of the grill on and the other side off.

Step 2: Prepare the fish. Season the cavity with the whole fish. Herbs, slices of citrus, chopped garlic, grated ginger, and lemongrass spears all make excellent and exciting stuffing.

Step 3: Grease the grill grates with a neutral oil and place your fish pieces over the heat, skin side down, if there is one. Get a nice sear on the skin and if it's a whole fish, turn once to sear the opposite side. Keep an eye as oil and fat will drip and cause flare-ups. When you have a nice sear on the skin, gently pull the fish to the side of the grill that is off and continue to cook using indirect heat until you get the doneness you desire. If this is not possible, finish cooking in an oven.

Step 4: Plate the fish with lemon slices and fresh herbs.

Poultry and Meat (Beef and Pork)

If you enjoy red meat, enjoy it in small amounts and only occasionally — see Section 11 for the protein flip. Look for cuts of meat that have very little visible fat and when choosing ground meat select one that is no more than 15% fat. Processed meats should be minimized or avoided altogether as these meats have the clearest relationship with poor health outcomes.

Healthful Cooking Methods

- Start with a lean cut of meat
- If there is visible fat, cut it off before cooking
- Skim fat after cooking — off the top of soups and stews
- If there is a need for oil (frying, searing), use a minimal amount
- Select a cooking method that:
  - Minimizes nutrient loss —
    - Cooking meat in a liquid base that will be consumed after cooking ensures that water-soluble nutrients that are released from the meat into the liquid are consumed
    - Don't cook on high heat
    - Don't cook for long periods of time
  - Prevent or limit the production of toxic compounds, which are caused by high heat, open flames, and overcooking or charring. See the chapter on Cooking, Nutrition, and Bioavailability for more information.
  - Adds nutrients
    - Cook with vegetables — add vegetables to stews, stir-fries, steaming, poaching and soups in a 3-to-1 ratio. For every quart of finished product, ¾ should consist of vegetables and ¼ of meat.
    - Add vegetables when roasting, sautéing, and grilling.

Dry Methods for Meat/Fish/Poultry

Roast Meat and Poultry

Roasting uses indirect dry heat to cook. The art of roasting meat is in the selection of the temperature (low and slow, high and fast, or somewhere in between), deciding to sear first, and/or to baste during cooking.

Step 1: Bring to room temperature before cooking (do not leave out for more than an hour or two). Season the meat while it is reaching room temperature with salt and pepper.

Step 2: Cook the meat — see Table 11 for guidance. Note: Always start with a preheated oven.

Table 11: Temperatures for Roasting Meat

Oven Temperature	Good For...	Outcome
Low (250F/125C and below) and slow	Tender cuts, tough cuts – rib roast (beef), boneless blade roast (pork), center rib roast (pork), leg of lamb	Dissolves tough collagen (often found in cheaper cuts of meat) into tender gelatin
Medium (350F/175C)	Most cuts	
High (400F/200C and above) and fast	Tender and small cuts of meat – tenderloin, top sirloin roast, rack of lamb	Helps to brown the outside of the meat
Alternate – start high and then drop the temperature		Can get a brown exterior

(McGee, 2004; Roasting Meat 101 | Cook's Illustrated, accessed 1/22)

Step 3: Remove from the oven and let it rest for at least a half hour (McGee, 2004). This allows for the after-heat to keep cooking the meat and to allow for the structure to become firmer, which will lock in the juices. The temperature of the meat can rise five or more degrees during the resting period.

Cutting meat across the grain of the muscle fibers creates a more tender piece of meat and it is easier to chew. See How to Cut Meat Against the Grain by Fine Cooking: https://www.finecooking.com/article/how-to-cut-meat-against-the-grain

Image: Searing

Pan Frying or Sautéing is best for thinner cuts of meat. It requires the transfer of heat from a hot metal pan, through a layer of oil (usually) to the meat itself. This cooking technique browns meat quickly which brings a new flavor to the profile.

Pan Roasting starts with panfrying to create a brown crust and then continues cooking meat in the oven. This technique can be used for thicker cuts of meat.

To Sear or Not to Sear? It depends. If you are trying to lock in the juices, that question was answered in the 1930s — searing does not lock in juices. What it does however is add a layer of flavor through browning, so if your goal is a tasty piece of meat, go ahead and sear.

Grilling meat involves cooking over a direct heat source which can be wood, coals, an open gas flame, or electric element. In order to avoid burning/charring meat it is best to brown quickly over a higher heat and then move the meat to a lower heat source to finish cooking (similar to pan frying).

Barbecuing is a slower cooking method in a closed chamber using a lower temperature than that used for grilling. The meat can be flavored by the type of wood used to create the fire.

Broiling involves cooking meat below a heat source. The same rules apply in regard to limiting the time under a high heat source — just until browned — and then moving to a lower heat source to continue cooking.

Table 12: Safe Minimum Cooking Temperatures

Food	Type	Internal Temperature
Ground meat and meat mixtures	Beef, pork, lamb, veal	160°F / 71°C
	Turkey, chicken	165°F / 74°C
Fresh beef, lamb, veal	Steaks, roasts, chops Rest time: 3 minutes	145°F / 63°C
Poultry	All poultry (breasts, whole bird, legs, thighs, wings, ground poultry, giblets and stuffing	165°F / 74°C
Pork and ham	Fresh pork, including fresh ham Rest time: 3 minutes	145°F / 63°C
	Precooked ham to reheat	165°F / 74°C
Eggs and egg dishes	Eggs	Cook until yolk and white are firm
	Egg dishes (e.g. quiche, frittata)	160°F /71°C

Food	Type	Internal Temperature
Leftovers and Casseroles	Leftovers and casseroles	165°F / 74°C
Seafood	Fish and fins	145°F / 63°C or until flesh is opaque and separates easily
	Shrimp, lobster, crab and scallops	Cook until flesh is pearly or white and opaque
	Clams, oysters, mussels	Cook until shells open during cooking

Copied from FoodSafety.gov (https://www.foodsafety.gov/food-safety-charts/safe-minimum-cooking-temperature). Last reviewed 3/11/22

Stir-Fry

Image: Beef Stir Fry

Figure 5: Build a Stir-Fry

Protein	Aromatics	Hard Vegetables	Quick Cooking Vegetables
Chicken	Ginger	Carrots	Asparagus
Fish	Shallots	Cauliflower	Bean sprouts
Meat	Scallions	Celery	Green leafy – kale, Bok choy, spinach
Seitan	Garlic	Broccoli	Mushrooms
Tofu		Green beans	Sugar snap peas
Tempeh		Cabbage	Water chestnuts

The secret to stir-frying is to cook over high heat for a brief amount of time using an oil that has a high smoke point. Making a stir-fry is a great way to introduce more vegetables into the diet as not much meat is needed (if at all).

1. **Choose an oil:** Peanut, safflower, canola, grape seed and sunflower (see the chapter on Fats and Oils for further information).
2. **Prepare the ingredients into bite-size pieces:** It is very important to have all ingredients ready to go because once the cooking process starts it happens quickly.

a. Cut vegetables into thinner, longer pieces (see the picture above) and the same size so that they cook at the same time.

b. Cut meat (against the grain for tenderness) for maximum surface area and even cooking.

3. **Identify the cooking time:** Separate ingredients into groups with similar cooking times. For example, the meat would be separated from vegetables, and within the vegetables there are those that are harder and take more time (carrots, broccoli, and green beans) versus those that cook quickly (mushrooms, and green leafy vegetables for example).

4. **Heat the wok or cast-iron pan and then add the oil:** Once the oil is glimmering it is ready.

a. Cook the meat first, remove from the pan into a bowl (to be added at the end so as not to overcook the meat). If using tofu, tempeh, or seitan, this step can be avoided as the tofu will cook at the same time as the vegetables. Stir often.

b. Cook the aromatics quickly making sure they do not burn. Once you can smell them, add the vegetables.

c. Cook the harder vegetables and when almost ready add the quicker cooking vegetables (and tofu). Stir often. Add flavor to the vegetables and then add the meat (if using) back in.

5. **Add flavor**: Choose any of the following and/or add your own favorites: Add, then taste, then add again if desired. If a thick sauce is desired (not necessary) mix 1 tablespoon of cornstarch with 3 to 4 tablespoons of water and add to the stir-fry.

a. Soy sauce or Tamari

b. Fish sauce, oyster sauce

c. Asian wine (Shaoxing)

d. Rice vinegar

e. Curry paste

f. Stock — beef, chicken, and vegetable

g. Toasted sesame oil

h. Coconut aminos

Moist Methods for Meat/Fish/Poultry (McGee, 2004)

Moist methods for cooking meats, fish, and poultry include stewing, braising, poaching and steaming. For all methods, a liquid water medium is used, which can be flavored.

Water used in these methods allows for an even and rapid distribution of heat, which should be kept below the boiling point (180°F/80°C). The water-based medium can impart flavor and be used as a sauce afterward. What moist methods cannot do however is brown meat as water never reaches a high enough temperature like oil does.

Image: Moist Cooking Methods for Protein

- **Stew** meat and poultry —
  - There is an option to pre-brown meat before cooking in the water/broth to add a layer of flavor.
  - Stewing allows for the addition of lots of vegetables
    - Nutrients are leached into the surrounding liquid so make sure to consume it.
  - A long slow cook is needed with tough pieces of meat. Note: the tough connective tissue must reach an internal heat of 160°F/71°C to 180°F/82°C for it to start to break down.
- **Braise** meat and poultry — the piece of meat is larger than that used for stewing and less liquid is required. The same rule applies to a tough piece of meat.
- **Steam** meat and poultry — this should be reserved for thin tender cuts of meat or poultry, or you run the risk of overcooking and drying it out. Herbs and spices can be added to the water. Another method is to wrap the piece of meat in something (banana leaf, corn husk, foil, cabbage leaf or parchment) to prevent the steam from drying it out.
- **Poach** meat and poultry. Poaching is not the same as boiling or simmering because of the temperature used:
  - Steaming occurs when water turns to steam above the boiling point, boiling occurs at 212°F/100°C, simmering at 185°F/85°C to 205°F/96°C, and poaching at 160°F/71°C to 180°F/82°C.
  - It is a gentle method — few if any bubbles rise up — and is usually reserved for eggs and fish.
  - The food is gently slipped into the hot liquid slowly using a spoon, tongs, or fork.

It is important to allow time after cooking for the meat, fish, poultry to cool so that it can absorb water as it cools. It should be **served around 120°F/50°C.**

Build a More Healthful Burger

- If using beef, purchase 90% lean (and grass-fed if available and affordable).
- Swap beef burgers for turkey, chicken, fish or vegetable-based burgers.
- Make a blended burger https://www.mushroomcouncil.org/foodservice/the-blend/.
- Build a burger bowl: Instead of a hamburger with a refined grain bun, saturated-fat-laden sauces, or cheese, choose to make a burger bowl instead. Add lettuce or other green to the

base, place 2 to 3 ounces of cooked ground meat in one section (divide it into pie slices), and add chopped tomatoes, pickles, onion, and sauteed mushrooms to the other sections.

Build a More Healthful Taco

Image: Healthier Taco

- Use less red meat, which can be accomplished by sautéing black beans (or another legume) with the hamburger meat, and/or adding puréed mushrooms. Or, switch from red meat to turkey, fish, chicken or plant-based meat.
- Add diced vegetables such as corn kernels and peppers.
- Add a lot of vegetables to the taco to the point of overflowing.

LEGUMES AND PLANT-BASED PROTEIN

Beans and legumes can be purchased either dried or canned. Working with dried beans does involve some planning ahead as they require soaking and a longer cooking time, however, the cooking process itself is not overly difficult. Dried beans can also be prepared and cooked in large batches and then frozen until they are ready to be used. Canned beans offer a convenient alternative, but be sure to rinse contents well before using to remove any additional sodium or other additives.

Adding legumes to meat dishes is a great cost-effective way to make a meal go further; plus, it adds a host of nutritional benefits like phytonutrients, fiber, vitamins and minerals.
- Add adzuki, garbanzo, or black beans to sautéed taco meat. After the meat is cooked, add cooked legumes and sauté for a minute or two. Add taco seasoning and continue to cook as directed. This can double the number of tacos for just pennies.
- Add any type of bean or a mixture of beans to soups and stews. You will want to soak the dried beans in water overnight before using, or rinse and add lentils as long as you will be cooking for over an hour. Note: **Do not add acid until the end** — vinegar, lime, or lemon juice — as that will **slow down the cooking process for legumes**.

Replace traditional recipes with a vegetable-protein option
- Make a tofu scramble instead of scrambled eggs

- Use tofu to thicken a smoothie instead of dairy

FLAVOR DEVELOPMENT

- Mix protein blends — substitute minced mushrooms (for up to 50% of the meat) and add leafy greens, peppers, and onions to ground meat to both enhance the flavor, as well as increase vegetable intake
- Utilize non-meat savory (umami) ingredients to mimic the savory-ness of meat — mushrooms, tomatoes, onions and soy sauce, for example
- Select cooking methods to increase the flavor and texture of the dish

SAFETY TIPS

The CDC's Four Steps to Food Safety lists the following safety tips for cooking with protein:

Clean: Wash your hands before working with any food.

Separate: Keep eggs, raw meat, poultry and seafood separate from other food.
- Use a dedicated cutting board reserved for raw meat, clean thoroughly after use.
- In the refrigerator keep raw meat on the lower shelf and separate from other food so that raw juices do not spill on the food below it.

Cook to the Right Temperature:

- 145 °F/63 °C — fish with fins
- 145 °F/63 °C — whole cuts of beef (and veal), lamb, pork (and ham)
- 160 °F/71 °C — ground meat
- 165 °F/74 °C — leftovers and casseroles; all poultry

Refrigerate: Bacteria can multiply when perishable food is exposed to temperatures between 40°F/4°C and 140°F/60°C (The Danger Zone). Refrigerate within two hours (and within one hour if the outside temperature is above 90°F/32°C).

COOKING WITH PLANT-BASED MEAT ALTERNATIVES

(This section is also found in the *Vegetarian Diet* chapter)

Soy-based meat alternatives include tofu and tempeh, while seitan is made from wheat gluten. These alternatives are complete proteins, making them a great vegetarian choice. On their own, there is not much flavor, but the great thing about these products is that they can easily pick up the flavor of the marinade.

Table 13: Plant-Based Meat Alternatives

Type of Product	Made From...	Flavor and Texture	Best Used for...
Tofu	Soybeans are boiled and curdled, then pressed	Very subtle, bean-like flavor, but it absorbs others flavors very well. Texture is creamy and varies from soft to extra firm.	Soft: Smoothies and sauces, raw desserts Medium: Soups Firm: Tofu scramble, stir-fry, baked (use when you want to retain the shape) Extra firm: Same as for firm, plus grilled and crumbled
Tofu — silken (Japanese tofu)	Cooked soybeans that are unpressed and not curdled or drained	Subtle taste and is much more delicate than regular tofu listed above. It has a custard-like texture.	Best used in sauces, desserts, smoothies, and salad dressings. It can also be used in baking to replace oil, eggs, or cream
Tempeh	Soybeans are cooked, fermented, and pressed into patties	Nutty flavor with a firm texture	Baked, grilled, stir-fried, barbeque, fried and in soups
Natto	Soybeans are soaked, cooked, and fermented with a rich source of probiotic	Strong fermented smell and gooey, stringy texture (takes getting used to)	Can be eaten from the package with special sauce and mustard, added to grains, or topped with an egg
Seitan	Wheat gluten that has been shaped and cooked	Savory flavor and chewy texture. Its texture is close to meat as it is almost all protein too.	Most like meat in texture. It can also pick up flavors very well. You can do anything with seitan that you can do with meat.

Successfully cooking with plant-based meat alternatives requires the addition of flavor, as by themselves the options have very little taste. What they lack in taste is more than made up for by their ability to absorb flavors like a sponge. You can turn a basic block of plant protein into anything. Listed below are examples of some liquids and spices that can be used to marinate plant-based proteins – the varieties are endless.

Table 14: Liquid Marinade Ingredients to Choose From

Sweet	Salty	Acid	Other
Orange, peach, or other fruit juice	Soy sauce	Lime juice	Heat — Sriracha
Maple syrup	Tamari	Lemon juice	Olive oil
Rice vinegar	Liquid aminos	Rice vinegar	Spices

Build a Marinade Spice Blend

Select a spice blend, which can transport the eater anywhere they want to go in the world. The basics are soy sauce, garlic powder, and onion powder. Feel free to experiment with the spices listed in Figure 6 below or other favorites.

- For crazy-delicious spice blends, read Ottolenghi's Flavor Cookbook.
- Skordo has some amazing ready-made blends too.

Figure 6: Spice Blends

Caribbean	Mexican	Thai	Italian
Allspice	Black pepper	Black pepper	Basil
Black pepper	Chili powder	Cayenne	Black pepper
Cinnamon	Cumin	Coriander	Garlic
Garlic	Garlic	Cumin	Oregano (Italian)
Ginger	Onion	Fenugreek	Sage
Nutmeg	Oregano (Mexican)	Ginger	Thyme
Red pepper flakes	Red pepper flakes	Mustard (dried)	
Smoked paprika	Sweet paprika	Turmeric	
Thyme			

Steps to Cooking With Tofu

Image: Cooking With Tofu

Step 1: Press to drain excess water from firm or extra firm tofu, or tempeh only. This will allow it to pick up more flavors and become crispy when fried or baked. This step is optional and can be skipped when in a hurry. Tofu can also be frozen for up to three months.

- Drain the excess water
- Place tofu on a plate and wrap in a dish towel or paper towel
- Top with a cutting board and add weight to it - a frying pan works great
- Let sit for up to 30 minutes, and then it is ready to use — don't press for more than four hours

Step 2: Marinate. This is a critical step unless the tofu is to be eaten straight from the package, thrown in smoothies, or added to soups. When tofu is cooked — baked, fried, grilled, stir-fried — marinate it first to add flavor.

- In a bowl or glass pan:
  - Add orange, lemon, or lime juice (or other liquid)
  - Add soy sauce (not much is needed)
  - Add spices
- Whisk together before adding sliced or cubed tofu or tempeh
- Let marinate for 30 minutes

Step 3: Select a cooking method:

- Bake at 400 °F/204 °C for 20 minutes on a dry baking sheet; flip halfway through
- Stir-fry in oil with vegetables
- Panfry with a tiny bit of oil; turn over when browned on one side. It is done when both sides are browned
- Place on a grill or BBQ and turn halfway through. Both sides should have brown grill marks
- Add to soups or stews but press first — there is no need to marinate it first as it will pick up the flavor of the soup

Steps to Cooking With Tempeh:

Image: Cooking With Tempeh

1. **Steam** one inch cubed or sliced tempeh for 10 minutes. This helps to soften the tempeh to allow flavors from a marinade to seep in.

2. **Marinate** in liquid (as listed previously for tofu) for 30 minutes. Save marinade for another time or to add some extra sauce when the tempeh is cooked. It can also make a great sauce for stir-fry.

3. **Select your cooking method:**
   a. **Bake** at 425 °F/218 °C for 20 minutes on parchment paper, turning over after 10 minutes.
   b. **Grill** on a lightly oiled grill for five to six minutes on each side depending on the thickness. The steaming step can be skipped as a tougher texture is needed to hold up to grilling.
   c. **Stir-fry** with vegetables in a wok (lightly oiled) until vegetables are crisp but tender.

Steps to Cooking With Seitan:

Image: Cooking with Seitan

Seitan is already cooked and just needs to be reheated. Unless it has been packaged in oil, it has very little carbohydrates and fat.

1. Open the package of premade seitan or make your own with vital wheat gluten (follow directions on package) and create the shape you are looking for.
   a. Crumbled to resemble hamburger meat — add a sloppy Joe sauce, and you are good to go
   b. Chunks can resemble beef stew meat and can be used in place of meat in stews and soups
   c. Lobes of seitan can be braised whole, like pot roast in a mushroom-based sauce
2. It is important to keep seitan moist so that it can pick up flavors. When it dries out, its texture changes to a tough, chewy piece of meat alternative

Image: Seitan Dishes

A word on the new, highly processed, plant-based meat alternatives: *Beyond Beef* and *Beyond Meat* are made with pea protein, and the *Impossible Burger* is made with soy protein. These options are considered highly processed plant-based alternatives to beef burgers. Most are high in saturated fat (from coconut oil – a saturated fat) and contain more sodium than beef burgers. Dr. Gardner at Stanford Prevention Research Center, with support from *Beyond Meat*, conducted an eight-week trial whereby approximately 30 participants ate two servings a day of Beyond Beef or two servings a day of mostly red meat products. He and his team measured a marker for cardiovascular disease — trimethylamine N-oxide (TMAO) — and found it was lower when the participants were eating the plant-based meat product, and so were levels of LDL cholesterol.

Our experts (mostly) agree — using plant-based processed alternatives can be a step in the right direction toward eating a whole food plant-based diet. There is concern about the absence of phytochemicals that a whole vegetable-made burger can provide versus these options made with a protein isolate made out of pea or soy. One of our experts reminded us that mock meat products have been used in Asia for centuries and are a part of their cuisine. For a great opinion piece, read Dr. Hu's opinion on Harvard's Nutrition Source.

When it comes to land use and the environment, there is no question that switching to a plant-based diet is healthier for the planet: Land Use of Foods per 1,000 Kilocalories.

SECTION 11:
SERVING PROTEIN

THE PROTEIN FLIP

Image: Protein Flip

The Protein Flip is a very useful document put together by the Culinary Institute of America (CIA) and Harvard T.H. Chan School of Public Health. The goal for menu offerings is to offer poultry/seafood/vegetarian options **40%** of the time, meat as a condiment **5%** of the time, meat at a celebratory occasion **5%** of the time, and **50%** of the time use the protein flip.

Examples of the protein flip are:
- Serve 2 ounces of meat, poultry, or seafood instead of 4 to 6+ ounces
- Protein can either be used as a side, a condiment, or mixed in with plant-based protein as the main focus (stir-fry, for example)
- Create blends of both plant and animal sources of protein for burgers, meatballs, pasta sauce, taco meat and more. Adjust the proportions; start by replacing one half of the animal protein with a plant source and continue to increase until either it becomes unpalatable to those that are eating it or until a full swap has been made (100% plant-based protein).

Animal Protein	Plants
Beef, veal	Carrots
Chicken	Grains – quinoa, farro, barley, buckwheat …
Lamb	Leafy greens
Pork	Legumes – lentils, beans
Turkey	Mushrooms
	Nuts

- Create tacos, pasta dishes, and rice bowls using plant-based protein sources and focusing on a wide array of flavors used around the world.
- Replace large dishes with small plant-forward plates — tapas or mezze for example.
- Rethink the mixed grill by serving a large portion of vegetables, some seafood, and a small amount of meat.

SECTION 12:

MENU PLANNING WITH PROTEIN

A 2021 Culinary Institute of America report found the following:
- One-quarter of consumers eat meat every day
- Millennials are the top consumers of daily animal and plant-based protein, but they are also the most open to eating a plant-forward diet
- Boomers are the least willing to purchase plant-based and plant-forward foods at a restaurant

- Many consumers believe that animal-based protein is the most healthful option

The CIA's Protein Plays: Foodservice Strategies for our Future is a great resource (https://www.ciaprochef.com/MOC/ProteinPlays.pdf/) .

Table 15 lists the recommended number of servings of protein each day for various age and gender groups, according to the Dietary Guidelines for Americans. Keep the total daily amount in mind when planning a meal or menu.

Table 15: Protein Servings Per Day

Age (years)	Amount Per Day in Ounce Equivalents*	Serving size
2 to 3	2 ounce eq	½ ounce eq = ½ egg; ½ ounce meat
4 to 8	4 ounce eq	4 to 6 years: 1 ounce eq = 1 tablespoon peanut butter; 1 egg; 1 ounce of meat or fish 7 to 8 years: 1 ½ to 2 ounce eq = 1 ½ to 2 tablespoons nut butter; 1 ½ to 2 ounce meat; ½ cup lentils; 2 eggs
Boys 9 to 13	5 ounce eq	
Boys 14 to 18	6 ½ ounce eq	
Girls 9 to 13	5 ounce eq	
Girls 14 to 18	5 ounce eq	2 to 3 ounce eq = 1 small chicken breast; 2 to 3 ounce meat; 1 small hamburger; ½ to ¾ cup lentils or other cooked dry bean (pinto, lima, navy, white and black beans).
Women 19 to 30	5 ½ ounce eq	
Women 31 to 50	5 ounce eq	
Women 51+	5 ounce eq	
Men 19 to 30	6 ½ ounce eq	
Men 31 to 50	6 ounce eq	
Men 51+	5 ½ ounce eq	

*1 ounce equivalent (ounce eq) = 1 ounce cooked beef, chicken, turkey, pork, lamb, fish, 1 egg, ½ ounce nuts or seeds, 1 tablespoon nut butter, ¼ cup cooked legumes (black, kidney, pinto or white beans, chickpeas, lentils, split peas), 1 ounce tempeh, 1 tablespoon hummus.

MENU PLANNING

When planning out meals for the week or meals for the day, it is helpful to think about the following concepts:

1. **Variety:** Select a combination of protein sources — both plant- and animal-based — throughout the day and week. Start by assessing the current situation: How many times a week and a day are animal-based protein sources served/eaten? From this information, you can begin to encourage your client/patient to make one change at a time (or you make the change in your dining room/restaurant) until they are following a more plant-forward diet.

2. **Plan the meal around the protein source:** Make a template of the protein sources throughout the week, like the one below. From there, add on an assortment of plant-based proteins, vegetables, fruits and grains. Using the protein goal outlined for a menu (discussed previously) and translating that into the 21 weekly meals, a week's worth of meals would include:
   - Poultry, fish and vegetarian options **(40% = 8 ½ meals)**
   - Celebratory meat **(5% = one meal on special occasions)**
   - Decreased amount of meat **(5% = one meal a week)**
   - Protein flip for 10 to 11 meals **(50% = 10 ½ meals)**

Table 16: A Week's Worth of Protein Sources for Meals

Day of the Week	Breakfast	Lunch	Dinner
Monday	Egg	Cheese	Turkey burger blend
Tuesday	Yogurt	Salad with legumes	Fish (taco)
Wednesday	Nuts/seeds	Rice bowl with 2 ounces salmon	Vegetarian meal
Thursday	Grains with milk	Legumes	2 ounces poultry per serving in a stir-fry
Friday	Egg	2 slices chicken on whole wheat bread	Bolognese on whole wheat pasta (with lots of grounded veggies and small amount of beef)
Saturday	Yogurt	Salad grain bowl with nuts	Legumes — veggie burger
Sunday	Nuts and seeds	Tuna fish salad	Chicken

3. **Less is more:** Think about serving no more than 2 ounces of animal-based protein per meal for the majority of meals. In order to be successful (the people you cook for enjoying their meal), begin by slowly decreasing the portion size of animal-based proteins while you increase vegetables and grains on the plate. Keep this up until you get pushback. At this time, it is important to talk to your client(s), customer, patient, to see if they are willing to continue decreasing animal-based protein in their diet. It is your job to make — or teach them how to make — the plant-forward dishes spectacularly delicious. It is their choice to decide how far they want to go.

SECTION 13:

PRACTICAL TIPS FOR PROTEIN INTAKE

Dietary patterns such as the Mediterranean Diet and the DASH Diet are clearly associated with positive health outcomes, and one thing both of these patterns have in common is a focus on plant-based protein foods. Here are some easy, practical ways to begin to increase plant-based proteins in the diet:

1. Sprinkle sunflower seeds or chopped nuts on a salad.
2. Add seeds or nuts to baked goods or pancakes.
3. Make a grain and bean salad as a side or main dish. Potential combinations could be quinoa with black beans or farro with garbanzo beans. Add in some chopped season veggies to complete the dish.
4. Snack on edamame (green soybeans) or hummus with veggies or pita.
5. Make a stir-fry with tofu or tempeh instead of meat or poultry.
6. Serve a high-protein grain such as farro or teff as a side dish instead of white rice or mashed potatoes.
7. Make your own trail mix of nuts, seeds, and dried fruit.
8. Add extra grains and beans to vegetable soup.

SUMMARY

Protein is an essential nutrient for health and can be obtained from plant and animal sources. While protein itself has a neutral effect on health outcomes (provided you're eating enough), other nutrients that accompany protein in food — fat, sodium, vitamins and minerals, fiber, additives and preservatives — will influence whether or not the source of protein is associated with either an increased or decreased risk of chronic disease.

What things should be considered when selecting protein sources that are health-promoting?
- First, choose protein from plants most often. Legumes, nuts, seeds and whole grains not only provide health benefits but also a host of other important nutrients and are typically very low in saturated fat and sodium. When choosing plant-based proteins, be sure to eat a wide variety to ensure all essential amino acids will be present in your diet.
- Second, if you choose to include animal sources of protein, make conscientious choices so that these foods are still health-promoting. Include a variety of seafood, and when choosing

poultry, remove the skin so as to limit saturated fat intake. Eggs are also a great source of high-quality protein.

- Third, if you enjoy red meat, enjoy it in small amounts and only occasionally. Look for cuts of meat that have very little visible fat and choose ground meat that is no more than 15% fat. Processed meats should be minimized or avoided altogether, as these meats have the clearest relationship with chronic disease risk.

Appendix 1: Recipes and How To

Image: Italian Chicken with Whole Wheat Pasta and Heirloom Tomatoes

Italian Chicken with Whole Wheat Pasta and Heirloom Tomatoes by Chef Russell

Yield   4 people
Time   30 minutes
Difficulty   Easy

Ingredients

- 10 ounce whole-wheat spaghetti, dry
- 4 ounces olive oil or olive oil blend (75/25 - Canola oil/Olive oil)
- 16 ounces chicken thighs, excess fat removed
- 2 each portabella mushroom
- 1 each Ronde De Nice squash or zucchini
- ½ itch yellow onion, medium
- 4 each garlic cloves, sliced
- 1.5 cups heirloom cherry tomatoes, cut in half
- 9 each basil leaves, julienned or chopped
- 1 cup white wine, Chardonnay or Riesling
- 4 ounces Pecorino Romano, grated
- 2 ounces extra virgin olive oil (EVOO), or flavored oil

Methods

1. Toss the chicken in 1 ounce of olive oil blend, salt, and black pepper
2. In a separate container toss the mushroom and zucchini with ½ ounce of olive oil blend, salt, and black pepper
3. Grill chicken and vegetables until fully cooked. Allow to cool to room temperature
4. Cut the chicken thighs into ¾ inch cubes. Also, cut the squash and mushroom the same size and set aside

5. Bring 3 quarts of water to a boil in a 4-quart pot; add a touch of salt and 2 tablespoons of olive oil to the water. Once the water comes to a boil add the spaghetti to the water stirring immediately to ensure the pasta does not stick to one another

6. Stir for 30 seconds and then stir occasionally until al dente. Al dente means: cooked but firm. Strain in a colander and rinse with cold water. Set aside

7. While the pasta is cooking, place 1 ounce of olive oil blend in a sauté pan over medium-high heat. Add the onions, sautéing for approximately 3 minutes, stirring constantly.

8. Add the garlic sautéing for 1 minute to allow the garlic to bloom or become fragrant.

9. Add the cubed chicken, squash, mushroom, heirloom tomato and basil, sautéing for 4 minutes.

10. Add the wine, allowing the wine to reduce by half, cooking for approximately 4 minutes

11. Toss in the pasta, allowing it to reheat for 1 minute; then add 3 ounces of cheese, folding in to melt with the pasta and other ingredients

12. Toss in the EVOO or finishing oil along with salt and pepper to taste

13. Separate into 4 plates and garnish with the remaining grated pecorino and a sprig of fresh basil

Turkey Taco Meat by Chef Russell

Image: Turkey Taco Meat

Ingredients

- ½ teaspoon morita chili powder
- 2 tablespoons chili powder
- 2 teaspoons cumin
- 1 teaspoon coriander
- 1 tablespoon Mexican oregano
- 1 teaspoon smoked paprika
- ½ teaspoon onion powder
- ½ teaspoon garlic powder
- ½ teaspoon Himalayan salt
- ½ teaspoon pepper, black
- 2 tablespoons olive oil
- 12 ounces ground turkey
- ½ cup chicken stock,

- 1 tablespoon apple cider vinegar
- 1 teaspoon maple syrup
- 2 tablespoons chopped cilantro

Methods

1. Gather all ingredients and equipment prior to beginning the recipe
2. Mix the two chili powders, cumin, coriander, oregano, paprika, onion, garlic, salt and pepper together in a small bowl; mix well
3. In a skillet, add the olive oil and heat over medium-high
4. Add the ground turkey cooking until fully cooked (no pink remaining). While cooking, continue to break up the meat to disperse any clumps. Cook for approximately 5 minutes
5. Add the spice mix and chicken stock
6. Reduce heat to simmer, stirring occasionally, until most of the liquid has been absorbed. About 10 minutes
7. Add the vinegar, maple syrup, and cilantro, allowing to cook for an additional 3 minutes

Marinara Sauce by Chef Russell

Image: Marinara Sauce

Ingredients

- 2 tablespoons extra virgin olive oil
- 1 cup yellow, chopped onions
- 2 tablespoons minced garlic
- ½ cup red wine
- 8 ounces tomato paste
- 1 cup water
- 24 ounces San Marzano stewed tomatoes with juice
- 1 teaspoon dried oregano
- Pinch of ground cinnamon
- ½ teaspoon crushed, red chili flakes
- 4 tablespoons fresh, chopped Italian parsley leaves
- 4 tablespoons chopped basil - including the stems

- ¼ teaspoons Himalayan salt,
- Pinch black pepper
- 1 tablespoon maple syrup, if needed based on flavor profile of tomatoes (if they are bitter or not sweet enough, add some maple syrup)

Preparation

- Gather all ingredients and equipment prior to beginning the recipe
- In a medium saucepan, heat the oil over medium-high heat
- Once the oil begins to shimmer, add the onions and sauté for 3 minutes
- Add the garlic sautéing for an additional minute to bloom or become fragrant
- Add the red wine, reducing to au sec (almost dry)
- Add the tomato paste, cooking until it begins to caramelize
- Add the water, allowing it to come to a boil
- Add the tomatoes, oregano, cinnamon, chili flakes; bring to a boil
- Reduce the temperature to simmer, allowing to cook for 1 and ½ hours
- Add water if necessary for consistency later in the cooking process
- Blend well with an immersion blender or blender
- Add the parsley, basil, salt and pepper
- Taste for sweetness adding the maple syrup if necessary
- It is best to make the sauce a day in advance to enhance the melding of flavor
- Cool to 70 degrees within 2 hours and 40 degrees within 6 hours; then put in the refrigerator
- Reheat to a boil prior to serving

REFERENCES

2015-2020 Dietary Guidelines | health.gov. Retrieved March 17, 2020, from https://health.gov/our-work/food-nutrition/2015-2020-dietary-guidelines/guidelines/

Alagawany, M., Elnesr, S. S., Farag, M. R., Abd El-Hack, M. E., Khafaga, A. F., Taha, A. E., Tiwari, R., Yatoo, Mohd. I., Bhatt, P., Khurana, S. K., & Dhama, K. (2019). Omega-3 and Omega-6 Fatty Acids in Poultry Nutrition: Effect on Production Performance and Health. Animals : An Open Access Journal from MDPI, 9(8). https://doi.org/10.3390/ani9080573

Arnett Donna K., Blumenthal Roger S., Albert Michelle A., Buroker Andrew B., Goldberger Zachary D., Hahn Ellen J., Himmelfarb Cheryl Dennison, Khera Amit, Lloyd-Jones Donald, McEvoy J. William, Michos Erin D., Miedema Michael D., Muñoz Daniel, Smith Sidney C., Virani Salim S., Williams Kim A., Yeboah Joseph, & Ziaeian Boback. (2019). 2019 ACC/AHA Guideline on the Primary Prevention of Cardiovascular Disease: A Report of the American College of Cardiology/American Heart Association Task Force on Clinical Practice Guidelines. Circulation, 140(11), e596–e646. https://doi.org/10.1161/CIR.0000000000000678

Beauchamp, G. K. (2009). Sensory and receptor responses to umami: An overview of pioneering work. The American Journal of Clinical Nutrition, 90(3), 723S-727S. https://doi.org/10.3945/ajcn.2009.27462E

Bernstein, A. M., Sun, Q., Hu, F. B., Stampfer, M. J., Manson, J. E., & Willett, W. C. (2010). Major dietary protein sources and risk of coronary heart disease in women. Circulation, 122(9), 876–883. https://doi.org/10.1161/CIRCULATIONAHA.109.915165

Blomstrand, E., Eliasson, J., Karlsson, H. K. R., & Köhnke, R. (2006). Branched-Chain Amino Acids Activate Key Enzymes in Protein Synthesis after Physical Exercise. The Journal of Nutrition, 136(1), 269S-273S. https://doi.org/10.1093/jn/136.1.269S

Bouvard, V., Loomis, D., Guyton, K. Z., Grosse, Y., Ghissassi, F. E., Benbrahim-Tallaa, L., Guha, N., Mattock, H., Straif, K., & International Agency for Research on Cancer Monograph Working Group. (2015). Carcinogenicity of consumption of red and processed meat. The Lancet. Oncology, 16(16), 1599–1600. https://doi.org/10.1016/S1470-2045(15)00444-1

Carson Jo Ann S., Lichtenstein Alice H., Anderson Cheryl A.M., Appel Lawrence J., Kris-Etherton Penny M., Meyer Katie A., Petersen Kristina, Polonsky Tamar, Van Horn Linda, & null null. (2020). Dietary Cholesterol and Cardiovascular Risk: A Science Advisory From the American Heart Association. Circulation, 141(3), e39–e53. https://doi.org/10.1161/CIR.0000000000000743

Chen, Q.-Y., Alarcon, S., Tharp, A., Ahmed, O. M., Estrella, N. L., Greene, T. A., Rucker, J., & Breslin, P. A. (2009). Perceptual variation in umami taste and polymorphisms in TAS1R taste receptor genes. The American Journal of Clinical Nutrition, 90(3), 770S-779S. https://doi.org/10.3945/ajcn.2009.27462N

CIA. (2016). The CIA challenges chefs to rethink the "protein portfolio" on their menus: The Institute releases "The Protein Flip," and protein plays signaling a new era for the foodservice industry. https://www.ciachef.edu/protein-portfolio-release

Coletta, J. M., Bell, S. J., & Roman, A. S. (2010). Omega-3 Fatty Acids and Pregnancy. Reviews in Obstetrics and Gynecology, 3(4), 163–171.

Daley, C. A., Abbott, A., Doyle, P. S., Nader, G. A., & Larson, S. (2010). A review of fatty acid profiles and antioxidant content in grass-fed and grain-fed beef. Nutrition Journal, 9, 10. https://doi.org/10.1186/1475-2891-9-10

Davoodi, S. H., Shahbazi, R., Esmaeili, S., Sohrabvandi, S., Mortazavian, A., Jazayeri, S., & Taslimi, A. (2016). Health-Related Aspects of Milk Proteins. Iranian Journal of Pharmaceutical Research : IJPR, 15(3), 573–591.

Dwyer, T., Hynes, K. L., Fryer, J. L., Blizzard, C. L., & Dalais, F. S. (2008). The lack of effect of isoflavones on high-density lipoprotein cholesterol concentrations in adolescent boys: A 6-week randomised trial. Public Health Nutrition, 11(9), 955–962. https://doi.org/10.1017/S1368980007000869

Farvid, M. S., Cho, E., Chen, W. Y., Eliassen, A. H., & Willett, W. C. (2015). Adolescent meat intake and breast cancer risk. International Journal of Cancer. Journal International Du Cancer, 136(8), 1909–1920. https://doi.org/10.1002/ijc.29218

FoodData Central. Retrieved March 28, 2020, from https://fdc.nal.usda.gov/

Fraser, G. E. (1992). A Possible Protective Effect of Nut Consumption on Risk of Coronary Heart Disease: The Adventist Health Study. Archives of Internal Medicine, 152(7), 1416. https://doi.org/10.1001/archinte.1992.00400190054010

Fuller, N. R., Sainsbury, A., Caterson, I. D., Denyer, G., Fong, M., Gerofi, J., Leung, C., Lau, N. S., Williams, K. H., Januszewski, A. S., Jenkins, A. J., & Markovic, T. P. (2018). Effect of a high-egg diet on cardiometabolic risk factors in people with type 2 diabetes: The Diabetes and Egg (DIABEGG) Study—randomized weight-loss and follow-up phase. The American Journal of Clinical Nutrition, 107(6), 921–931. https://doi.org/10.1093/ajcn/nqy048

Goh, Y. M., & Lim, K. M. (2004). Effects of cooking methods on the n-3 PUFA content of PUFA-enriched eggs. 332–333. http://psasir.upm.edu.my/id/eprint/65113/

Goyal, A., Sharma, V., Upadhyay, N., Gill, S., & Sihag, M. (2014). Flax and flaxseed oil: An ancient medicine & modern functional food. Journal of Food Science and Technology, 51(9), 1633–1653. https://doi.org/10.1007/s13197-013-1247-9

Gribble, M. O., Karimi, R., Feingold, B. J., Nyland, J. F., O'Hara, T. M., Gladyshev, M. I., & Chen, C. Y. (2016). Mercury, selenium and fish oils in marine food webs and implications for human health. Journal of the Marine Biological Association of the United Kingdom. Marine Biological Association of the United Kingdom, 96(1), 43–59. https://doi.org/10.1017/S0025315415001356

Guasch-Ferre, M., Liu, X., Malik, V., Sun, Q., Willett, W., Manson, J., Rexrode, K., Li, Y., Hu, F., & Bhupathiraju, S. (2017). Nut Consumption and Risk of Cardiovascular Disease | Journal of the American College of Cardiology. Journal of the American College of Cardiology, 70(20), 2519–2532.

Guasch-Ferre, M., Satija, A., Blondin, S., Janiszewski, M., & Emlen, E. (2019). Meta-Analysis of Randomized Controlled Trials of Red Meat Consumption in Comparison With Various Comparison Diets on Cardiovascular Risk Factors. Circulation, 139(15), 1828–1845.

Hamilton-Reeves, J. M., Vazquez, G., Duval, S. J., Phipps, W. R., Kurzer, M. S., & Messina, M. J. (2010). Clinical studies show no effects of soy protein or isoflavones on reproductive hormones in men: Results of a meta-analysis. Fertility and Sterility, 94(3), 997–1007. https://doi.org/10.1016/j.fertnstert.2009.04.038

Here's the Shocking Number of Peanuts You Eat Every Year | National Peanut Board. (2016). National Peanut Board. https://nationalpeanutboard.org/news/heres-the-shocking-number-of-peanuts-you-eat-every-year.htm

Higgs, J. D. (2000). The changing nature of red meat: 20 years of improving nutritional quality. Trends in Food Science & Technology, 11(3), 85–95. https://doi.org/10.1016/S0924-2244(00)00055-8

Holscher, H. D., Guetterman, H. M., Swanson, K. S., An, R., Matthan, N. R., Lichtenstein, A. H., Novotny, J. A., & Baer, D. J. (2018). Walnut Consumption Alters the Gastrointestinal Microbiota, Microbially Derived Secondary Bile Acids, and Health Markers in Healthy Adults: A Randomized Controlled Trial. The Journal of Nutrition, 148(6), 861–867. https://doi.org/10.1093/jn/nxy004

Howe, P., Buckley, J., & Meyer, B. (2007). Long-chain omega-3 fatty acids in red meat. Nutrition & Dietetics, 64(s4), S135–S139. https://doi.org/10.1111/j.1747-0080.2007.00201.x

Hu, F. B., Stampfer, M. J., Manson, J. E., Rimm, E. B., Colditz, G. A., Rosner, B. A., Speizer, F. E., Hennekens, C. H., & Willett, W. C. (1998). Frequent nut consumption and risk of coronary heart disease in women: Prospective cohort study. BMJ : British Medical Journal, 317(7169), 1341–1345.

Hu, F. B., Stampfer, M. J., Rimm, E. B., Manson, J. E., & Ascherio, A. (1999). A Prospective Study of Egg Consumption and Risk of Cardiovascular Disease in Men and Women. JAMA, 281(15), 1387. https://doi.org/10.1001/jama.281.15.1387

Institute of Medicine. (2006). Dietary Reference Intakes: The Essential Guide to Nutrient Requirements. National Academies Press.

Jakobsen, J., & Knuthsen, P. (2014). Stability of vitamin D in foodstuffs during cooking. Food Chemistry, 148, 170–175. https://doi.org/10.1016/j.foodchem.2013.10.043

Jenkins, D. J. A., Kendall, C. W. C., Augustin, L. S. A., Mitchell, S., Sahye-Pudaruth, S., Blanco Mejia, S., Chiavaroli, L., Mirrahimi, A., Ireland, C., Bashyam, B., Vidgen, E., de Souza, R. J., Sievenpiper, J. L., Coveney, J., Leiter, L. A., & Josse, R. G. (2012). Effect of Legumes as Part of a Low Glycemic Index Diet on Glycemic Control and Cardiovascular Risk Factors in Type 2 Diabetes Mellitus: A Randomized Controlled Trial. Archives of Internal Medicine, 172(21), 1653. https://doi.org/10.1001/2013.jamainternmed.70

Jenkins, D. J. A., Mirrahimi, A., Srichaikul, K., Berryman, C. E., Wang, L., Carleton, A., Abdulnour, S., Sievenpiper, J. L., Kendall, C. W. C., & Kris-Etherton, P. M. (2010). Soy Protein Reduces Serum Cholesterol by Both Intrinsic and Food Displacement Mechanisms. The Journal of Nutrition, 140(12), 2302S-2311S. https://doi.org/10.3945/jn.110.124958

Kalita, S., Khandelwal, S., Madan, J., Pandya, H., Sesikeran, B., & Krishnaswamy, K. (2018). Almonds and Cardiovascular Health: A Review. Nutrients, 10(4). https://doi.org/10.3390/nu10040468

Karwowska, M., & Kononiuk, A. (2020). Nitrates/Nitrites in Food—Risk for Nitrosative Stress and Benefits. Antioxidants, 9(3). https://doi.org/10.3390/antiox9030241

Khan, M. A. K., & Wang, F. (2009). Mercury-selenium compounds and their toxicological significance: Toward a molecular understanding of the mercury-selenium antagonism. Environmental Toxicology and Chemistry, 28(8), 1567–1577. https://doi.org/10.1897/08-375.1

Killinger, K. M., Calkins, C. R., Umberger, W. J., Feuz, D. M., & Eskridge, K. M. (2004). A comparison of consumer sensory acceptance and value of domestic beef steaks and steaks from a branded, Argentine beef program,. Journal of Animal Science, 82(11), 3302–3307. https://doi.org/10.2527/2004.82113302x

Koh, W.-P., Wu, A. H., Wang, R., Ang, L.-W., Heng, D., Yuan, J.-M., & Yu, M. C. (2009). Gender-specific Associations Between Soy and Risk of Hip Fracture in the Singapore Chinese Health Study. American Journal of Epidemiology, 170(7), 901–909. https://doi.org/10.1093/aje/kwp220

Layman, D. K., Anthony, T. G., Rasmussen, B. B., Adams, S. H., Lynch, C. J., Brinkworth, G. D., & Davis, T. A. (2015). Defining meal requirements for protein to optimize metabolic roles of amino acids12345. The American Journal of Clinical Nutrition, 101(6), 1330S-1338S. https://doi.org/10.3945/ajcn.114.084053

Leaf, A. (2007). Prevention of sudden cardiac death by n-3 polyunsaturated fatty acids. Journal of Cardiovascular Medicine, 8, S27. https://doi.org/10.2459/01.JCM.0000289270.98105.b3

Leung Yinko, S. S. L., Stark, K. D., Thanassoulis, G., & Pilote, L. (2014). Fish Consumption and Acute Coronary Syndrome: A Meta-Analysis. The American Journal of Medicine, 127(9), 848-857.e2. https://doi.org/10.1016/j.amjmed.2014.04.016

Lichtenstein, A. H. (1998). Soy Protein, Isoflavones and Cardiovascular Disease Risk. The Journal of Nutrition, 128(10), 1589–1592. https://doi.org/10.1093/jn/128.10.1589

Lin, C.-Y., Kuo, H.-Y., & Wan, T.-C. (2014). Effect of Free-range Rearing on Meat Composition, Physical Properties and Sensory Evaluation in Taiwan Game Hens. Asian-Australasian Journal of Animal Sciences, 27(6), 880–885. https://doi.org/10.5713/ajas.2013.13646

Ložnjak, P., & Jakobsen, J. (2018). Stability of vitamin D3 and vitamin D2 in oil, fish and mushrooms after household cooking. Food Chemistry, 254, 144–149. https://doi.org/10.1016/j.foodchem.2018.01.182

Marangoni, F., Corsello, G., Cricelli, C., Ferrara, N., Ghiselli, A., Lucchin, L., & Poli, A. (2015). Role of poultry meat in a balanced diet aimed at maintaining health and wellbeing: An Italian consensus document. Food & Nutrition Research, 59. https://doi.org/10.3402/fnr.v59.27606

McAfee, A. J., McSorley, E. M., Cuskelly, G. J., Moss, B. W., Wallace, J. M. W., Bonham, M. P., & Fearon, A. M. (2010). Red meat consumption: An overview of the risks and benefits. Meat Science, 84(1), 1–13. https://doi.org/10.1016/j.meatsci.2009.08.029

McGee, H. (2004). On Food and Cooking: The Science and Lore of the Kitchen (1st edition). Scribner Books.

Messina, M. (2016). Soy and Health Update: Evaluation of the Clinical and Epidemiologic Literature. Nutrients, 8(12), 754. https://doi.org/10.3390/nu8120754

Messina, M., & Lane, B. (2007). Soy protein, soybean isoflavones and coronary heart disease risk: Where do we stand? Future Lipidology, 2(1), 55–74. https://doi.org/10.2217/17460875.2.1.55

Messina, M., & Messina, V. (2010). The Role of Soy in Vegetarian Diets. Nutrients, 2(8), 855–888. https://doi.org/10.3390/nu2080855

Messina, M., & Redmond, G. (2006). Effects of Soy Protein and Soybean Isoflavones on Thyroid Function in Healthy Adults and Hypothyroid Patients: A Review of the Relevant Literature. Thyroid, 16(3), 249–258. https://doi.org/10.1089/thy.2006.16.249

Micha, R., Michas, G., & Mozaffarian, D. (2012). Unprocessed red and processed meats and risk of coronary artery disease and type 2 diabetes—An updated review of the evidence. Current Atherosclerosis Reports, 14(6), 515–524. https://doi.org/10.1007/s11883-012-0282-8

Miki, A., Hashimoto, Y., Matsumoto, S., Ushigome, E., Fukuda, T., Sennmaru, T., Tanaka, M., Yamazaki, M., & Fukui, M. (2017). Protein Intake, Especially Vegetable Protein Intake, Is Associated with Higher Skeletal Muscle Mass in Elderly Patients with Type 2 Diabetes. Journal of Diabetes Research, 2017, 7985728. https://doi.org/10.1155/2017/7985728

Mínguez-Alarcón, L., Afeiche, M. C., Chiu, Y.-H., Vanegas, J. C., Williams, P. L., Tanrikut, C., Toth, T. L., Hauser, R., & Chavarro, J. E. (2015). Male soy food intake was not associated with in vitro fertilization outcomes among their partners attending a fertility center. Andrology, 3(4), 702–708. https://doi.org/10.1111/andr.12046

Nachvak, S. M., Moradi, S., Anjom-Shoae, J., Rahmani, J., Nasiri, M., Maleki, V., & Sadeghi, O. (2019). Soy, Soy Isoflavones, and Protein Intake in Relation to Mortality from All Causes, Cancers, and Cardiovascular Diseases: A Systematic Review and Dose-Response Meta-Analysis of Prospective Cohort Studies. Journal of the Academy of Nutrition and Dietetics, 119(9), 1483-1500.e17. https://doi.org/10.1016/j.jand.2019.04.011

Negro, M., Giardina, S., Marzani, B., & Marzatico, F. (2008). Branched-chain amino acid supplementation does not enhance athletic performance but affects muscle recovery and the immune system. J Sports Med Phys Fitness, 48(3), 347–351.

NHLBI. DASH Eating Plan | National Heart, Lung, and Blood Institute (NHLBI). Retrieved January 30, 2020, from https://www.nhlbi.nih.gov/health-topics/dash-eating-plan

Nimalaratne, C., Schieber, A., & Wu, J. (2016). Effects of storage and cooking on the antioxidant capacity of laying hen eggs. Food Chemistry, 194, 111–116. https://doi.org/10.1016/j.foodchem.2015.07.116

Ninomiya, K. (2015). Science of umami taste: Adaptation to gastronomic culture. Flavour, 4(1), 13. https://doi.org/10.1186/2044-7248-4-13

Norat, T., Bingham, S., Ferrari, P., Slimani, N., Jenab, M., Mazuir, M., Overvad, K., Olsen, A., Tjønneland, A., Clavel, F., Boutron-Ruault, M.-C., Kesse, E., Boeing, H., Bergmann, M. M., Nieters, A., Linseisen, J., Trichopoulou, A., Trichopoulos, D., Tountas, Y., … Riboli, E. (2005). Meat, fish, and colorectal cancer risk: The European Prospective Investigation into cancer and nutrition. Journal of the National Cancer Institute, 97(12), 906–916. https://doi.org/10.1093/jnci/dji164

Oken, E., & Bellinger, D. C. (2008). Fish consumption, methylmercury and child neurodevelopment. Current Opinion in Pediatrics, 20(2), 178–183. https://doi.org/10.1097/MOP.0b013e3282f5614c

Onneken, P. (2018). Salvia Hispanica L (Chia Seeds) as Brain Superfood—How Seeds Increase Intelligence. Glob J Health Sci, 10(7), 69–72.

Orlich, M. J., & Fraser, G. E. (2014). Vegetarian diets in the Adventist Health Study 2: A review of initial published findings1234. The American Journal of Clinical Nutrition, 100(1), 353S-358S. https://doi.org/10.3945/ajcn.113.071233

Pan, A., Sun, Q., Bernstein, A. M., Manson, J. E., Willett, W. C., & Hu, F. B. (2013). Changes in Red Meat Consumption and Subsequent Risk of Type 2 Diabetes: Three Cohorts of US Men and Women. JAMA Internal Medicine, 173(14). https://doi.org/10.1001/jamainternmed.2013.6633

Pan, A., Sun, Q., Bernstein, A. M., Schulze, M. B., Manson, J. E., Stampfer, M. J., Willett, W. C., & Hu, F. B. (2012). Red Meat Consumption and Mortality: Results from Two Prospective Cohort Studies. Archives of Internal Medicine, 172(7), 555–563. https://doi.org/10.1001/archinternmed.2011.2287

Pan, A., Sun, Q., Bernstein, A. M., Schulze, M. B., Manson, J. E., Willett, W. C., & Hu, F. B. (2011). Red meat consumption and risk of type 2 diabetes: 3 cohorts of US adults and an updated meta-analysis123. The American Journal of Clinical Nutrition, 94(4), 1088–1096. https://doi.org/10.3945/ajcn.111.018978

Pannucci, T. State of the American Diet—A Selection of Data Describing Current Dietary Intakes. 33.

Polak, R., Phillips, E. M., & Campbell, A. (2015). Legumes: Health Benefits and Culinary Approaches to Increase Intake. Clinical Diabetes : A Publication of the American Diabetes Association, 33(4), 198–205. https://doi.org/10.2337/diaclin.33.4.198

Preis, S. R., Stampfer, M. J., Spiegelman, D., Willett, W. C., & Rimm, E. B. (2010). Dietary protein and risk of ischemic heart disease in middle-aged men123. The American Journal of Clinical Nutrition, 92(5), 1265–1272. https://doi.org/10.3945/ajcn.2010.29626

Raliou, M., Wiencis, A., Pillias, A.-M., Planchais, A., Eloit, C., Boucher, Y., Trotier, D., Montmayeur, J.-P., & Faurion, A. (2009). Nonsynonymous single nucleotide polymorphisms in human tas1r1, tas1r3, and mGluR1 and individual taste sensitivity to glutamate. The American Journal of Clinical Nutrition, 90(3), 789S-799S. https://doi.org/10.3945/ajcn.2009.27462P

Réhault-Godbert, S., Guyot, N., & Nys, Y. (2019). The Golden Egg: Nutritional Value, Bioactivities, and Emerging Benefits for Human Health. Nutrients, 11(3), 684. https://doi.org/10.3390/nu11030684

Rehm, C. D., & Drewnowski, A. (2017). Replacing American snacks with tree nuts increases consumption of key nutrients among US children and adults: Results of an NHANES modeling study. Nutrition Journal, 16. https://doi.org/10.1186/s12937-017-0238-5

Richter, C. K., Skulas-Ray, A. C., Champagne, C. M., & Kris-Etherton, P. M. (2015). Plant protein and animal proteins: Do they differentially affect cardiovascular disease risk? Advances in Nutrition (Bethesda, Md.), 6(6), 712–728. https://doi.org/10.3945/an.115.009654

Roasting Meat 101 | Cook's Illustrated. Retrieved January 4, 2022, from http://www.cooksillustrated.com/how_tos/5544-roasting-meat-101

Rohrmann, S., Overvad, K., Bueno-de-Mesquita, H. B., Jakobsen, M. U., Egeberg, R., Tjønneland, A., Nailler, L., Boutron-Ruault, M.-C., Clavel-Chapelon, F., Krogh, V., Palli, D., Panico, S., Tumino, R., Ricceri, F., Bergmann, M. M., Boeing, H., Li, K., Kaaks, R., Khaw, K.-T., … Linseisen, J. (2013). Meat consumption and mortality—Results from the European Prospective Investigation into Cancer and Nutrition. BMC Medicine, 11, 63. https://doi.org/10.1186/1741-7015-11-63

Salmon, C. P., Knize, M. G., & Felton, J. S. (1997). Effects of marinating on heterocyclic amine carcinogen formation in grilled chicken. Food and Chemical Toxicology, 35(5), 433–441. https://doi.org/10.1016/S0278-6915(97)00020-3

Santanachote, P. Is Store-Bought Rotisserie Chicken Good for You? Consumer Reports. Retrieved June 5, 2021, from https://www.consumerreports.org/chicken/is-store-bought-rotisserie-chicken-good-for-you/

Shigemura, N., Shirosaki, S., Sanematsu, K., Yoshida, R., & Ninomiya, Y. (2009). Genetic and Molecular Basis of Individual Differences in Human Umami Taste Perception. PLoS ONE, 4(8), e6717. https://doi.org/10.1371/journal.pone.0006717

Signal to Noise Special Edition: GMOs and Our Food. Science in the News. Retrieved January 24, 2022, from https://sitn.hms.harvard.edu/signal-to-noise-special-edition-gmos-and-our-food/

Sinha, R., Cross, A. J., Graubard, B. I., Leitzmann, M. F., & Schatzkin, A. (2009). Meat intake and mortality: A prospective study of over half a million people. Archives of Internal Medicine, 169(6), 562–571. https://doi.org/10.1001/archinternmed.2009.6

Souza, P. R., Marques, R. M., Gomez, E. A., Colas, R. A., De Matteis, R., Zak, A., Patel, M., Collier, D. J., & Dalli, J. (2020). Enriched Marine Oil Supplements Increase Peripheral Blood Specialized Pro-Resolving Mediators

Concentrations and Reprogram Host Immune Responses. Circulation Research, 126(1), 75–90. https://doi.org/10.1161/CIRCRESAHA.119.315506

Stamler, J., Liu, K., Ruth, K. J., Pryer, J., & Greenland, P. (2002). Eight-year blood pressure change in middle-aged men: Relationship to multiple nutrients. Hypertension (Dallas, Tex.: 1979), 39(5), 1000–1006. https://doi.org/10.1161/01.hyp.0000016178.80811.d9

Stradley, L. (2015, April 30). Marinating Meat Guidelines. What's Cooking America? https://whatscookingamerica.net/marinatingsafely.htm

Sugizaki, C. S. A., & Naves, M. M. V. (2018). Potential Prebiotic Properties of Nuts and Edible Seeds and Their Relationship to Obesity. Nutrients, 10(11). https://doi.org/10.3390/nu10111645

The EAT-Lancet Commission on Food, Planet, Health. EAT. Retrieved June 13, 2020, from https://eatforum.org/eat-lancet-commission/

Tuttle, K. R., Milton, J. E., Packard, D. P., Shuler, L. A., & Short, R. A. (2012). Dietary Amino Acids and Blood Pressure: A Cohort Study of Patients With Cardiovascular Disease. American Journal of Kidney Diseases, 59(6), 803–809. https://doi.org/10.1053/j.ajkd.2011.12.026

Uribarri, J., Woodruff, S., Goodman, S., Cai, W., Chen, X., PYZIK, R., YONG, A., STRIKER, G. E., & VLASSARA, H. (2010). Advanced Glycation End Products in Foods and a Practical Guide to Their Reduction in the Diet. Journal of the American Dietetic Association, 110(6), 911-16.e12. https://doi.org/10.1016/j.jada.2010.03.018

U.S. Department of Agriculture and U.S. Department of Health and Human Services. (2020). Dietary Guidelines for Americans, 2020-2025 (9th Edition; p. 164).

USDA & HHS. (2015). Dietary Guidelines for Americans 2015-2020. U.S. Department of Health and Human Services and U.S. Department of Agriculture. https://health.gov/dietaryguidelines/2015/guidelines/

van den Brandt, P. A., & Schouten, L. J. (2015). Relationship of tree nut, peanut and peanut butter intake with total and cause-specific mortality: A cohort study and meta-analysis. International Journal of Epidemiology, 44(3), 1038–1049. https://doi.org/10.1093/ije/dyv039

Van Horn Linda, Carson Jo Ann S., Appel Lawrence J., Burke Lora E., Economos Christina, Karmally Wahida, Lancaster Kristie, Lichtenstein Alice H., Johnson Rachel K., Thomas Randal J., Vos Miriam, Wylie-Rosett Judith, & Kris-Etherton Penny. (2016). Recommended Dietary Pattern to Achieve Adherence to the American Heart Association/American College of Cardiology (AHA/ACC) Guidelines: A Scientific Statement From the American Heart Association. Circulation, 134(22), e505–e529. https://doi.org/10.1161/CIR.0000000000000462

van Vliet, S., Burd, N. A., & van Loon, L. J. C. (2015). The Skeletal Muscle Anabolic Response to Plant- versus Animal-Based Protein Consumption. The Journal of Nutrition, 145(9), 1981–1991. https://doi.org/10.3945/jn.114.204305

Williams, P. (2007). Nutritional composition of red meat. Nutrition & Dietetics, 64(s4), S113–S119. https://doi.org/10.1111/j.1747-0080.2007.00197.x

Wolfe, R. R., Cifelli, A. M., Kostas, G., & Kim, I.-Y. (2017). Optimizing Protein Intake in Adults: Interpretation and Application of the Recommended Dietary Allowance Compared with the Acceptable Macronutrient Distribution Range123. Advances in Nutrition, 8(2), 266–275. https://doi.org/10.3945/an.116.013821

World Cancer Research Fund/American Institute for Cancer Research. (2018). Diet, Nutrition, Physical Activity and Cancer: A Global Perspective. Continuous Update Project Expert Report 2018. dietandcancerreport.org

Wu, A. H., Yu, M. C., Tseng, C.-C., & Pike, M. C. (2008). Epidemiology of soy exposures and breast cancer risk. British Journal of Cancer, 98(1), 9–14. https://doi.org/10.1038/sj.bjc.6604145

Yu, J., Bi, X., Yu, B., & Chen, D. (2016). Isoflavones: Anti-Inflammatory Benefit and Possible Caveats. Nutrients, 8(6). https://doi.org/10.3390/nu8060361

FATS & OILS

~

By Rima Kleiner MS, RDL, LDN
and Deborah Kennedy PhD
with
The Expert Chef Panel

"Fat gives things flavor."
Quote by Julia Child

ISTORICALLY, DIETARY FAT HAS arguably been the most misunderstood macronutrient. From our once plant-foraging ancestors who learned to carve spears for animal hunting, to royalty who feasted on fatty foods, from the 1980s fat phobia to the high-fat keto diet craze, fats have been loved, loathed, and vilified over the centuries. Regardless of its current popularity or notoriety, fat is essential for proper development and good health. The conventional thought that eating fat in food causes people to be fat has been debunked. However, the portion and ratio of various fats — unsaturated fat, saturated fat, and trans fat — remains important to health.

Fat has been a part of the human diet for thousands of years. There is even some research to suggest that eating fat from animals may have caused our early ancestors to become, well, human. Because the human brain demands significantly more energy than other bodily systems, humans consumed a higher quality diet — meaning more calories and more fat, specifically long-chain polyunsaturated fatty acids — than other similar-sized primates. Another evolutionary note is that the human digestive system also developed the ability to digest and metabolize the more complex and longer fatty acid chains.

Fats are the most efficient form of energy storage. They are essential to optimal brain and body development as well as proper growth. In fact, the brain needs specific unsaturated fatty acids obtained by the diet — alpha-linolenic acid, arachidonic acid, and cervonic acid for example — to reach maximum health and function although it is not a source of energy for the brain (Bourre, 2004).

Fat in food imparts an amazing flavor profile and brings out the flavor of other compounds in a dish as well. Eating or cooking with little to no fat is like watching a 3-D movie without the special glasses. This chapter will lay out which fats to cook with and how to use them wisely to both promote health and elevate flavor.

SECTION 1:
FAT AND OIL CHARACTERISTICS

Lipid is a general term used for fats and oils that are derived from either plant or animal sources. Fat is a title often reserved for lipids that are solid at room temperature and mostly come from animal sources — some exceptions being palm and coconut oil. Oils are liquid at room temperature and come from high-oil vegetable sources that are pressed. A rule of thumb is that lipids that are liquid at room temperature are generally more healthful than those that are solid.

Lipids are essential for a variety of life-sustaining functions such as insulating the body, protecting organs, boosting absorption of phytochemicals and fat-soluble nutrients (vitamins A, D, E and K) and helping to produce important hormones. Table 1 lists edible sources of fats and oils.

Table 1: Edible Fats and Oils

Fats	Oils
Beef • Drippings • Suet • Tallow • Tail Fat	Fish • Cod liver oil • Shark liver oil
Pork • Fat back – lardo, salt pork, salo, szalonna • Lard • Lardon • Pork belly – bacon, pancetta, tocino • Speck	Vegetable Oils • Coconut oil • Corn oil • Cottonseed oil • Olive oil • Palm and palm kernel oil • Peanut oil • Rapeseed — canola oil, colza oil • Safflower oil • Soybean oil • Sunflower oil

Fats	Oils
Poultry • Chicken fat • Duck fat • Schmaltz	Nuts • Almond oil • Argan oil • Cashew oil • Hazelnut oil • Macadamia oil • Marula oil • Mongongo oil • Pecan oil • Pine oil • Pistachio oil • Walnut oil
Other Animal Fats • Blubber – muktuk, whale oil	Fruit and Seeds • Ambadi seed oil • Avocado oil • Castor oil • Grapeseed oil • Linseed oil • Mustard oil • Olive oil • Perilla oil • Poppy seed oil • Pumpkin oil • Rice bran oil • Sesame seed oil • Tea seed oil • Watermelon seed oil
Dairy • Butter • Clarified butter – ghee, smen	
Vegetable • Borneo tallow • Cacao butter • Margarine • Shea butter	

Just like the macronutrients protein and carbohydrate, fats are composed of carbon, hydrogen, and oxygen molecules, but they are arranged differently than in proteins and carbohydrates. Fats also differ in that they provide 9 kcal/gram whereas carbohydrates and proteins deliver 4 kcal/gram. Fat in foods provides satiety and fullness, which may help to curb overeating.

Most dietary fats are triglycerides (TG) that are a blend of three fatty acids attached to a glycerol backbone. When consumed, the dietary fat is digested into free fatty acids and glycerol. These components enter the enterocyte (intestinal cell) where they are repackaged into TGs. TGs (also known as triacylglycerol) are then either used by the body or are stored in fat cells.

TYPES OF FATS

Fatty acids are the basic units of dietary fats and are found in plant and animal foods. These fatty acid chains can differ in carbon length and degree of saturation. Whether in solid or liquid form, fats and oils are not soluble in water and are a blend of both saturated and unsaturated fatty acids. Fatty acids can be segmented by both the degree of saturation (unsaturated or saturated) and by the length of the fatty acid chain:

- Short-chain fatty acids (SCFA) have less than six carbon atoms in the aliphatic tail.
- Medium-chain fatty acids (MCFA) have six to 12 carbon atoms.
- Long-chain fatty acids (LCFA) have 13 to 21 carbon atoms (e.g., lard has 17 carbons in the aliphatic tail).
- Very long-chain fatty acids (VLCFA) have 22 or more carbon atoms.

**Figure 1: A Listing of Saturated Fatty Acids
Based on the Length of the Carbon Chain**

Saturated Fatty Acids

Saturated fatty acids (SFAs) have all of the carbon atoms attached to a hydrogen atom in a single bond on the fatty acid chain. In other words, the fatty acid is fully saturated with carbon-hydrogen bonds and is straight or rigid, so the saturated fatty acid tails can pack tightly together. This results in a fat that is solid at room temperature has a higher melting point and is shelf-stable.

Foods that are high in SFAs include butter, lard, full-fat dairy products, and meat. However, there are some tropical vegetable oils that are higher in SFAs, like coconut, palm, and palm kernel oils. Due to their stability, SFAs tend to be used more in processed foods, ready-to-eat products, baked goods, and frozen foods. Palm and coconut oils are not considered a part of the "oils" considered healthful in the Dietary Guidelines for Americans 2020-2025 because of the high amount of saturated fat that they contain compared to other oils (Dietary Guidelines for Americans, 2020-2025).

SFAs have historically been associated with an increased risk of heart disease, although a current meta-analysis of 43 studies casts doubt on that (Zhu et al., 2019) as neither total fat nor saturated fat intake was associated with cardiovascular disease (CVD) whereas consumption of trans fatty acids increased CVD. Despite the controversy, health experts continue to recommend:

- **Replacing SFAs with polyunsaturated fatty acids** — not carbohydrates — to reduce the risk of heart disease (Nettleton et al., 2017)
- **Keeping SFA intake to 5% to 6%** (The Facts on Fat, 2015) **or less than 10%** (Dietary Guidelines for Americans, 2020-2025) **of total energy intake.**

It is important to note, however, that SFAs are not a single nutrient and that the health impacts of SFAs may depend on the length of the fatty acid chains. While the jury is still out on exactly how harmful SFAs are, we do know that some SFAs are associated with arterial plaque buildup and cardiovascular disease when compared to unsaturated fatty acids from plant sources (Zong et al., 2016). A 2017 article by Frank Sacks et al., — Dietary Fats and Cardiovascular Disease: A Presidential Advisory From the American Heart Association — discusses the reasoning behind replacing saturated fats with unsaturated fats in the diet for lowering the rates of cardiovascular disease (Sacks et al., 2017). A nuance behind this recommendation is that individuals should consume a diet consisting of a variety of plant-based oils in order to consume adequate omega-3 and omega-6 fatty acids.

> "Approximately 5 percent of total calories inherent to the nutrient-dense foods in the Healthy U.S.-Style Dietary Pattern are from saturated fat from sources such as lean meat, poultry, and eggs; nuts and seeds; grains; and saturated fatty acids in oils. As such, there is little room to include additional saturated fat in a healthful dietary pattern while staying within limits for saturated fat and total calories" (Dietary Guidelines for Americans, 2020-2025).

The top three contributors of saturated fatty acids in the U.S. diet are **cheese, beef, and milk**. The most common saturated fatty acids in the average U.S. diet are stearic acid, palmitic acid, myristic acid, and lauric acid (Zong et al., 2016). Stearic acid tends to be the most common SFAs found in foods, such as beef tallow, cocoa butter, coconut oil, and palm kernel oil. Unlike other SFAs, stearic acid does not appear to increase LDL or total cholesterol levels and is believed to have a neutral — or no effect — on blood cholesterol levels (Grundy, 1994; van Rooijen & Mensink, 2020). While the exact mechanism is not entirely understood, it is believed that the body can quickly convert some stearic acid into oleic acid, an unsaturated fatty acid. Regardless, caution is needed as lauric acid, myristic acid, palmitic acid, and stearic acid have been shown to be positively associated with coronary artery disease in two large cohort studies during a 24 to 28 year follow-up (Zong et al., 2016).

The type of fat in whole dairy products is two-thirds saturated fats. In addition, both red meat and dairy have very little polyunsaturated fats.

Are palm and coconut oil considered healthful fats?

When trans fats were removed from the food supply in 2018, manufacturers replaced partially hydrogenated oils with palm, palm kernel, and coconut oil. Both coconut oils and palm kernel oils, of which about 80% of the fatty acids are saturated, may cause the liver to make more cholesterol than the body needs (*Control Your Cholesterol*). Both are medium-chain fatty acids, which means they tend to be more quickly digested and used as energy by cells more efficiently than longer-chain fatty acids. As such, the DGA 2020-2025 does not consider either oil a healthful alternative when compared to other plant oils (*Dietary Guidelines for Americans, 2020-2025*). In addition, because coconut oil raises LDL cholesterol levels, the Presidential Advisory from the American Heart Association advises against the use of coconut and tropical oils (Sacks et al., 2017, *The American Heart Association Diet and Lifestyle Recommendations*). In conclusion, despite the hype, replacing an animal-based source of saturated fat with a plant-based source of saturated fat still raises LDL levels and therefore cannot be considered a healthful oil.

Unsaturated Fatty Acids

Unsaturated fatty acids have at least one double bond between neighboring carbon atoms; therefore, the fatty acid has fewer — or is not totally saturated with — hydrogen molecules. Unsaturated fatty acids that have one carbon double bond are called monounsaturated fatty acids (MUFAs). Those with multiple carbon double bonds are called polyunsaturated fatty acids (PUFAs). The double carbon bond of unsaturated fatty acids allows for bending, so the fatty acid tails of unsaturated fats cannot pack tightly together. Food products that are high in unsaturated fatty acids are typically liquid at room temperature and less stable.

Monounsaturated Fatty Acids

Monounsaturated fatty acids (MUFAs) are missing only one hydrogen pair, so there is just one double bond. Foods that are rich in MUFAs include avocados, olives, nuts and seeds, peanut butter and oils like olive oil, peanut oil, canola oil and sesame oils.

Polyunsaturated Fatty Acids

Polyunsaturated fatty acids (PUFAs) are missing two or more hydrogen pairs, meaning that there are two or more double bonds. Foods that are rich in PUFAs include oils of fatty fish (like salmon, mackerel, trout and herring), walnuts, sunflower seeds, flaxseed, soybeans, and soybean and sunflower oils.

Research shows that unsaturated fatty acids contribute to a favorable health profile and are recommended in place of SFAs and trans fats (Siri-Tarino et al., 2015). Unsaturated fatty acids also play a prominent role in healthful eating patterns, like the Mediterranean diet.

Where the double bonds lie on the fatty acid chain determines whether they are omega-3 or omega-6 fatty acids. For example, omega-3 fatty acids have a double bond on the 3rd carbon from the end of the carbon chain, whereas the double bond is found on the 6th carbon from the end in omega-6 fatty acids.

Essential Fatty Acids

Omega-3 and omega-6 fatty acids are both considered essential fatty acids (EFA) because the body is not able to synthesize them on its own and it is essential that they be consumed in the diet. There are several types of omega-3 fatty acids, but the omega-3s of primary concern are alpha-linolenic (ALA), docosahexaenoic acid (DHA), and eicosapentaenoic acid (EPA). (Larsen et al., 2010; Stephen et al., 2010)

While the body cannot manufacture ALA, DHA, or EPA, it can use ALA from plant-based foods to synthesize small amounts of EPA and DHA (normally found in marine-based foods). However, the body's ability to convert ALA to EPA and DHA is so inefficient that it is recommended that individuals get EPA and DHA directly from foods, like seafood and algae. There are numerous health benefits conferred from EFAs that are discussed below.

Table 2: Sources of Omega-3 and Omega-6 Fatty Acids

Class of EFA	Name	Food Sources
Omega-3	Alpha-linolenic acid (ALA)	Canola, soybean, and walnut oil; chia, flax, and hemp seeds; green leafy vegetables
Omega-3	Stearidonic acid (SDA)	Hemp seeds and oil
Omega-3	Eicosapentaenoic Acid (EPA)	Fatty fish (salmon, mackerel, sardines, trout), oysters, shrimp, krill and algae oil
Omega-3	Docosahexaenoic Acid (DHA)	Fatty fish (salmon, sardines, trout, seabass), oysters, krill and algae oil
Omega-6	Linoleic acid (LA)	Vegetable, nut, and seed oils
Omega-6	Arachidonic Acid (AA)	Poultry, eggs, meat

Benefits of EPA and DHA

Both EPA and DHA are recommended by the American Heart Association for individuals with high triglycerides and coronary artery disease – the recommendation is to eat fish at least twice a week (Fish and Omega-3 Fatty Acids). In a systematic review, marine oil (both DHA and EPA) has been shown to prevent cardiovascular and coronary events, and cardiac death (Delgado-Lista et al., 2012). In a more recent review (86 randomized clinical trials (RCTs) with over 162,000 participants), the certainty of evidence was found to be only moderate and low for Omega-3 fats slightly decreasing coronary heart disease mortality and events, and in reducing triglycerides (mostly from supplement trials) (Abdelhamid et al., 2020).

EPA and DHA are anti-inflammatory and help to reduce chronic inflammation, but they work in different ways. In a small randomized trial of older adults, DHA was shown to decrease gene expression of pro-inflammatory protein among other effects but EPA was shown to improve the balance of pro- and anti-inflammatory proteins (So et al., 2021). In addition, both EPA and DHA reduce neuroinflammation but only EPA had a positive effect on mood disorders (Devassy et al., 2016).

Benefits of DHA

The health benefits of DHA are different but just as important as for EPA. Because of the spatial composition of DHA, this omega-3 fatty acid is larger than EPA. The size of DHA allows for greater movement, which helps keep cell membranes, especially those in the brain, more fluid (Stillwell & Wassall, 2003). DHA is also critical for healthy nerves and the retina (Querques et al., 2011). The large size and continuous sweeping of DHA may also help to break up large lipids and make it more difficult for cancer cells to survive (Dierge et al., 2021).

Additionally, DHA lowers triglycerides, increases HDL cholesterol, lowers heart rate and inhibits platelet function leading to an attenuated risk of developing cardiovascular disease (Innes & Calder, 2018).

Benefits of Omega-6 fatty Acids

Omega-6 EFAs used to be thought of as pro-inflammatory, but current research has not supported that. In fact Omega-6 fatty acids can also be anti-inflammatory (Innes & Calder, 2018). In a recent meta-analysis, higher levels of LA were significantly associated with lower risks of total CVD, cardiovascular mortality, and ischemic stroke, and higher levels of AA were also associated with a lower risk of CVD (Marklund et al., 2019). While the jury is still out regarding the most healthful amount of omega-6 fatty acids, individuals should aim to consume these EFAs from plant-based sources such as nuts and seeds rather than from fatty meats or processed foods. For more information read No Need to Avoid Healthy Omega-6 Fats by Harvard Health Publishing.

Trans Fat

Most of the trans fatty acids (TFA) found in the food supply are chemically made. Interestingly, TFAs are chemically unsaturated fatty acids, meaning there are double bonds between neighboring carbons. However, unlike unsaturated fatty acids, the two hydrogen atoms attached to the double carbon bond are positionally trans, or on opposite sides of the double bond. This causes TFAs to act more like saturated fatty acids and can be packed tightly together. TFAs are solid at room temperature and more stable than other unsaturated fatty acids.

While some TFAs do exist in nature (typically in the rumen of cows and sheep), the majority of trans fats in the human diet are artificially created during processing. This process, known as hydrogenation, chemically turns an unsaturated fatty acid into more of an SFA by adding hydrogens to unsaturated fatty acid chains. Manufacturers began using this process because it was an inexpensive way to make processed foods with highly desirable traits in terms of consistency, taste, and shelf life.

However, hydrogenated TFAs were found to have a very negative impact on health. Science demonstrated that TFAs raise LDL (or bad) cholesterol and lower HDL (or good) cholesterol levels and have been clearly linked to a higher risk of developing heart disease, type 2 diabetes, and other chronic health conditions (Mozaffarian et al., 2006). In 2015, FDA banned the use of TFAs, or partially hydrogenated oils, in processed foods and gave food manufacturers until

2018 to comply (Seattle & Washington 98104-1008, 2015). While trans fat in the food supply has drastically decreased, there is still room within these regulations for small amounts of hydrogenated oils to be used – imported foods for example – but in general, we don't need to worry about them anymore.

Cholesterol

Cholesterol is a waxy substance in the blood that is necessary for building cells. There are two sources of cholesterol. First, cholesterol is naturally produced in the body and is made in amounts sufficient for cell-building. Second, dietary cholesterol is consumed in animal foods, such as meat, poultry, and full-fat dairy products. Most foods that are rich in cholesterol are also high in saturated fats, with the exception of shrimp and eggs (Soliman, 2018).

Image of HDL and LDL Cholesterol

Image: HDL and LDL Cholesterol

There are two primary types of cholesterol found in the body — low-density lipoprotein (LDL) and high-density lipoprotein (HDL). LDL is often referred to as "bad" cholesterol, and HDL is often considered "good" cholesterol. Too much LDL and/or too little HDL can contribute to the gradual buildup of plaque in the arteries and can increase the risk for heart disease.

The previous recommendation to limit intake of dietary cholesterol to 300 mg maximum per day was not included in the 2015 Dietary Guidelines for Americans because dietary cholesterol alone is not responsible for increased blood cholesterol levels. For every 100 mg/dL increase in dietary cholesterol, circulating LDL increases by only 1.9 mg/dL (Vincent et al., 2019). The focus has shifted to reducing saturated fat and by doing so, one is reducing dietary cholesterol as well. To summarize, **the best way to decrease blood LDL cholesterol is to replace saturated fat in the diet with #1 polyunsaturated fats and #2 monounsaturated fats** (Micha & Mozaffarian, 2010).

SECTION 2:

RECOMMENDATION FOR FAT AND OIL INTAKE

Since the first edition USDA Dietary Guidelines for Americans (DGA) in 1980, advice about fat intake has been included. The advice from 1980 to 1995 basically remained the same — avoid too much total fat, saturated fat, and cholesterol. The DGA 2005-2010 recommended keeping total fat calories to between 20% and 35% of all calories with most fat coming from unsaturated fat (National Academies of Sciences et al., 2017). This was the only edition of the DGAs where a minimum and maximum amount of fat intake was proposed. The advice to consume less than 10% of calories from saturated fat started in 2005 and continues with the most current DGA 2020-2025 (Dietary Guidelines for Americans, 2020-2025). To see specific recommendations for fats and oils from 1980 to 2020, see Appendix A.

Unsaturated fatty acids and oils confer many health benefits and should be part of a healthful diet. On the other hand, TFAs do not provide health benefits and should be consumed minimally, if at all, which shouldn't be hard to do as TFAs were taken out of the food supply in 2018. Finally, saturated fats should be replaced with unsaturated fats wherever possible.

Because all dietary fats, including oils, contain more calories per gram than carbohydrates and proteins, nutrition experts advocate consuming even healthful fats in moderation. The following are key recommendations for dietary fats and oils (Kaushik et al., 2009; Sacks et al., 2017; Zong et al., 2016).
* Limit calories from SFAs to less than 10% of total daily calories
* Replace saturated fats with unsaturated fats — both PUFAs and MUFAs – found in seafood, nuts, seeds, avocados, olives, and vegetable oils (limit tropical oils), whole grains, and plant-based protein.
* Choose lean cuts of meat and poultry and low fat or fat-free dairy products.
* Don't replace fats with refined carbohydrates.

Table 3: Recommended Limits of Saturated Fat
from Total Daily Calories Per Calorie Levels

Total Daily Calorie Intake	Limit on Saturated Fat Intake
1,000 kcal	10 g or less
1,200 kcal	12 g or less
1,400 kcal	14 g or less
1,600 kcal	16 g or less

Total Daily Calorie Intake	Limit on Saturated Fat Intake
1,800 kcal	18 g or less
2,000 kcal	20 g or less
2,200 kcal	22 g or less
2,400 kcal	24 g or less
2,600 kcal	26 g or less

While the importance of dietary fat is well-documented, the data for the level at which chronic disease occurs due to total fat intake is insufficient to establish an Adequate Intake (AI) or Estimated Average Requirement (EAR). Because there is no EAR, a Recommended Dietary Allowance (RDA) cannot be established for dietary fats. However, it is often recommended to consume a low ratio of omega-6 to omega-3 fatty acids to reduce chronic disease risk (Simopoulos, 2002). To put that recommendation into perspective – a typical Western diet delivers about fifteen to sixteen times more omega-6 fats than omega-3 fats, and anthropological evidence suggests humans evolved consuming a diet with a one to one ratio (Simopoulos, 2006). **The goal is no to stop consuming plant based sources of omega-6 fats but to replace saturated fat with unsaturated fat; select plant based sources of omega-6 fats; and increase the amount of omega-3 fats consumed to bring the ratio back into balance (what that exact ratio is, is not as important as making sure sources of both healthful fats – omega-6 and omega-3 – are consumed).**

FAT CONSUMPTION AMONG AMERICANS

According to USDA (2015–2020 Dietary Guidelines for Americans - Health.Gov, 2015) and NHANES (Jacqueline D. Wright et al., 2003) data, Americans across all age groups — including children and adults — consume too little unsaturated oils and far exceed limits of solid fats or SFAs. While children of all ages — particularly children under age 6 years — appear to consume the highest amounts of SFAs, intake above the recommended limits remains consistent throughout all life stages and between genders.

Average Intake of Oils and Fats (DGA 2015-2020)

Image: Average Intake of Oils and Saturated Fats

Recent research shows that approximately 42% to 65% of American adults consume more than the recommended 10% of total calories from saturated fat (Liu et al., 2017). In order to meet dietary fat recommendations, individuals are encouraged to replace SFA intake (from processed foods, fatty meats, butter, full-fat dairy products, fried foods, baked goods and processed foods like potato chips) with unsaturated fats, especially PUFAs found in walnuts and other nuts, flaxseed and other seeds, fatty fish, olives, olive oil, other plant oils (soy, canola, sunflower and corn for example), and avocados.

Thanks to decades of conflicting data surrounding dietary fats, it is no wonder that Americans consume the wrong types of fat. Years of dietary guidance that focused on eating little to no fat and replacing fats with carbohydrates was then followed by advice to eat more healthful fats and fewer "low-fat" carbohydrate products, which only served to confuse consumers even more. In fact, studies have examined the history of consumer confusion around dietary fats.

In 2009, 65% of consumers thought a low-fat diet was healthful, 59% thought fat should be avoided and 38% said they avoid foods containing fat (Diekman & Malcolm, 2009). Not much has changed over the years as a survey of over 1,200 consumers in 2018 showed that the majority (54%) thought a low-fat diet — when compared to medium- and high-fat diets — was the most healthful (Lusk, 2019).

SECTION 3:

THE HEALTH BENEFITS
OF FATS AND OILS

Table 4: Sources of Healthful and Unhealthful Fats

Healthful Sources of Fat	Unhealthful Sources of Fat
Fish	Fat from red and processed meat
Nuts and seeds – e.g., flaxseeds	Fat in whole fat dairy products
Plants	Partially hydrogenated oils

Despite decades of a negative image, dietary fats provide many health benefits. The benefits, however, depend on the type — and amount — of fat consumed. Eaten in moderation, unsaturated fats confer a variety of health benefits. On the other hand, trans fats provide no health benefits and are associated with negative health outcomes. When it comes to saturated fat however recent evidence suggests that saturated fat by itself is not as harmful as was once thought; what is harmful however is what food replaces saturated fat in the diet (Siri-Tarino et al., 2010, 2015).

Unsaturated fats provide a myriad of health benefits and are essential to optimal health. Here are just a few health benefits of unsaturated fats and oils:

- Brain and eye development — fat not only makes up every cell membrane, but it also makes up the insulating layer around each nerve cell, called myelin. Myelin is important for helping nerves communicate quickly and efficiently. The need for dietary fats begins even before birth. More than half of the human brain and retina are comprised of the omega-3 fatty acids (DHA and AA). Because humans do not make omega-3 fatty acids, it is imperative that pregnant and breastfeeding women consume adequate omega-3s to promote optimal baby brain and eye development. Studies show that expectant women who regularly consumed omega-3s during pregnancy had children who reached developmental milestones like crawling and recognizing faces sooner than pregnant women who did not consume omega-3s (Davidson et al., 2011).
- Cell membrane formation — free fatty acids affect not only the fluidity of the cell membrane but the function of the cell itself through its influence on membrane protein functioning and the ability for a cell signal to propagate (Ibarguren et al., 2014). A healthful cell membrane made up of unsaturated fat is more fluid and helps cells function properly, while the presence of saturated fatty acids creates a solid-like, inflexible area in the cell membrane (Shen et al., 2017).
- Heart health — unsaturated fats, specifically omega-3s and omega-6s, help to improve blood lipid profile and reduce chronic inflammation, both of which help to combat cardiovascular disease.
- Hormone production — fats and cholesterol are integral components of hormones and other substances. Hormones are the chemical messengers that help to control appetite, weight, mood and other important functions. Fats are especially important for hormone production in adolescence or teen years, and in midlife and later when certain hormones decline with age.
- Absorption and transport of fat-soluble vitamins — vitamins A, D, E and K –and carotenoids. Without adequate amounts of dietary fat, these important vitamins may not be efficiently absorbed or transported in the body.
- Organ protection — fat helps protect and cushion many of our vital organs, such as the heart, kidneys, liver and intestines.
- Source of energy — fat becomes the last fuel resource for our body when energy resources run low.

SECTION 4:

FAT AND OIL INTAKE AND HEALTH OUTCOMES

With all of its important health benefits, unsaturated dietary fats are essential to optimal health. Consuming too little dietary fat can compromise many of these functions. On the other hand, too much dietary fat can also counter many of these health benefits.

A diet rich in solid or saturated fats — found primarily in fatty meats, full-fat dairy products, lard, butter, bakery items, processed snack foods, fast foods, fried foods and tropical vegetable oils — raises total and LDL cholesterol levels (Micha & Mozaffarian, 2010). While some recent studies have shown that SFAs may not be quite as detrimental as once thought, experts continue to agree that replacing SFA with PUFAs and MUFAs and limiting SFAs to less than 10% of daily calories still provide the biggest health benefits (Siri-Tarino et al., 2010). A diet rich in MUFAs and PUFAs is particularly important in various medical conditions and/or life stages as discussed below.

PREGNANCY AND CHILD DEVELOPMENT

Studies show that a diet rich in MUFAs and PUFAs is particularly critical for optimal brain, eye, and body development in the fetus and functioning for mom during pregnancy, as well as in infancy and childhood (Davidson et al., 2011). Specifically:

- Brain and eye development during pregnancy, infancy, and early childhood — essential unsaturated fatty acids like omega-3s contribute to optimal brain and eye health when consumed by the mother during pregnancy and lactation and by the child during infancy and early childhood (Madden et al., 2009).
- Cognitive and behavioral milestones — high amounts of omega-3s during pregnancy are associated with higher verbal intelligence scores, optimal prosocial behavior, and fine motor and communication skills (Hibbeln et al., 2007).
- Neurocognitive conditions — low intakes of omega-3s during pregnancy are associated with a higher risk of the child having neurocognitive conditions, such as depression or attention-deficit hyperactivity disorder (ADHD) (Golding et al., 2009).
- Asthma — children who consume inadequate amounts of omega-3s, especially EPA, in their diet are at a higher risk for developing asthma (Yang et al., 2013).

It is recommended that **children under the age of two years old consume saturated fat** for proper brain and eye development. After age two years, however, saturated fat is not necessary for development. In fact, the Dietary Guidelines for Americans states that there is no dietary need or requirement for anyone over the age of two years to consume saturated fat and recommend that saturated fat sources be replaced with unsaturated fats, especially PUFAs (2015–2020 Dietary Guidelines for Americans - Health.Gov, 2015). The evidence is clear that no amount of trans fat is healthy as trans fat has been shown to increase inflammation, heart disease, stroke and diabetes.

CARDIOVASCULAR HEALTH

Consuming a diet rich in PUFAs and MUFAs and low in SFAs and TFAs may help reduce the risk of developing heart disease and preventing death from cardiovascular disease. These benefits reach across the lifespan.

- Benefits to heart health are most significant when SFAs and trans fats are replaced by PUFAs and MUFAs, not when replaced with refined carbohydrates (which has been linked to higher triglycerides and, thereby, increased risk of heart disease) (Hernáez et al., 2019).
- A recent Cochrane review of randomized clinical trials found that reducing saturated fat for two years reduced cardiovascular events (Hooper et al., 2020)
- EPA, in particular, has been shown to help reduce the risk of heart disease in individuals without a history of heart disease risk (Lee et al., 2008).
- A diet rich in omega-3s has been associated with a reduced risk of older adults dying from a stroke (Goodarz Danaei et al., 2009).
- Low intakes of omega-3s and high intakes of trans fat were two of the risk factors most strongly related to overall mortality (Goodarz Danaei et al., 2009).

Cholesterol and Heart Health

It was once believed that your blood cholesterol level was directly linked to the amount of cholesterol that you ate. We now know that this is true only for a small subset of people called "responders"; for most of us, however, our cholesterol level is influenced not just by dietary fat but also by the intake of refined carbohydrates.

Our bodies produce sufficient amounts of cholesterol for cell-building and other important roles. When we consume too many SFAs and trans fats, blood cholesterol levels increase, plus too much refined carbohydrates can lead to a decrease in HDL and an increase in triglycerides as well (Parks & Hellerstein, 2000; Siri & Krauss, 2005).

While recent research has shown that dietary cholesterol has less of an impact on blood cholesterol than previously thought, the National Academy of Medicine continues to recommend consuming as little (or no) dietary cholesterol as possible (Medicine, 2002). The

Dietary Guidelines for Americans recommends consuming as few SFAs as possible, zero industrial TFAs, and limiting intake of refined carbohydrates to help keep blood cholesterol levels in check (2015–2020 Dietary Guidelines for Americans - Health.Gov, 2015).

> In summary, to lower LDL cholesterol and prevent heart disease, focus on consuming polyunsaturated fats (the best choice) and monounsaturated fats. Unhealthful choices include animal fats, palm oil, coconut oil, and trans fat.

BRAIN HEALTH

Consuming a Mediterranean-style diet that includes unsaturated fats and omega-3 fats from seafood may help to slow age-related cognitive decline, improve brain function, and reduce the risk of dementia and Alzheimer's disease (Martínez-Lapiscina et al., 2013). Other research findings include:

- A Mediterranean-style diet high in DHA-rich foods may help improve cognitive function in adults (Martínez-Lapiscina et al., 2013)
- EPA and DHA may help to slow the loss of cognitive brain function or neurological disease with age-related brain atrophy (Pottala et al., 2014)
- Replacing some meat meals with omega-3 rich fish meals may help reduce the likelihood of developing dementia (Albanese et al., 2009)

CANCER

There is some research to suggest that diets rich in PUFAs and MUFAs may reduce the risk of cancer and a diet rich in SFAs may increase the risk for cancer, but further research is still needed (Othman, 2007). What is clear with regards to cancer and dietary fats is that a Mediterranean-style diet with moderate intakes of MUFAs and PUFAs and low intakes of SFAs and TFAs may help with maintaining a healthful weight (Huo et al., 2015; Kastorini et al., 2011), which has been shown to help reduce the risk of certain cancers, including breast and colon cancer.

DIABETES

Research looking at the impact of dietary fats on the development of type 2 diabetes is relatively new, conflicting, and more research is needed. In a pooled analysis of 20 prospective cohort studies representing over 39,000 individuals, Wu et al. concluded that intake of the omega-6 fatty acid (linoleic acid) has long-term benefits for preventing type 2 diabetes (Wu et al., 2017).

While more research is needed in this area, a diet that replaces SFAs and TFAs with MUFAs and PUFAs has been found to help maintain a healthful weight and lower the risk of cardiovascular disease, both of which are important for helping to prevent diabetes (Kaushik et al., 2009). A Mediterranean-style diet rich in MUFAs and PUFAs has been associated with a reduced risk of developing gestational diabetes (Assaf-Balut et al., 2019).

GASTROINTESTINAL HEALTH

Diet is believed to impact gut microbiota, but the extent to which this occurs is not yet fully understood. More research is needed to determine whether dietary fats play a role in altering the gut microbiome (Wolters et al., 2019).

MENTAL HEALTH

Preliminary research suggests that omega-3 fatty acids may help reduce the risk of depression, schizophrenia, youth mood disorders and disordered eating such as anorexia, however, the science is not yet conclusive and more research needs to be done in this area (Hibbeln & Gow, 2014). There is promising research showing a positive association between a diet rich in omega-3 fatty acids and a reduced risk of postnatal depression in new mothers (Bozzatello et al., 2016). The chapter on Psychology, Food and Mood goes into this in-depth.

OBESITY

The role of dietary fats on body weight may be beneficial. Existing research suggests that replacing SFAs with MUFAs and PUFAs, particularly, may help promote weight maintenance and/or weight loss (Estruch et al., 2019; Makhoul et al., 2011).

Fun Fact: When someone loses weight, where does fat go? Most of it is exhaled as carbon dioxide, and the rest is turned into water and excreted in sweat or urine.

IMMUNITY

Some research suggests that there is a positive association between omega-3 fatty acids, particularly PUFAs, and the reduced risk for autoimmune diseases. Other research also suggests that PUFAs may help reduce the need for certain anti-inflammatory medications. This is a promising area, but more research is needed to look specifically at certain autoimmune conditions and the impact of dietary fats on inflammatory diseases (Li et al., 2019).

SECTION 5:

DIETS FOCUSED ON FAT CONTENT

THE KETOGENIC DIET

The ketogenic diet (also known as the keto diet) has been around since the 1920s. It originally was developed as a diet to help reduce the risk of seizures in individuals with epilepsy. The ketogenic diet has recently risen in popularity as a weight loss diet.

While there is no official ketogenic diet formula for weight loss, the premise of the diet is to consume mostly fat and proteins and few carbohydrates. After three to four days of consuming less than 50 grams of carbohydrates (which is about the amount in one banana and one slice of whole wheat bread), the body goes into a state of ketosis. Ketosis means the body begins to use protein and fat — instead of carbohydrates — for fuel. This diet is intended to be a short-term option to help spur weight loss. Most studies have not looked at the long-term effects of the ketogenic diet for weight loss, and more research is needed (Masood & Uppaluri, 2020).

It has been demonstrated, however, that following a ketogenic diet can lead to multiple nutrient deficiencies even if the individual consumes nutrient-dense foods while on the diet. Deficiencies include vitamin K, linolenic acid, water-soluble vitamins (except B_{12}) and most importantly fiber (Crosby et al., 2021). Go to the chapter on the Ketogenic Diet for more information.

THE LOW-FAT DIET

The theory behind a low-fat diet is that replacing calorie-laden fat (9 kcal/gram) with carbohydrates and protein (both are 4 kcal/gram) will lead to a reduction in calories, resulting in weight loss. The low-fat diet became very popular in the 1970s and 1980s when fat was considered a villain. Instead of replacing fat with whole grains, fruits, and vegetables, many individuals increased their intake of simple carbohydrates and sugar, which led to both weight gain and chronic disease associated with weight gain.

A low-fat diet is defined as a diet where no more than 30% of calories come from fat. This amount still gives room for healthful fat in the diet. The key to a healthful low-fat diet is to replace fat-calories with nutrient-dense foods like fruits, vegetables, plant-based protein sources and whole grains. Examples of low-fat diets are listed in Table 5. The amount of total fat in each of these diets ranges from a low of 10% or less to a high of 28%.

Table 5: Ranking of Diets by 39 Nutrition Experts

The Diet	Amount of Fat	Ranking of Best Diet Overall and Best for Weight Loss[*] (out of 39)	Nutrient Score on a Scale of 0 to 5[**]
Ornish	No more than 10% calories from fat	9th overall 6th for weight loss	4.2/5
Jenny Craig	28% total fat and 8% saturated fat	12th overall 5th for weight loss	3.9/5
Macrobiotics	17% total fat 0 saturated fat	25th overall 26th for weight loss	3.1/5
Engine 2	23% total fat 0.02% saturated fat	19th overall 9th for weight loss	3.4/5
Therapeutic Lifestyle Changes (TLC)	Saturated fat cut to less than 7% daily calories	5th overall 22nd for weight loss	4.5/5

[*]US News and World Report 2021 convened 24 national nutrition experts to rank 39 diets
[**]A score from one to five was assigned for nutritional completeness (5 =complete)

The American Heart Association no longer recommends a low-fat diet; they recommend a diet with moderate fat intake and a focus on healthful fats (Recent Study Adds Weight to the Low-Carb vs. Low-Fat Debate, 2014). The AHA describes a healthful eating pattern as one that includes a variety of fruits and vegetables, whole grains, non-tropical vegetable oils, nuts, seeds, fatty fish, skinless poultry, lean meat, eggs, beans and fat-free or low-fat dairy products (The American Heart Association Diet and Lifestyle Recommendations).

THE ATKINS DIET

The Atkins Diet is high in fat, moderate in protein and low in carbohydrates (Astrup et al., 2004). Similar to the ketogenic diet, the Atkins Diet is intended to promote a state of ketosis through a diet rich in fat and protein and very low in carbohydrates. Unlike the ketogenic diet, the Atkins Diet slowly allows for the increase of carbohydrates to about 100 grams per day in the long term. The gradual addition of carbohydrate-rich foods helps to prevent blood sugar and insulin spikes, thereby ultimately helping to promote weight loss. In his later years Atkins modified his diet to include healthful fats and vegetables.

Proponents of the Atkins Diet claim the diet comes with many health benefits, such as improved blood sugar, blood cholesterol and triglyceride levels. Some science does support that the Atkins Diet helps reduce the risk of heart disease (Dansinger et al., 2005; Gardner et al., 2007; Jenkins et al., 2014), whereas other studies shows that a high-fat diet like Atkins may in fact increase risk of heart disease, especially in certain individuals (Lagiou et al., 2012). More studies are needed to show whether health benefits are maintained over the long term.

An interesting history of low carb diets can be found at https://dieteticallyspeaking.com/the-history-of-low-carb/.

Take away:
- Fat is not a villain
- The type of fat consumed is important — less saturated and more polyunsaturated
- When a macronutrient is excluded from the diet — fats for example — protein and or carbohydrate intake must increase significantly
- Most individuals do not substitute healthful whole grains for the decrease in fats, but see a low-fat diet as a license to eat more refined carbohydrates
- Stick to a whole food way of eating (like the Mediterranean diet) for long term health instead of partaking in a restrictive "diet"
- There are many ways to lose weight, and it is the ability to sustain the weight loss that is unknown at this time. See the chapter on Overweight/Obesity for more information

---

SECTION 6:

CLINICAL AND CULINARY COMPETENCIES FOR FAT

Clinical Recommendations (2015-2020 Dietary Guidelines | Health.Gov; Dietary Guidelines for Americans, 2020-2025; U.S. Department of Health and Human Services and U.S. Department of Agriculture, 2005):
1. Limit calories from SFAs to less than 10% of total daily calories starting at age two
2. Replace SFAs with PUFAs and MUFAs found in seafood, nuts, seeds, avocados, olives, and vegetable oils (limit tropical oils)
3. Consume less than 300 mg per day of dietary cholesterol
4. Avoid trans fatty acid intake as much as possible
5. Choose lean cuts of meat and poultry and low-fat or fat-free dairy products

CLINICAL COMPETENCIES

1. Define fats and oils and their energy contribution
2. Relate the importance of fats and oils for overall health

3. Define and list essential fatty acids
4. Explain the difference between saturated and unsaturated fat and their risks/benefits
5. Differentiate between healthful and unhealthful sources of fats
6. Compare and contrast diets for weight loss defined by their fat content – low and high-fat diets
7. Describe the risks and benefits of consuming various fats and oils
8. List the recommended servings of fats and oils per day based on age
9. List the amount of total fat, saturated fat, cholesterol, and trans fat recommended in one's daily diet
10. Define nutrient content claims related to fat

CULINARY COMPETENCIES FOR FATS AND OILS

Messaging from the Menus of Change 2020
Choose Healthier Oils   *Go Good Fat, Not Low Fat*

SHOPPING AND STORING COMPETENCIES

1. Demonstrate how to shop for healthful fats and oils
2. Purchase the most healthful cuts of meat, poultry, and fish
3. Describe how to identify different types of fat in a product
4. Select authentic olive oil
5. Demonstrate how to store fats and oils

COOKING/PREPARING/SERVING COMPETENCIES
STOCKING THE KITCHEN COMPETENCIES

1. Stock a variety of oils
   a. Monounsaturated – extra virgin olive oil, for example
   b. Polyunsaturated – sunflower seed oil, for example
   c. Omega 3 fatty acids
   d. Solid fats
2. Stock a variety of flavorful, healthful high-fat ingredients
   a. Yogurt
   b. Avocadoes
   c. Nuts and Seeds
3. Stock oils with various flavor profiles
   a. Strong flavored oils (e.g., toasted sesame oil and peanut oil)

b. Infused oils (e.g., orange or oregano-infused oils)
c. Neutral oils (e.g., corn, safflower, canola, and grapeseed oil)

FLAVOR DEVELOPMENT COMPETENCIES

1. Describe how fats and oils affect flavor and texture
2. Demonstrate healthful cooking techniques that influence flavor and texture using various oils and fats
3. Describe how various cooking methods affect the flavor profile of various foods

COOKING COMPETENCIES

1. List the various functions that fat and oil plays in cooking and preparation methods
2. Prepare a healthful salad dressing
3. Prepare a healthful creamy sauce
4. Demonstrate various cooking techniques for preparing animal-based protein
5. Demonstrate how to decrease the fat content in food
6. Select the appropriate oil for various cooking temperatures
7. Bake a lower-fat version of a bakery item

SERVING COMPETENCIES

1. Model eating healthful fats and oils
2. Display the proper serving sizes of fats and oils
3. Utilize healthful fats in meals and menu planning

SAFETY COMPETENCIES

1. Identify rancid fats and oils
2. Identify when to throw out oil
3. Defend why it is not healthful to cook oil above its smoke point

SECTION 7:

FATS AND OILS AT THE STORE

ON THE LABEL

Image: Fat on the Label

The Nutrition Facts label provides consumers with useful information for choosing products that are lower in saturated and trans fats. In May 2016, the FDA set forth new rules for the Nutrition Facts label to reflect the science showing a clear link between diet and the risk of chronic disease (Nutrition, 2021). These changes include updating the label to reflect the evolving science on dietary fats, specifically that the **amount of dietary fat consumed may have less of an impact than the types of dietary fat of consumed**. The updated label includes information on SFAs and TFAs.

NUTRIENT CONTENT CLAIMS

Nutrient content claims for fat include the following (AHA, 2020):

Table 6: Nutrient Content Claims for Fat

Nutrient Content Claim	Means One Serving Contains:
Fat free	Less than 0.5 g of fat and no ingredient that is fat
Low fat	3 g of fat or less (and not more than 30% of calories from fat for meals and main dishes)
Reduced fat or less fat	At least 25% less fat than the regular product
Low in saturated fat	1 g or less of saturated fat, and 15% or less of the calories coming from saturated fat (10% or less for meals and main dishes)
Lean	Less than 10 g of fat, 4.5 g of saturated fat, and 95 mg of cholesterol
Extra lean	Less than 5 g of fat, 2 g of saturated fat, and 95 mg of cholesterol

Nutrient Content Claim	Means One Serving Contains:
Light or lite	At least 50% less fat than the regular product (or 1/3 fewer calories if less than 50% of calories are from fat)
Cholesterol free:	Less than 2 mg per serving
Low cholesterol:	20 mg or less per serving
Reduced cholesterol or less cholesterol	The product has at least 25% less cholesterol than the regular version

Light or lite does not mean anything unless you know the amount of fat in the full-fat product. One-half of a large amount of fat can still be a high-fat product.

QUALIFIED HEALTH CLAIMS

The FDA recently authorized the use of qualified health claims on products containing healthful fats, like essential unsaturated fatty acids.

Nuts received the first qualified health claim for the impact of unsaturated fatty acids on heart health. The following qualified health claim can be used on tree nut packages:
- "Scientific evidence suggests but does not prove that eating 1.5 ounces per day of most nuts, as part of a diet low in saturated fat and cholesterol, may reduce the risk of heart disease. [See nutrition information for fat content.]" (Nutrition, 2019a)

More recently, seafood products can now include a qualified health claim about the impact of the omega-3 fatty acids EPA and DHA on heart health. However, the manufacturer must include how much EPA and DHA are in a serving of this food. The qualified health claim is as follows:
- "Supportive but not conclusive research shows that consumption of EPA and DHA omega-3 fatty acids may reduce the risk of coronary heart disease. One serving of [name of food] provides [x] grams of EPA and DHA omega-3 fatty acids. [See nutrition information for total.]

AT THE STORE

Supermarket shelves are full of choices, and it is easy to become confused when shopping for healthful fat products. The Nutrition Facts and product ingredients labels are the place to look for products that contain beneficial fats. First, check the Nutrition Facts label to see whether — or how much — the product contains SFAs or TFAs. Aim for no TFAs and little to no SFAs. Secondly, scan the ingredients list and limit products that contain tropical oils like palm and coconut (high in SFAs).

Choose foods that contain higher amounts of unsaturated fats, like MUFAs and PUFAs, in place of foods high in saturated fats. These foods tend to contain a healthful fat profile:

- **Avocados** — this fruit is rich in monounsaturated omega-6s, which help to increase beneficial HDL cholesterol. Avocados also contain dietary fiber, potassium, B vitamins and vitamins C and E. Choose avocados that are firm but yield to a gentle press. Use mashed avocado in place of mayonnaise on sandwiches, add to egg burritos or toss in a fruit smoothie.

- **Seafood** — fish and shellfish contain polyunsaturated omega-3s which are known for their heart, brain, and eye benefits. Seafood also provides protein, selenium, vitamin D, iron and B vitamins. The Dietary Guidelines for Americans recommends eating a variety of seafood **at least twice a week** to meet nutrient needs. Frozen and canned seafood provides nutrients similar to fresh fish and shellfish, so choose varieties you enjoy. Some popular choices include salmon, shrimp, halibut, trout, mackerel, tuna, herring, sardines, anchovies and scallops. The FDA advises that pregnant and breastfeeding women and children should avoid the following higher-mercury species: king mackerel, shark, swordfish, tilefish, orange roughy, marlin, and bigeye tuna (found in sushi) (Nutrition, 2019b). It is important to be aware of the mercury content in fish and how much one is consuming but no species are off-limits for all other consumers. Whatever species you choose, try grilling, sautéing, baking, roasting, broiling, poaching, or steaming your seafood for the best flavor and health benefits.

- **Nuts and seeds** — nuts and seeds and their butters provide a healthful combination of MUFAs and PUFAs. Plus, nuts and seeds contain protein, dietary fiber, vitamins like vitamin E, and minerals like selenium and magnesium. Eating 1.5 ounces of nuts at least five days each week has been associated with improved heart and brain health (Martínez-Lapiscina et al., 2013). There are many kinds of nuts — like walnuts, almonds, hazelnuts, pecans, and pistachios — and seeds, like chia, flax, pumpkin, sunflower, and hemp. To get 1.5 ounces of nuts and seeds in your diet, add crushed nuts to oatmeal, nut butter to smoothies, seeds to salads, or snack on raw. Watch the salt content of nuts and seeds, opting for low-salt or no-salt versions.

- **Olives** — this little fruit is rich in MUFAs and antioxidants. There are many varieties of both green and black olives. Try adding olives to tomato-based sauces, cook alongside fish or poultry, dice and spread on sandwiches, or enjoy on their own as a snack.

- **Vegetable Oils** — like olive, canola, sunflower, peanut, and corn oils — contain a combination of MUFAs and PUFAs. Limit consumption of tropical oils like palm, palm kernel, and coconut oils, which contain a higher percentage of saturated than unsaturated fats. Replace highly saturated spreads like butter and oils like palm, palm kernel, and coconut with heart-healthful unsaturated oils.

- **Olive oil** — choose the first pressed virgin olive oil for most of your needs; you can purchase the lighter versions to cook with. Extra virgin olive oil (EVOO) and virgin olive oil are made without heat (called cold-pressed) or chemicals. EVOO means the olives were only pressed once to get the oil. The first pressing will release most of the nutrients into the oil; the more you press the olive the fewer nutrients go into the oil and flavor decreases.

- **Corn, canola, and soybean oil** – these three vegetable oils usually come from plants that have been genetically modified. In fact, the majority of the corn and soybean products in the United States are made from genetically modified corn and soybeans. You won't know which products are genetically modified because manufacturers do not have to put that on the label, yet. You can assume it is GMO if it does not say organically grown (even then you cannot be sure). If you want to avoid GMOs, make sure that you buy organic soybean, corn, and canola products. Environmental Working Groups 2014 Shopper's Guide to Avoiding GMO Food (https://www.ewg.org/consumer-guides/ewgs-2014-shoppers-guide-avoiding-gmo-food) lists several reasons why individuals may choose to avoid GMO foods in general:
  - GMO crops require an increase in pesticide use.
  - The use of GMO crops has created the production of more toxic pesticides, which produces 'superweeds'.

While the World Health Organization and The American Medical Association have determined that GMO foods are safe for consumers, the environmental impact is still significant (AMA, 2012; Food, Genetically Modified). This may be reason enough for some consumers to avoid GMO's but they do not need to base their fears on health risks.

For a great review of the science, Harvard University summarized the science in their blog - Signal to Noise Special Edition: GMO's and Our Food. (https://sitn.hms.harvard.edu/signal-to-noise-special-edition-gmos-and-our-food/)

Table 7: Amount of Fat in Dairy and Meat Products

Food or Beverage	Grams of Fat per Serving
8 oz whole milk yogurt	8 grams
8 oz low fat yogurt	4 grams
1 oz Mozzarella cheese (whole milk)	6 grams
1 oz Mozzarella cheese (part skim)	4 ½ grams
3 oz hamburger (70% lean)	15 grams
3 oz hamburger (95% lean)	6 ½ grams
Chicken white meat (100 grams)	4 ½ grams
Chicken dark meat (100 grams)	9 ½ grams
1 cup whole milk	8 grams
1 cup 2 % milk	5 grams
1 cup 1 % milk	2 grams

(USDA and ARS, 2020)

- Dairy — Reduce the intake of saturated fat from dairy by choosing low-fat or fat-free milks, cheese, and yogurts.
- Poultry—Choose turkey or chicken without skin to reduce saturated fat. White meat also has less fat than brown meat in turkey and chicken.
- Red meat — Choose leaner cuts of beef and pork like sirloin, tenderloin, and 93% or higher lean ground beef to reduce saturated fat intake from meat.

Table 8: Lean Cuts of Beef

Lean Cuts of Beef	Extra Lean Cuts of Beef
Round steak	Eye of round roast
95% lean ground beef	Top round steak
Chuck shoulder roast	Mock tender steak
Arm pot roast	Bottom round roast
Shoulder steak	
Strip steak	
Tenderloin steak	
T-bone steak	

- Pork: Choose pork tenderloin instead of the loin or butt.
- Other meats: Other lean meats include lean game, such as rabbits, venisons, and alligators.

Should I eat butter or margarine?

While butter was the original spread of choice, margarine has actually been around since it was created in the mid-1800s. It wasn't until the 1920s and '30s that margarine gained prominence in the U.S. Because butter was expensive and high in SFAs, margarine quickly became a competitor with butter during the war years. Decades later, however, margarine came under scrutiny because it contained TFAs, which were discovered to both raise LDL "bad" and lower HDL "good" cholesterol levels. Along with this discovery and the eventual ban of TFAs, margarine manufacturers removed TFAs. For the most healthful spread, try using extra-virgin olive oil, avocado, or a stanol-based spread shown to help improve cholesterol levels. See the chapter on Dairy for more information.

SECTION 9:
FATS, OILS, AND SUSTAINABILITY

The sustainability of fats and oils depends largely on the origin of the product, environmental impacts – climate-related emissions (greenhouse gasses), waste, water and land use, soil, and pollution – and processing; thus, much variation and complexities exist (World Bank Group, 2015).

Oils

Over the past 25 years, global oil crops have expanded with major impacts on the amount of land used, now utilizing about 30 percent of all cropland globally, with palm, soy, and rapeseed accounting for 80 percent (Meijaard et al., 2020). The current and projected growth in the world population and concurrent shifts in diets globally will propel a continued increased demand for cooking oil. Although the prevalent use of plant oils for biofuels has an important impact on sustainability, particularly the use of palm, soybean, and rape (canola), this section will focus only on oils produced for human consumption.

Environmental Impacts

Environmental impacts occur across all steps of growing and producing vegetable oils.

1. **Agriculture** reflects all impacts of growing the product (seed, nut, or fruit), from fertilizer and pesticide production for the crops to land use and energy inputs.
2. Oil is extracted from seeds or nuts that have been cleaned and ground into a course meal. **Oil seed extraction** usually requires a solvent and cleaning agent called hexane, which is categorized as an EPA hazard that may be unhealthy for workers due to inhalation exposure. Alternatively, some oils are expeller (mechanical) or cold-pressed. For example, extra virgin olive oil production uses pressure to extract without heat, which keeps health benefits intact.
3. **Refining** includes a series of steps to produce a bland, stable oil. These processes may use significant amounts of water for cooling, chemical neutralization, washing and de-odorizing. Processing facilities also use energy to heat water and produce steam, refrigeration, and compressed air. Finally, wastewater from these facilities may have a high nutrient load, thus they are sources of methane and nitrous oxide.
4. **Packaging and transport** vary depending on the product and final destination.
5. **By-products.** The production of vegetable oils often results in significant quantities of organic solid waste, residues and other by-products. When these by-products are used for

animal feed, fertilizers or commercially viable products or even biodiesel, the environmental impact of the oil itself is generally lessened because it's distributed across other products. When they are discarded, they add to a larger environmental footprint.

Image: Area of Land Needed to Produce Oil

Choosing Sustainable Oils

The most widely used vegetable on earth is palm oil and the World Wide Fund for Nature (WWF) developed a Palm Oil Buyers Scorecard 2020 to assist buyers in selecting palm oil from sellers who are being responsible and using sustainability practices.

Every oil has significant environmental impacts across the various production steps, though **the agricultural stage is the most influential** overall. Nuts or seeds grown on high-yielding trees may require fewer inputs over time than annual crop production. For example, palm oil production uses far less land than other monocrops — one-fifth of that of canola oil and one-eighth of soybean oil; however, the clearing of land for palm trees is responsible for high greenhouse gas emissions (Palm-Oil-and-Global-Warming). Soil degradation should also be considered as well as heavy use of pesticides and fertilizers. Table 9 outlines a few issues unique to the production of specific oils. The fat from dairy products has a large environmental impact as well as greenhouse gas emissions.

**Table 9: Environmental Impact of Oils and
the Percent of Genetically Modified Organisms (GMO)***

Oil	Environmental Impact**	GMO%
Soybean	Contributes significantly to deforestation; production is driven by demand for animal feed.	94%
Canola	Vulnerable to disease and require heavy fertilizer. Grown as mono crops, so they often require extensive clearing of land.	95%
Sunflower	Generally has lower greenhouse gas footprint but may use more water than some oils and have higher processing costs.	0%
Coconut	Often requires clearing of important habitats, such as coastal mangroves, and loss of species. In addition, coconut farmers are typically low wage earners.	0%

Oil	Environmental Impact**	GMO%
Corn	Grown as a monocrop requiring nitrogen fertilizer; a highly refined oil.	92%
Olive	The growing demand has impacted production methods, shifting toward less traditional methods that lend to more soil degradation and habitat loss.	0%
Avocado	Linked to extensive land clearing and water use.	0%
Peanut	Requires a lot of land and water for production; however, as a nitrogen fixer, promotes healthful soil and can be intercropped for improved productivity of other crops	0%

*GMO

** (FAOSTAT; Poore & Nemecek, 2018; Rochmyaningsih; Schmidt, 2015)

What about Butter?

The production of butter from dairy milk follows a much different process than plant oils. Butter has more than three times the greenhouse gas emissions footprint and uses more water and land than plant-based spreads/margarines, which is largely attributed to the feeding and raising of cows for milk. Some margarines contain palm oil, which has unique environmental impacts, as mentioned above (Liao et al., 2020).

Tips for Shopping

Choosing the most sustainable oil can be difficult because of the complexity and variability in production methods, as well as the transparency in the food chain. Here are a few tips for making the best choice:

• For vegetable oils, choose organic when possible
• Look for naturally refined or unrefined oils
• Choose cold-pressed if available
• Consider fair trade for oils typically produced in lower-income countries, such as coconut oil
• Purchase CSPO palm oils. Use WWF scorecard to compare products
• (Palm_oil_buyers_scorecards).

To save money, use a less expensive neutral oil when cooking and at the end, add a touch of extra virgin olive oil for flavor.

SECTION 10:

FATS AND OILS IN THE KITCHEN

Dietary fats affect the appearance (e.g., fatty streaks in steak), odor, taste, and physical properties (e.g., thickness of beverages, oiliness, creaminess) of food (Mattes, 2009). Because of these qualities, it becomes possible for individuals to estimate the amount of fat in a food or beverage by how it looks, smells, and tastes.

Essential properties of fat that are important to be aware of in the kitchen are the following:
1. Lipids and water do not mix: To combine these two ingredients takes work and an emulsifier.
2. There is no sharp defined melting point for fats. Each fat molecule melts slowly within a range of temperatures, which varies depending on the type of fat molecule.
3. Fats can reach a smoke point at which it breaks down into gaseous products. At this point the flavor is ruined and toxic compounds are formed.

ON THE TONGUE

Humans are born with an innate preference for the taste of sweetness, which promotes an infant's interest in trying new foods. However, humans are not pre-wired to like the taste of fat. Experts theorize that humans began eating fatty foods out of evolutionary demands when they had to eat more energy-dense foods to survive. As a person ages, most develop an affinity for fat, but the level of affinity varies greatly. The degree to which an individual likes or even desires fat likely stems from many factors, including genetic predisposition, metabolic needs, emotional factors, behavior, and even cultural or socioeconomic factors (Drewnowski & Almiron-Roig, 2010).

Historically, it was believed that human taste buds could not detect the taste of fat and that fat in foods contributed only to the texture and flavor release of foods, not taste per se. Recently, however, research has suggested that fatty acids do have a taste and that, in isolation, the taste tends to range from bitter to rancid. Emerging research suggests that medium-chain and long-chain fatty acids have a taste that is characteristically different from the better-known tastes — sweet, sour, salty, and bitter. However, there may be some overlap between the taste of umami and the taste of fatty acids. Interestingly, scientists believe that as the fatty acid chain length increases, the fat sensation or taste gets more bitter (Running et al., 2015).

Despite fat's bitter taste on its own, fat combined with sugar or salt creates an undeniable sensory appeal. In addition to fat being a taste enhancer, fat also contributes properties that cause a product or food to become thicker and creamier and, for some individuals, impossible to refuse. In fact, scientists believe that the fat-sugar combination elicits the release of dopamine, a neurotransmitter related to motivation and reward brain circuitry. Dopamine is released as soon as a food high in fat and sugar touches the tongue, and the brain is rewarded with a "hedonic" or pleasure sensation. In individuals who frequently overeat these foods, there is an overload of dopamine to the brain. Eventually, the body compensates by desensitizing itself, which means that some then require higher amounts of "hedonic" foods to be consumed in order to reach the previous threshold. There is emerging science showing that the hunger hormone, ghrelin, may also play a role in the fatty food-dopamine release mechanism (Volkow et al., 2002).

IN THE PANTRY

- Sources of omega-3 fatty acids:
  - Seafood (salmon, tuna, sardines, and other fatty fish)
  - Walnuts
  - Flax seeds
  - Organic canola oil
- Sources of monounsaturated fats:
  - Avocado
  - Extra virgin olive oil (use cold-pressed EVOO)
- Polyunsaturated fats that are good sources of omega-6 fats are mostly plant-based oils:
  - Safflower oil
  - Grapeseed oil
  - Flaxseed oil
  - Sunflower oil
  - Soybean oil
- Solid fats
  - Ghee
  - Butter
- High-fat ingredients (to use strategically and not in excess in order to bring out the flavor in a dish)
  - Nuts and seeds
  - Cheese
  - Eggs
  - Smoked meats like bacon and pancetta (use sparingly)
  - Yogurt — substitute Greek yogurt for the whole fat version

- o Cream: <u>dairy</u> varieties — sour cream, whipping cream, and vegetable varieties — coconut cream
  - o Avocados
- A variety of oils: Have on hand higher-quality oils that come packed with their own flavor for use on salads and cold dishes. Save the neutral oils for cooking as they don't impart any distinguishable flavor to the dish.
  - Flavorful oils — extra virgin olive oil, peanut, and toasted sesame seed oil
  - Infused oils – orange, lemon and/or lemon infused oils (there are dozens to choose from or create)
  - Neutral oils — corn, safflower, canola, and grapeseed oil

STORING FATS

Fats can go bad — turn rancid — when exposed to heat, light, and high temperatures. When a fat or oil becomes rancid, it will give off an unpleasant odor — similar to crayons — and have an off-putting flavor. Unsaturated fats (most vegetable oils that are liquid at room temperature) are more susceptible to damage from air. Store in an airtight container, away from direct light, and in a relatively cool place.

FLAVOR DEVELOPMENT

"Fat is essential for achieving the full spectrum of flavors and textures of good cooking" (Samin Nosrat, 2017 page 60). When it comes to flavor, fat affects flavor in a multitude of ways.

- Fat has its own flavor: Fat is considered as the sixth basic taste.
- Fat is a carrier for other flavors. Without it, certain flavors would not be picked up.
- Fat brings out and alters the entire flavor profile of the dish — not unlike salt.
- Fat coats the tongue and, in doing so, allows for aromatic ingredients to remain for longer periods of time, thus promoting the experience of flavor.
- Fat allows for browning, which will impart flavors to the food.
- Fat can transform the texture of food, lending a pleasant mouthfeel experience.
- Fat cuts the zing of acid in food – e.g., oil and vinegar dressing.

Taste Test. Sample various varieties of olive oil, from the very light pale yellow to the deep green. Close your eyes and pay attention to the subtle flavors of the deeper-colored olive oils. You may pick up on a grassy, peppery, or buttery aspect, or other subtle flavors. When it hits the back of your palette, a distinguishing bitter taste and a slight burn arises, or at least it should. That's when you know you have the real thing — EVOO and not some other cheaper oil being sold as the real thing.

Choosing the right olive oil is as unique to one's taste buds as is choosing a wine. Individuals need to try various ones until they find one that they prefer. Save the more expensive, better-tasting olive oils as a finishing touch to a dish and use the cheaper versions to cook with.

When it comes to selecting the type of oil needed for a dish, first decide if the oil is needed to impart a flavor to the dish — sesame oil in Thai dishes, or EVOO in salads for example. If not, select an oil with a neutral flavor. If the oil is to be heated, make sure it can withstand the heat by knowing its smoke point — the temperature at which the fat begins to break down and start smoking — found in Table 10. In general, plant-based oils do better at higher temperatures than animal fats, and refined vegetable oils can withstand a higher temperature before smoking than unrefined oils.

ROLE OF FAT IN COOKING AND PREPARATION

Fat in cooking and food preparation provides not only flavor and texture, but also contributes to a food's structure and consistency, plus it is a heat conductor. Fat inhibits gluten formation and assists the leavening process. It also adds moisture and helps to create a tender consistency.

The following is a list of the main functions that fats play in food
1. Flavor: Refer to the section above for a thorough description of fat's role in flavor.
2. Texture:
   a. Words like **silkiness**, richness, smooth, boldness, and succulent, are often used when describing the texture and flavor of dishes that use fat to enhance the flavors.
   b. Cooking in fat also allows for a **crispy** texture to be created by providing a much higher cooking temperature on the surface of food.
   c. Layering fat throughout pastry dough creates a **flaky** crust.
3. Transfer Heat: Fats used in cooking can reach a temperature beyond the boiling point of water, plus oils and melted fats act as a conductor dispersing even temperature around the food being cooked. These two qualities of fats allow food to develop a crisp outer texture and amazing flavor due to browning reactions. It also allows the food being cooked to reach a temperature (300 °F/149 °C to 500 °F/260 °C) above the boiling point of water (212 °F/100 °C).
4. Emulsification: Normally, water and fat would separate in a mixture, but if an emulsifier is present, it will hold the two in the solution. Two common emulsifiers used in the kitchen are mustard (used in vinaigrettes) and egg yolks (used to make hollandaise sauce and mayonnaise).
5. Exterior Appearance: When frying food in oil, the exterior becomes crisp while the interior remains tender and moist. The exterior starch portion of battered chicken or vegetables, for example, dries out as moisture is released from within and the hot oil creates a crispy crust.

Fat can play many roles in creating a dish. It can be:

1. A main ingredient — the fat interlaced within a steak, or the butter layers in puff pastry for example.
2. A medium in which food is cooked — frying chicken tenders in a frying pan or sautéing broccoli in olive oil and garlic (you do not need a lot of oil, just enough to coat the bottom of the pan).
3. A seasoning — buttered toast, mayonnaise on a sandwich, and drizzling olive oil on top of crusty bread.
4. A finishing touch — a drop of pesto or toasted sesame oil with fresh herbs on top of a bowl of soup. Finish a dish with an oil that can be seen as it will increase the flavor profile.

While fats are important in creating out-of-this-world dishes, the type and amount used can be manipulated to create healthful meals. Choosing liquid over solid forms of fat, finishing a dish with a bit of fat instead of adding it throughout, and removing excess fat before and after cooking are all techniques that can lead to a more healthful fat profile.

The type of fat that is used is much more important than the amount (CIA, 2000)

Table 10: Fats, Their Flavor Profile, and Smoke Point

Type of Oil	Smoke Point[a]	Flavor	Uses	Note
Walnut oil	320 °F/ 160 °C	Slight walnut taste	A finishing oil	Drizzle over soups, salads, and vegetables
Coconut oil	350 °F/ 177 °C	Powerful coconut flavor	Baking and light sautéing	Has a creamy and buttery feel to it
Canola oil (refined)	400 °F/ 204 °C	Neutral	Stir fry, deep frying	Pressed from the rapeseed plant
Vegetable oil	400 °F/ 204 °C	Neutral	Stir fry, deep frying	Is a blend of oils that are usually neutral in taste
Sesame oil	410 °F/ 210 °C	Sesame flavor	Stir fry, light sautéing	Great to add to finish soups, salad dressing, etc.
Grapeseed oil	420 °F/ 216 °C	Neutral	Sautéing, baking, and emulsification	Plays nice with other flavors and is a great emulsifying agent
Peanut oil	440° F/ 227 °C	Nutty scent and powerful peanut flavor	Stir fry, deep fry, sautéing	Be careful as you don't want to serve to anyone with a peanut allergy

Type of Oil	Smoke Point[a]	Flavor	Uses	Note
Sunflower oil	440 °F/ 227 °C	Neutral	Frying, baking, roasting	92% of U.S. corn is genetically engineered[b]
Corn oil (refined)	450 °F/ 232 °C	Neutral	Roasting, baking, stir fry, deep frying, sautéing	
Palm oil and palm kernel oil	450°F/ 232°C	neutral	Frying, baking	In order to neutralize its flavor, a chemical solvent is used. EVOO can be heated to 400°F
Light olive oil	465 °F/ 241 °C to 470 °F/243 °C	Neutral	Frying, sautéing, deep frying and baking	
Soybean oil	495 °F/ 257 °C	Neutral	Roasting, baking, stir fry, deep frying, sautéing	94% of U.S. soybeans is genetically engineered[b]
Safflower oil	510 °F/ 266 °C	Neutral	Sautéing and deep frying	
Avocado oil	520 °F/ 271 °C	Delicate avocado taste	Sautéing and finishing oil	Drizzle over cooked vegetables

Access on 12/8/2019:
a http://www.cookingforengineers.com/article/50/Smoke-Points-of-Various-Fats and
b https://www.centerforfoodsafety.org/issues/311/ge-foods/about-ge-foods

---

Culinary Tip: Once an oil starts to smoke, throw it away as harmful chemicals are formed once it reaches its smoke point.

BAKING

Baking and Butter

Using butter in baking is pretty standard, but there are substitutes that can be employed by understanding the role that butter plays in baking. Creaming butter and sugar (a typical first step in cakes, cookies, loaves, etc.) ensures an even rising and rich texture in baked goods. Oil can be substituted for butters in most recipes; however, the product may be dense or flat. To combat this, add a liquid sweetener, a solid fat, and an emulsifier to the oil base. Liquid sweeteners could include honey, agave, maple syrup, molasses, etc. Solid fats include peanut butters, almond butters, avocado, etc. The classic emulsifier is eggs, which requires using the yolks with the oil base and the whites with the remainder of the ingredients. These steps should produce a very similar product to butter in baked goods.

Cookies are an easier baked item for substituting the butter for oil. Replacing the butter with oil, liquid sweetener, and nut butter will create a shortbread-like product. Replacing butter with oil, egg yolks, and a sweetener will create a more cakey, soft, and chewy cookie.

Other substitutions:
- Eggs: Reduce yolks and, if binding is the main function, replace whole eggs with whites. If yolks are needed, reduce the amount: replace four eggs with two whole eggs and two egg whites.
- Fat tenderizes baked goods. Tenderize low-fat baked goods by using cake flour instead of all-purpose flour, or whole-wheat pastry flour in place of regular whole-wheat flour.
- Layers of phyllo pastry moistened with canola oil (or browned butter) and egg whites in place of puff pastry.
- Fruit purées add moisture (fig, applesauce, prune, banana, avocado, pear or apple butter) and are a good replacement for some fat (up to 30%) in a carrot cake, muffins, brownies, quick breads, etc.
- To reduce eggs, ¼ applesauce or banana purée can replace an egg if other leaveners are in use.
- Yolk-less soufflés with vegetable, meat, or fruit purées.
- Substitute cocoa (10% to 24% fat) for chocolate (36% to 60% fat).
- In place of traditional layer cakes that contain fat and whole eggs, try Dacquoise layers instead (baked meringue layers with ground toasted nuts), filled with a low-fat alternative.
- To add fiber and protein to baked goods, add a handful of cooked lentils or black beans
- Less fat, more flavor, better baking by King Arthur Baking Company

Replacing Whole Dairy in Recipes

- Thickened skim milk (2 tablespoons cornstarch added to 1 cup skim milk, stir, and wait for it to thicken) in soups or sauces for whole milk or cream.
- Evaporated skim milk for heavy cream, if robust flavors are available to mask its canned flavor (e.g., roasted garlic, chilies, and cumin in a southwest style soup).
- Chilled evaporated skim milk can be whipped for use in frozen mousses.
- Fromage blanc or pressed low-fat cottage cheese in place of ricotta or cream cheese.
- Low-fat yogurt or skim buttermilk for whole milk or cream (adjust for tartness).
- Replace whipped cream as a topping with drained low-fat vanilla yogurt.
- Italian meringue (uses pasteurized whites) in place of pastry cream or whipped cream as a topping or filling.

- Puréed low-fat cottage cheese sweetened and flavored with vanilla in place of crème anglaise.

MIXTURES WITH FAT AS THE MAIN INGREDIENT

Image: Salad Dressings

There are several varieties of salad dressings — the popular vinaigrette and the creamy salad dressing.

Image: Vinaigrettes

A typical vinaigrette is three parts oil to one part vinegar. Plant-based oils are a healthful part of a diet, but if a client is reducing overall fat intake, try the following recipes that use less fat:
- Use less oil and replace it with water: two parts oil, one part water, and one part vinegar
- Use flavored vinegars, which need less oil to impart a flavorful bite
- Use stronger flavored oils so that not as much oil is needed: walnut, sesame oil, virgin olive oil
- For a quick and easy salad dressing, whisk together one part lemon juice to one part oil, add garlic, salt, and pepper to taste

Image: Creamy Dressing

- Instead of using sour cream or mayonnaise for a creamy base for dressing, replace with the following:

- ○ Low-fat unflavored yogurt
- ○ Mustard
- ○ Tahini paste
- ○ Puréed silken tofu
- ○ An avocado
- ○ Cashew nuts

RECIPE: Chef's Russell's Quick Silken Tofu Vegan Ranch Dressing

Ingredients

- 1 pound silken tofu
- ¼ cup non-dairy milk (oat, rice, cashew, soy, etc...)
- 2 tablespoons green onions, chopped
- 2 tablespoons parsley, chopped
- 1 teaspoon garlic, chopped
- ¼ teaspoon onion powder
- ¼ teaspoon dill, dry
- 3 tablespoons lemon juice
- 1 tablespoon vinegar, red wine, or champagne

Methods

1. Gather all ingredients and equipment prior to beginning the recipe
2. In a blender, blend the tofu and non-dairy milk until velvety
3. Add all remaining ingredients pulsing the blender until fully incorporated

Chef's note: Pulsing the dressing at the end to incorporate the ingredients instead of blending until smooth will allow the ingredients to mix well without changing the color of the dressing to green.

Image: Infused Oils

To increase the flavor of a dish or food (slice of tomato, salad, or asparagus, for example), make an infused oil. These oils are super simple to make, but caution is needed when you use fresh instead of dry ingredients.

- Dried ingredients — place dry ingredients in a bottle or container of oil (dried or toasted herbs). Let sit for a couple of days before using it to let the flavors of the spices infuse into the oil. Store in a cool, dry place.
- Fresh ingredients — raw garlic, ginger, horseradish, shallots, orange or lemon zest for example can be used to infuse oil but it needs to be kept refrigerated and used within a week.

Image: Sauces

To thicken a sauce, blend any of the following (instead of cream and butter) into the mixture:
- Raw cashews
- Steamed cauliflower or boiled potatoes
- Soy yogurt or tofu

Instead of using creamy sauces to increase the flavor profile, reach instead for:
- Salsas, chutneys, coulis (light puréed fruit or sauce), jams, vegetable reductions, and drizzles of infused oils
- Use umami flavors to bring depth to a sauce, dried mushrooms, sundried tomatoes, nutritional yeast flakes, anchovy paste, and then lots of herbs and spices
- Add caramelized onions to soups, purée them into dressings, or add on top of grilled meat

Recipes to try:
- Stonyfield Farm's Penne With Yogurt Alfredo
- An Oat and Parsnip Bechamel Sauce for Pasta

COOKING MEAT WITH AN EYE ON FAT

Image: Remove Fat

Step 1: Select the cut of meat

Choose leaner cuts of meat as described in Table 8 for beef cuts; plus, lean meats also include poultry with the skin removed (if ground choose 90% or (%% lean), and pork labeled "loin" or "round."

Step 2: The preparation

Adding flavor before the cooking process will produce a tastier product. Poultry skin can be left on while roasting or sautéing (to preserve moisture) but removed before serving. If meat is being marinated or braised, remove the skin first so that fat is not emulsified in the cooking liquid.

Step 3: Choose a cooking method

Try any of the following: broil, grill, roast (on a rack), steam, sous vide, poach, braise, papillote — cooking in parchment or foil pouches. These are covered in the Protein chapter.

Step 4: Finishing step

For foods in a liquid base like stews or soups, skim the fat off before serving. Cool leftovers in the refrigerator. The fat will rise to the surface in a solid form, which is easy to remove.

A Note From Chef KJ: *I think it's important to start with the product that is going to give you the desired outcome, while still being the most healthful choice. For example, if you're making a chicken salad, you might as well use a boneless, skinless breast as it's the most healthful and best choice for the dish. However, if you are braising a piece of beef, you can't use a lean cut of meat off a bone because your final product will be dry and tasteless. Braising a fattier cut of meat and then leaving the meat submerged in the liquid to cool completely will benefit your dish in two ways; first, the meat will absorb the moisture and remain very tender and moist and, two, when the fat solidifies, it creates a cap on the surface you can remove in one go.*

Using lean cuts of meat and marinating is a great way to reduce fat while still maintaining flavor and texture. Marinated flank steak, chicken breasts, salmon steaks, whole fish, etc., on the BBQ is a great, low-fat option. Roasting in the oven is another low-fat cooking option, but I would suggest keeping some fat in your product during roasting to preserve flavor and moisture. Baked chicken thighs are a nice example of a product that has some fat naturally, but loses some in the roasting process and remains tender and moist.

Pan-searing in a small amount of oil and finishing in the oven is another option to use a small amount of fat during cooking.

Poaching and steaming are two methods of cooking that are so rarely used but are a great way to gently cook proteins and use basically no additional fats. Making a very flavorful court bouillon base to poach in is very important to ensure you have a flavorful final product. A base of water, white wine (if you want), lemon juice, leeks, onions, black peppercorns, bay leaves, cloves, allspice, celery, carrots, fresh parsley, fresh dill or any combination of those above is a great base to poach fish, chicken, and seafood.

Remedies for Adding Too Much Fat to a Dish

Image: Remedies for Removing Fat

Skim it: As shown in the picture, skim the fat off the top layer of cooled soups and stews.

Add more to it: Rebalance a dish that has too much fat by adding more ingredients by volume. This automatically dilutes the amount of fat per serving. Add solid ingredients (for example, add more potatoes, vegetables, or rice to a soup or stew); or liquids (more broth) to the soup.

Pat it: When frying food, place it on a paper towel to absorb the excess grease. The next time you get a takeout pizza, lay a paper towel on the slice. You will be astounded by the amount of grease the paper towel picks up.

COOKING WITH AN EYE ON ESSENTIAL FATTY ACIDS

Fats degrade when exposed to light, air, and heat. In regards to cooking, heat becomes the focus. In general, when cooking food immersed in fats and oil, some of that oil will be absorbed by the food, and some of the fat within the food can also migrate to the cooking oil.

When cooking tuna – EPA and DHA were preserved when tuna was cooked (baked) or microwaved, whereas 100% was lost when canned and 80% was lost with frying (Stephen et al., 2010). To preserve essential fatty acids avoid frying or cooking fish on high heat (Larsen et al., 2010; Stephen et al., 2010).

Similar results were found with eggs, whereby the amount of Omega 3 fatty acids decreased with increased heat and cooking time (Chen et al., 2021; Ren et al., 2013).

SECTION 10:

SERVING AND MENU PLANNING

3 teaspoons = 1 tablespoon

Table 11: Servings of Fats/Oils Per Day

Age of Child (years)	Amount per Day	Serving Size
2 to 3	3 teaspoons	½ teaspoon
4 to 8	4 teaspoons	1 teaspoon
Girls 9 to 13	5 teaspoons	2 teaspoons
Boys 9 to 13	5 teaspoons	
Girls 14 to 18	5 teaspoons	
Boys 14 to 18	5 teaspoons	2 to 3 teaspoons
Women 19 to 30	6 teaspoons	
Women 31 to 50	6 teaspoons	
Women 51+	5 teaspoons	
Men 19 to 30	5 teaspoons	
Men 31 to 50	7 teaspoons	
Men 51+	6 teaspoons	
	6 teaspoons	

When it comes to menu planning, think about cooking with and serving fats from plant-based oils, fish, nuts, and seeds. Use the culinary techniques discussed in this chapter to create flavorful dishes without resorting to the easy addition of butter and salt. The Menus of Change Principles Report recommends not worrying about using too much fat but to "go 'good fat,' not 'low fat' " and to "choose healthier oils." It is important to create meals that consumers will enjoy, and there are a lot of unsaturated fat sources to choose from. Figure two depicts the unnecessary addition of calories from unhealthful fats and sugar. One does not have to sacrifice taste and resort to added solid fat and sugar to create a delicious end product.

Figure 2: Example of Calories in Food Choices With & Without the Addition of Solid Fats & Sugar

SECTION 11:

PRACTICAL TIPS TO IMPROVE FAT AND OIL CONSUMPTION

1. Use fat where it will count the most — add a small amount toward the end of cooking; drizzle a small amount of olive oil on soups, salads, and salsas.
2. Use less oil by blanching or steaming vegetables beforehand and then quickly sautéing with a small amount of oil.
3. Brown butter (beurre noisette) is used to increase its flavor, so less is needed.
4. Substitute avocado as a spread on bread instead of butter.
5. Save the expensive first-pressed olive oil for finishing a dish and use less expensive varieties of oil for cooking.
6. Replace fats/oils with a small amount of lean, flavorful meat like smoked turkey or chicken.
7. Dried mushrooms, roasted eggplant, sun-dried tomatoes and smoked chilies are also great replacements for fats in a dish.
8. When using lean meat, marinade it first or add a natural sweetener like honey or an umami ingredient to improve the flavor and mouthfeel.
9. So many dishes are low in fat and tasty already. Hearty salads with a small amount of grilled protein, some whole grains, and just a pop of excitement like crumbled cheese, dried fruits, toasted nuts, and fresh herbs can be so satisfying and tasty.
10. Instead of frying, coat a baking pan in oil and bake breaded chicken for a crispy bite.
11. For a sandwich spread, use hummus, pesto, or a drizzle of olive oil, plus include fresh herbs and pickled vegetables for an extra punch of flavor.

SUMMARY

The overall messaging around fat has changed from "choose low fat" to "choose healthful fats." Research shows that unsaturated fatty acids, like PUFAs and MUFAs, can help to promote optimal health during all life stages. Saturated fat intake should be limited, and trans fat should be avoided. This is easier to do by limiting the intake of food purchased outside the home, as many are made with saturated fats.

The right type of fat is essential for optimal brain health and health in general as it is embedded into the wall of all cells within the body. Fat helps with satiety, and it is also crucial for flavor development and promoting a nice mouthfeel. Learning how to cook with fats and oils, and how to build flavor is essential for being able to eat a diet with a healthful fat profile.

APPENDIX A: The USDA DGA Guidelines for Fats and Oils From 1980 to 2020

USDA 1980:
- Avoid too much fat, saturated fat, and cholesterol

USDA 1985:
- Avoid too much fat, saturated fat, and cholesterol

USDA 1990:
- Choose a diet low in fat, saturated fat, and cholesterol

USDA 1995:
- Choose a diet low in fat, saturated fat, and cholesterol.

USDA 2000:
- Choose a diet that is low in saturated fat and cholesterol and moderate in total fat

The USDA DGA 2005 went into detail about what is too much:
- Consume less than 10 percent of calories from saturated fatty acids and less than 300 mg/day of cholesterol, and keep trans fatty acid consumption as low as possible.
- Keep total fat intake between 20 to 35 percent of calories, with most fats coming from sources of polyunsaturated and monounsaturated fatty acids, such as fish, nuts, and vegetable oils.
- When selecting and preparing meat, poultry, dry beans, and milk or milk products, make choices that are lean, low fat, or fat free.
- Limit intake of fats and oils high in saturated and/or trans fatty acids, and choose products low in such fats and oils.

DGA 2010 continued with the specificity and total fat amount was removed. It included:
- Consume less than 10 percent of calories from saturated fatty acids by replacing them with monounsaturated and polyunsaturated fatty acids.
- Consume less than 300 mg per day of dietary cholesterol.
- Keep trans fatty acid consumption as low as possible by limiting foods that contain synthetic sources of trans fats, such as partially hydrogenated oils, and by limiting other solid fats.
- Reduce the intake of calories from solid fats and added sugars.

- Increase intake of fat-free or low-fat milk and milk products, such as milk, yogurt, cheese, or fortified soy beverages.
- Replace protein foods that are higher in solid fats with choices that are lower in solid fats and calories and/or are sources of oils.
- Use oils to replace solid fats where possible

DGA 2015:
- Limit calories from added sugars and saturated fats, and reduce sodium intake
- A healthy eating pattern includes fat-free or low-fat dairy, including milk, yogurt, cheese, and/or fortified soy beverages
- A healthy eating pattern includes oils
- A healthy eating pattern limits saturated fats and trans fats,
- Consume less than 10 percent of calories per day from saturated fats.

DGA 2020:
- Oil – from vegetable oils and oils in food, such as seafood and nuts – is a core element that makes up a healthy eating pattern
- Saturated fat intake at less than 10% or less of calories per day starting at age 2
- The National Academies recommends that trans fat and dietary cholesterol consumption to be as low as possible without compromising the nutritional adequacy of the diet

REFERENCES

2015-2020 Dietary Guidelines | health.gov. Retrieved March 15, 2020, from https://health.gov/our-work/food-nutrition/2015-2020-dietary-guidelines/guidelines/

2015–2020 Dietary Guidelines for Americans—Health.gov. (2015). https://health.gov/dietaryguidelines/2015/

Abdelhamid, A. S., Brown, T. J., Brainard, J. S., Biswas, P., Thorpe, G. C., Moore, H. J., Deane, K. H., Summerbell, C. D., Worthington, H. V., Song, F., & Hooper, L. (2020). Omega-3 fatty acids for the primary and secondary prevention of cardiovascular disease. The Cochrane Database of Systematic Reviews, 3, CD003177. https://doi.org/10.1002/14651858.CD003177.pub5

AHA. (2020). Food Packaging Claims. Www.Heart.Org. https://www.heart.org/en/healthy-living/healthy-eating/eat-smart/nutrition-basics/food-packaging-claims

Albanese, E., Dangour, A. D., Uauy, R., Acosta, D., Guerra, M., Guerra, S. S. G., Huang, Y., Jacob, K. S., Llibre de Rodriguez, J., Noriega, L. H., Salas, A., Sosa, A. L., Sousa, R. M., Williams, J., Ferri, C. P., & Prince, M. J. (2009). Dietary fish and meat intake and dementia in Latin America, China, and India: A 10/66 Dementia Research Group population-based study. The American Journal of Clinical Nutrition, 90(2), 392–400. https://doi.org/10.3945/ajcn.2009.27580

Assaf-Balut, C., García de la Torre, N., Calle-Pascual, A. L., St. Carlos Study Group, Calle-Pascual, A. L., Torre, N. G. de la, Durán, A., Jiménez, I., Rubio, M. Á., Herraíz, M. Á., Izquierdo, N., Pérez, N., Garcia, A. S., Dominguez, G. C., Torrejón, M. J., Cuadrado, M. Á., Assaf-Balut, C., Del Valle, L., Bordiú, E., ... All members of St Carlos Study Group have read and agreed with the content of the last version of manuscript. Each member named has participated actively and sufficiently in the case reported and fulfilled all conditions as authors. (2019). Detection, treatment and prevention programs for gestational diabetes mellitus: The St Carlos experience. Endocrinologia, Diabetes Y Nutricion. https://doi.org/10.1016/j.endinu.2019.06.007

Astrup, A., Meinert Larsen, T., & Harper, A. (2004). Atkins and other low-carbohydrate diets: Hoax or an effective tool for weight loss? Lancet (London, England), 364(9437), 897–899. https://doi.org/10.1016/S0140-6736(04)16986-9

Bourre, J. M. (2004). Roles of unsaturated fatty acids (especially omega-3 fatty acids) in the brain at various ages and during ageing. The Journal of Nutrition, Health & Aging, 8(3), 163–174.

Bozzatello, P., Brignolo, E., De Grandi, E., & Bellino, S. (2016). Supplementation with Omega-3 Fatty Acids in Psychiatric Disorders: A Review of Literature Data. Journal of Clinical Medicine, 5(8). https://doi.org/10.3390/jcm5080067

Chen, X., Liang, K., & Zhu, H. (2021). Effects of cooking on the nutritional quality and volatile compounds in omega-3 fatty acids enriched eggs. Journal of the Science of Food and Agriculture, n/a(n/a). https://doi.org/10.1002/jsfa.11717

Crosby, L., Davis, B., Joshi, S., Jardine, M., Paul, J., Neola, M., & Barnard, N. D. (2021). Ketogenic Diets and Chronic Disease: Weighing the Benefits Against the Risks. Frontiers in Nutrition, 8, 702802. https://doi.org/10.3389/fnut.2021.702802

Dansinger, M. L., Gleason, J. A., Griffith, J. L., Selker, H. P., & Schaefer, E. J. (2005). Comparison of the Atkins, Ornish, Weight Watchers, and Zone diets for weight loss and heart disease risk reduction: A randomized trial. JAMA, 293(1), 43–53. https://doi.org/10.1001/jama.293.1.43

Davidson, P. W., Cory-Slechta, D. A., Thurston, S. W., Huang, L.-S., Shamlaye, C. F., Gunzler, D., Watson, G., van Wijngaarden, E., Zareba, G., Klein, J. D., Clarkson, T. W., Strain, J. J., & Myers, G. J. (2011). Fish consumption and prenatal methylmercury exposure: Cognitive and behavioral outcomes in the main cohort at 17 years from the Seychelles child development study. NeuroToxicology, 32(6), 711–717. https://doi.org/10.1016/j.neuro.2011.08.003

Delgado-Lista, J., Perez-Martinez, P., Lopez-Miranda, J., & Perez-Jimenez, F. (2012). Long chain omega-3 fatty acids and cardiovascular disease: A systematic review. The British Journal of Nutrition, 107 Suppl 2, S201-213. https://doi.org/10.1017/S0007114512001596

Devassy, J. G., Leng, S., Gabbs, M., Monirujjaman, M., & Aukema, H. M. (2016). Omega-3 Polyunsaturated Fatty Acids and Oxylipins in Neuroinflammation and Management of Alzheimer Disease12. Advances in Nutrition, 7(5), 905–916. https://doi.org/10.3945/an.116.012187

Diekman, C., & Malcolm, K. (2009). Consumer Perception and Insights on Fats and Fatty Acids: Knowledge on the Quality of Diet Fat. Annals of Nutrition and Metabolism, 54(Suppl. 1), 25–32. https://doi.org/10.1159/000220824

Dierge, E., Debock, E., Guilbaud, C., Corbet, C., Mignolet, E., Mignard, L., Bastien, E., Dessy, C., Larondelle, Y., & Feron, O. (2021). Peroxidation of n-3 and n-6 polyunsaturated fatty acids in the acidic tumor environment leads to ferroptosis-mediated anticancer effects. Cell Metabolism, 33(8), 1701-1715.e5. https://doi.org/10.1016/j.cmet.2021.05.016

Dietary Guidelines for Americans, 2020-2025. 164.

Drewnowski, A., & Almiron-Roig, E. (2010). Human Perceptions and Preferences for Fat-Rich Foods. In J.-P. Montmayeur & J. le Coutre (Eds.), Fat Detection: Taste, Texture, and Post Ingestive Effects. CRC Press/Taylor & Francis. http://www.ncbi.nlm.nih.gov/books/NBK53528/

Estruch, R., Martínez-González, M. A., Corella, D., Salas-Salvadó, J., Fitó, M., Chiva-Blanch, G., Fiol, M., Gómez-Gracia, E., Arós, F., Lapetra, J., Serra-Majem, L., Pintó, X., Buil-Cosiales, P., Sorlí, J. V., Muñoz, M. A., Basora-Gallisá, J., Lamuela-Raventós, R. M., Serra-Mir, M., Ros, E., & PREDIMED Study Investigators. (2019). Effect of a high-fat Mediterranean diet on bodyweight and waist circumference: A prespecified secondary outcomes analysis of the PREDIMED randomised controlled trial. The Lancet. Diabetes & Endocrinology, 7(5), e6–e17. https://doi.org/10.1016/S2213-8587(19)30074-9

FAOSTAT. Retrieved January 17, 2022, from https://www.fao.org/faostat/en/#data/QC

Fish and Omega-3 Fatty Acids. Www.Heart.Org. Retrieved January 17, 2022, from https://www.heart.org/en/healthy-living/healthy-eating/eat-smart/fats/fish-and-omega-3-fatty-acids

Gardner, C. D., Kiazand, A., Alhassan, S., Kim, S., Stafford, R. S., Balise, R. R., Kraemer, H. C., & King, A. C. (2007). Comparison of the Atkins, Zone, Ornish, and LEARN diets for change in weight and related risk factors among overweight premenopausal women: The A TO Z Weight Loss Study: a randomized trial. JAMA, 297(9), 969–977. https://doi.org/10.1001/jama.297.9.969

Golding, J., Steer, C., Emmett, P., Davis, J. M., & Hibbeln, J. R. (2009). High levels of depressive symptoms in pregnancy with low omega-3 fatty acid intake from fish. Epidemiology (Cambridge, Mass.), 20(4), 598–603. https://doi.org/10.1097/EDE.0b013e31819d6a57

Goodarz Danaei, Eric L. Ding, Dariush Mozaffarian, Ben Taylor, Jürgen Rehm, Christopher J. L. Murray, & Majid Ezzati. (2009). The Preventable Causes of Death in the United States: Comparative Risk Assessment of Dietary, Lifestyle, and Metabolic Risk Factors. https://journals.plos.org/plosmedicine/article?id=10.1371/journal.pmed.1000058

Grundy, S. M. (1994). Influence of stearic acid on cholesterol metabolism relative to other long-chain fatty acids. The American Journal of Clinical Nutrition, 60(6 Suppl), 986S-990S. https://doi.org/10.1093/ajcn/60.6.986S

Hernáez, Á., Sanllorente, A., Castañer, O., Martínez-González, M. Á., Ros, E., Pintó, X., Estruch, R., Salas-Salvadó, J., Corella, D., Alonso-Gómez, Á. M., Serra-Majem, L., Fiol, M., Lapetra, J., Gómez-Gracia, E., de la Torre, R., Lamuela-Raventós, R.-M., & Fitó, M. (2019). Increased Consumption of Virgin Olive Oil, Nuts, Legumes, Whole Grains, and Fish Promotes HDL Functions in Humans. Molecular Nutrition & Food Research, 63(6), e1800847. https://doi.org/10.1002/mnfr.201800847

Hibbeln, J. R., Davis, J. M., Steer, C., Emmett, P., Rogers, I., Williams, C., & Golding, J. (2007). Maternal seafood consumption in pregnancy and neurodevelopmental outcomes in childhood (ALSPAC study): An observational cohort study. The Lancet, 369(9561), 578–585. https://doi.org/10.1016/S0140-6736(07)60277-3

Hibbeln, Joseph. R., & Gow, R. V. (2014). Omega-3 Fatty Acid and Nutrient Deficits in Adverse Neurodevelopment and Childhood Behaviors. Child and Adolescent Psychiatric Clinics of North America, 23(3), 555–590. https://doi.org/10.1016/j.chc.2014.02.002

Hooper, L., Martin, N., Jimoh, O. F., Kirk, C., Foster, E., & Abdelhamid, A. S. (2020). Reduction in saturated fat intake for cardiovascular disease. The Cochrane Database of Systematic Reviews, 5, CD011737. https://doi.org/10.1002/14651858.CD011737.pub2

Huo, R., Du, T., Xu, Y., Xu, W., Chen, X., Sun, K., & Yu, X. (2015). Effects of Mediterranean-style diet on glycemic control, weight loss and cardiovascular risk factors among type 2 diabetes individuals: A meta-analysis. European Journal of Clinical Nutrition, 69(11), 1200–1208. https://doi.org/10.1038/ejcn.2014.243

Ibarguren, M., López, D. J., & Escribá, P. V. (2014). The effect of natural and synthetic fatty acids on membrane structure, microdomain organization, cellular functions and human health. Biochimica et Biophysica Acta (BBA) - Biomembranes, 1838(6), 1518–1528. https://doi.org/10.1016/j.bbamem.2013.12.021

Innes, J. K., & Calder, P. C. (2018). The Differential Effects of Eicosapentaenoic Acid and Docosahexaenoic Acid on Cardiometabolic Risk Factors: A Systematic Review. International Journal of Molecular Sciences, 19(2), 532. https://doi.org/10.3390/ijms19020532

Jacqueline D. Wright, Chia-Yih Wang, Jocelyn Kennedy-Stephenson, & R. Bethene Ervin. (2003). Advance Data From Vital and Health Statistics. 334, 4.

Jenkins, D. J. A., Wong, J. M. W., Kendall, C. W. C., Esfahani, A., Ng, V. W. Y., Leong, T. C. K., Faulkner, D. A., Vidgen, E., Paul, G., Mukherjea, R., Krul, E. S., & Singer, W. (2014). Effect of a 6-month vegan low-carbohydrate ('Eco-Atkins') diet on cardiovascular risk factors and body weight in hyperlipidaemic adults: A randomised controlled trial. BMJ Open, 4(2), e003505. https://doi.org/10.1136/bmjopen-2013-003505

Kastorini, C.-M., Milionis, H. J., Esposito, K., Giugliano, D., Goudevenos, J. A., & Panagiotakos, D. B. (2011). The effect of Mediterranean diet on metabolic syndrome and its components: A meta-analysis of 50 studies and 534,906 individuals. Journal of the American College of Cardiology, 57(11), 1299–1313. https://doi.org/10.1016/j.jacc.2010.09.073

Kaushik, M., Mozaffarian, D., Spiegelman, D., Manson, J. E., Willett, W. C., & Hu, F. B. (2009). Long-chain omega-3 fatty acids, fish intake, and the risk of type 2 diabetes mellitus. The American Journal of Clinical Nutrition, 90(3), 613–620. https://doi.org/10.3945/ajcn.2008.27424

Lagiou, P., Sandin, S., Lof, M., Trichopoulos, D., Adami, H.-O., & Weiderpass, E. (2012). Low carbohydrate-high protein diet and incidence of cardiovascular diseases in Swedish women: Prospective cohort study. BMJ (Clinical Research Ed.), 344, e4026. https://doi.org/10.1136/bmj.e4026

Larsen, D., SiewYoung, Q., & Eyres, L. (2010). Effect of cooking method on the fatty acid profile of New Zealand King Salmon (Oncorhynchus tshawytscha). Food Chemistry, 119(2), 785–790.

Lee, J. H., O'Keefe, J. H., Lavie, C. J., Marchioli, R., & Harris, W. S. (2008). Omega-3 Fatty Acids for Cardioprotection. Mayo Clinic Proceedings, 83(3), 324–332. https://doi.org/10.4065/83.3.324

Li, X., Bi, X., Wang, S., Zhang, Z., Li, F., & Zhao, A. Z. (2019). Therapeutic Potential of ω-3 Polyunsaturated Fatty Acids in Human Autoimmune Diseases. Frontiers in Immunology, 10. https://doi.org/10.3389/fimmu.2019.02241

Liao, X., Gerichhausen, M. J. W., Bengoa, X., Rigarlsford, G., Beverloo, R. H., Bruggeman, Y., & Rossi, V. (2020). Large-scale regionalised LCA shows that plant-based fat spreads have a lower climate, land occupation and water scarcity impact than dairy butter. The International Journal of Life Cycle Assessment, 25(6), 1043–1058. https://doi.org/10.1007/s11367-019-01703-w

Liu, A. G., Ford, N. A., Hu, F. B., Zelman, K. M., Mozaffarian, D., & Kris-Etherton, P. M. (2017). A healthy approach to dietary fats: Understanding the science and taking action to reduce consumer confusion. Nutrition Journal, 16(1), 53. https://doi.org/10.1186/s12937-017-0271-4

Lusk, J. L. (2019). Consumer beliefs about healthy foods and diets. PLoS ONE, 14(10), e0223098. https://doi.org/10.1371/journal.pone.0223098

Madden, S. M. M., Garrioch, C. F., & Holub, B. J. (2009). Direct Diet Quantification Indicates Low Intakes of (n-3) Fatty Acids in Children 4 to 8 Years Old. The Journal of Nutrition, 139(3), 528–532. https://doi.org/10.3945/jn.108.100628

Makhoul, Z., Kristal, A. R., Gulati, R., Luick, B., Bersamin, A., O'Brien, D., Hopkins, S. E., Stephensen, C. B., Stanhope, K. L., Havel, P. J., & Boyer, B. (2011). Associations of obesity with triglycerides and C-reactive protein are attenuated in adults with high red blood cell eicosapentaenoic and docosahexaenoic acids. European Journal of Clinical Nutrition, 65(7), 808–817. https://doi.org/10.1038/ejcn.2011.39

Marklund, M., Wu, J. H. Y., Imamura, F., Del Gobbo, L. C., Fretts, A., de Goede, J., Shi, P., Tintle, N., Wennberg, M., Aslibekyan, S., Chen, T.-A., de Oliveira Otto, M. C., Hirakawa, Y., Eriksen, H. H., Kröger, J., Laguzzi, F., Lankinen, M., Murphy, R. A., Prem, K., ... null, null. (2019). Biomarkers of Dietary Omega-6 Fatty Acids and Incident Cardiovascular Disease and Mortality. Circulation, 139(21), 2422–2436. https://doi.org/10.1161/CIRCULATIONAHA.118.038908

Martínez-Lapiscina, Clavero, P., Toledo, E., Estruch, R., Salas-Salvadó, J., San Julián, B., Sanchez-Tainta, A., Ros, E., Valls-Pedret, C., & Martinez-Gonzalez, M. Á. (2013). Mediterranean diet improves cognition: The PREDIMED-NAVARRA randomised trial. Journal of Neurology, Neurosurgery, and Psychiatry, 84(12), 1318–1325. https://doi.org/10.1136/jnnp-2012-304792

Masood, W., & Uppaluri, K. R. (2020). Ketogenic Diet. In StatPearls. StatPearls Publishing. http://www.ncbi.nlm.nih.gov/books/NBK499830/

Mattes, R. D. (2009). Is There a Fatty Acid Taste? Annual Review of Nutrition, 29, 305–327. https://doi.org/10.1146/annurev-nutr-080508-141108

Medicine, I. of. (2002). Dietary Reference Intakes for Energy, Carbohydrate, Fiber, Fat, Fatty Acids, Cholesterol, Protein, and Amino Acids. https://doi.org/10.17226/10490

Meijaard, E., Abrams, J. F., Juffe-Bignoli, D., Voigt, M., & Sheil, D. (2020). Coconut oil, conservation and the conscientious consumer. Current Biology: CB, 30(13), R757–R758. https://doi.org/10.1016/j.cub.2020.05.059

Micha, R., & Mozaffarian, D. (2010). Saturated Fat and Cardiometabolic Risk Factors, Coronary Heart Disease, Stroke, and Diabetes: A Fresh Look at the Evidence. Lipids, 45(10), 893–905. https://doi.org/10.1007/s11745-010-3393-4

Mozaffarian, D., Katan, M. B., Ascherio, A., Stampfer, M. J., & Willett, W. C. (2006). Trans fatty acids and cardiovascular disease. The New England Journal of Medicine, 354(15), 1601–1613. https://doi.org/10.1056/NEJMra054035

National Academies of Sciences, E., Division, H. and M., Board, F. and N., & Americans, C. to R. the P. to U. the D. G. for. (2017). Redesigning the Process for Establishing The Dietary Guidelines for Americans. In Redesigning the Process for Establishing the Dietary Guidelines for Americans. National Academies Press (US). https://www.ncbi.nlm.nih.gov/books/NBK469839/

Nettleton, J. A., Brouwer, I. A., Geleijnse, J. M., & Hornstra, G. (2017). Saturated Fat Consumption and Risk of Coronary Heart Disease and Ischemic Stroke: A Science Update. Annals of Nutrition & Metabolism, 70(1), 26–33. https://doi.org/10.1159/000455681

Nutrition, C. for F. S. and A. (2019a). FDA Completes Review of Qualified Health Claim Petition for Macadamia Nuts and the Risk of Coronary Heart Disease. FDA. http://www.fda.gov/food/cfsan-constituent-updates/fda-completes-review-qualified-health-claim-petition-macadamia-nuts-and-risk-coronary-heart-disease

Nutrition, C. for F. S. and A. (2019b). Advice about Eating Fish. FDA. http://www.fda.gov/food/consumers/advice-about-eating-fish

Nutrition, C. for F. S. and A. (2021). Changes to the Nutrition Facts Label. FDA. https://www.fda.gov/food/food-labeling-nutrition/changes-nutrition-facts-label

Othman, R. (2007). Dietary Lipids and Cancer. The Libyan Journal of Medicine, 2(4), 180–184. https://doi.org/10.4176/070831

Palm-oil-and-global-warming.pdf. Retrieved January 17, 2022, from https://www.ucsusa.org/sites/default/files/legacy/assets/documents/global_warming/palm-oil-and-global-warming.pdf

Palm_oil_buyers_scorecards. Retrieved January 17, 2022, from https://wwf.panda.org/discover/our_focus/food_practice/sustainable_production/palm_oil/scorecards/

Parks, E. J., & Hellerstein, M. K. (2000). Carbohydrate-induced hypertriacylglycerolemia: Historical perspective and review of biological mechanisms. The American Journal of Clinical Nutrition, 71(2), 412–433. https://doi.org/10.1093/ajcn/71.2.412

Poore, J., & Nemecek, T. (2018). Reducing food's environmental impacts through producers and consumers. Science, 360(6392), 987–992. https://doi.org/10.1126/science.aaq0216

Pottala, J. V., Yaffe, K., Robinson, J. G., Espeland, M. A., Wallace, R., & Harris, W. S. (2014). Higher RBC EPA + DHA corresponds with larger total brain and hippocampal volumes: WHIMS-MRI study. Neurology, 82(5), 435–442. https://doi.org/10.1212/WNL.0000000000000080

Querques, G., Forte, R., & Souied, E. H. (2011). Retina and Omega-3. Journal of Nutrition and Metabolism, 2011, 748361. https://doi.org/10.1155/2011/748361

Recent study adds weight to the low-carb vs. Low-fat debate. (2014, September 18). Www.Heart.Org. https://www.heart.org/en/news/2018/05/01/recent-study-adds-weight-to-the-lowcarb-vs-lowfat-debate

Ren, Y., Perez, T. I., Zuidhof, M. J., Renema, R. A., & Wu, J. (2013). Oxidative Stability of Omega-3 Polyunsaturated Fatty Acids Enriched Eggs. Journal of Agricultural and Food Chemistry, 61(47), 11595–11602. https://doi.org/10.1021/jf403039m

Rochmyaningsih, D. Claim that coconut oil is worse for biodiversity than palm oil sparks furious debate. Science. Retrieved January 17, 2022, from https://www.science.org/content/article/claim-coconut-oil-worse-biodiversity-palm-oil-sparks-furious-debate

Running, C. A., Craig, B. A., & Mattes, R. D. (2015). Oleogustus: The Unique Taste of Fat. Chemical Senses, 40(7), 507–516. https://doi.org/10.1093/chemse/bjv036

Sacks, F. M., Lichtenstein, A. H., Wu, J. H. Y., Appel, L. J., Creager, M. A., Kris-Etherton, P. M., Miller, M., Rimm, E. B., Rudel, L. L., Robinson, J. G., Stone, N. J., & Van Horn, L. V. (2017). Dietary Fats and Cardiovascular Disease: A Presidential Advisory From the American Heart Association. Circulation, 136(3), e1–e23. https://doi.org/10.1161/CIR.0000000000000510

Samin Nosrat. (2017). Salt Fat Acid Heat (1st ed.). Simon and Schuster.

Schmidt, J. H. (2015). Life cycle assessment of five vegetable oils. Journal of Cleaner Production, 87, 130–138. https://doi.org/10.1016/j.jclepro.2014.10.011

Seattle, F. S. N. 1012 F. A. F. F., & Washington 98104-1008. (2015, June 16). FDA Finalizes Decision to Ban Artificial Trans Fat. Food Safety News. https://www.foodsafetynews.com/2015/06/fda-finalizes-decision-to-ban-trans fat/

Shen, Y., Zhao, Z., Zhang, L., Shi, L., Shahriar, S., Chan, R. B., Paolo, G. D., & Min, W. (2017). Metabolic activity induces membrane phase separation in endoplasmic reticulum. Proceedings of the National Academy of Sciences, 114(51), 13394–13399. https://doi.org/10.1073/pnas.1712555114

Simopoulos, A. P. (2002). The importance of the ratio of omega-6/omega-3 essential fatty acids. Biomedicine & Pharmacotherapy = Biomedecine & Pharmacotherapie, 56(8), 365–379. https://doi.org/10.1016/s0753-3322(02)00253-6

Simopoulos, A. P. (2006). Evolutionary aspects of diet, the omega-6/omega-3 ratio and genetic variation: Nutritional implications for chronic diseases. Biomedicine & Pharmacotherapy, 60(9), 502–507. https://doi.org/10.1016/j.biopha.2006.07.080

Siri, P. W., & Krauss, R. M. (2005). Influence of dietary carbohydrate and fat on LDL and HDL particle distributions. Current Atherosclerosis Reports, 7(6), 455–459. https://doi.org/10.1007/s11883-005-0062-9

Siri-Tarino, P. W., Chiu, S., Bergeron, N., & Krauss, R. M. (2015). Saturated Fats Versus Polyunsaturated Fats Versus Carbohydrates for Cardiovascular Disease Prevention and Treatment. Annual Review of Nutrition, 35, 517–543. https://doi.org/10.1146/annurev-nutr-071714-034449

Siri-Tarino, P. W., Sun, Q., Hu, F. B., & Krauss, R. M. (2010). Meta-analysis of prospective cohort studies evaluating the association of saturated fat with cardiovascular disease. The American Journal of Clinical Nutrition, 91(3), 535–546. https://doi.org/10.3945/ajcn.2009.27725

So, J., Wu, D., Lichtenstein, A. H., Tai, A. K., Matthan, N. R., Maddipati, K. R., & Lamon-Fava, S. (2021). EPA and DHA differentially modulate monocyte inflammatory response in subjects with chronic inflammation in part via plasma specialized pro-resolving lipid mediators: A randomized, double-blind, crossover study. Atherosclerosis, 316, 90–98. https://doi.org/10.1016/j.atherosclerosis.2020.11.018

Soliman, G. A. (2018). Dietary Cholesterol and the Lack of Evidence in Cardiovascular Disease. Nutrients, 10(6), 780. https://doi.org/10.3390/nu10060780

Stephen, N. M., Jeya Shakila, R., Jeyasekaran, G., & Sukumar, D. (2010). Effect of different types of heat processing on chemical changes in tuna. Journal of Food Science and Technology, 47(2), 174–181. https://doi.org/10.1007/s13197-010-0024-2

Stillwell, W., & Wassall, S. R. (2003). Docosahexaenoic acid: Membrane properties of a unique fatty acid. Chemistry and Physics of Lipids, 126(1), 1–27. https://doi.org/10.1016/s0009-3084(03)00101-4

The American Heart Association Diet and Lifestyle Recommendations. Www.Heart.Org. Retrieved October 27, 2021, from https://www.heart.org/en/healthy-living/healthy-eating/eat-smart/nutrition-basics/aha-diet-and-lifestyle-recommendations

The Facts on Fat. Retrieved January 13, 2022, from https://www.heart.org/-/media/files/healthy-living/company-collaboration/inap/fats-white-paper-ucm_475005.pdf

U.S. Department of Health and Human Services and U.S. Department of Agriculture. (2005). DGA 2005. https://health.gov/dietaryguidelines/dga2005/document/html/chapter6.htm

USDA and ARS. (2020). USDA National Nutrient Database for Standard Reference. FoodData Central. https://fdc.nal.usda.gov/fdc-app.html#/?query=ndbNumber:18075

van Rooijen, M. A., & Mensink, R. P. (2020). Palmitic Acid Versus Stearic Acid: Effects of Interesterification and Intakes on Cardiometabolic Risk Markers—A Systematic Review. Nutrients, 12(3), 615. https://doi.org/10.3390/nu12030615

Vincent, M. J., Allen, B., Palacios, O. M., Haber, L. T., & Maki, K. C. (2019). Meta-regression analysis of the effects of dietary cholesterol intake on LDL and HDL cholesterol. The American Journal of Clinical Nutrition, 109(1), 7–16. https://doi.org/10.1093/ajcn/nqy273

Volkow, N. D., Wang, G.-J., Fowler, J. S., Logan, J., Jayne, M., Franceschi, D., Wong, C., Gatley, S. J., Gifford, A. N., Ding, Y.-S., & Pappas, N. (2002). "Nonhedonic" food motivation in humans involves dopamine in the dorsal striatum and methylphenidate amplifies this effect. Synapse (New York, N.Y.), 44(3), 175–180. https://doi.org/10.1002/syn.10075

Wolters, M., Ahrens, J., Romaní-Pérez, M., Watkins, C., Sanz, Y., Benítez-Páez, A., Stanton, C., & Günther, K. (2019). Dietary fat, the gut microbiota, and metabolic health—A systematic review conducted within the MyNewGut project. Clinical Nutrition (Edinburgh, Scotland), 38(6), 2504–2520. https://doi.org/10.1016/j.clnu.2018.12.024

Worl Bank Group. (2015). Environmental, Health, And Safety Guidelines For Vegetable Oil Production And Processing. https://www.ifc.org/wps/wcm/connect/6a6f9bc9-09dc-4d89-a003-82ee3749ad4c/FINAL_Feb+2015_Vegetable+Oil+Processing+EHS+Guideline.pdf?MOD=AJPERES&CVID=kU6XfbQ

Wu, J. H. Y., Marklund, M., Imamura, F., Tintle, N., Ardisson Korat, A. V., de Goede, J., Zhou, X., Yang, W.-S., de Oliveira Otto, M. C., Kröger, J., Qureshi, W., Virtanen, J. K., Bassett, J. K., Frazier-Wood, A. C., Lankinen, M., Murphy, R. A., Rajaobelina, K., Del Gobbo, L. C., Forouhi, N. G., ... Cohorts for Heart and Aging Research in Genomic Epidemiology (CHARGE) Fatty Acids and Outcomes Research Consortium (FORCE). (2017). Omega-6 fatty acid biomarkers and incident type 2 diabetes: Pooled analysis of individual-level data for 39 740 adults from 20 prospective cohort studies. The Lancet. Diabetes & Endocrinology, 5(12), 965–974. https://doi.org/10.1016/S2213-8587(17)30307-8

Yang, H., Xun, P., & He, K. (2013). Fish and fish oil intake in relation to risk of asthma: A systematic review and meta-analysis. PloS One, 8(11), e80048. https://doi.org/10.1371/journal.pone.0080048

Zhu, Y., Bo, Y., & Liu, Y. (2019). Dietary total fat, fatty acids intake, and risk of cardiovascular disease: A dose-response meta-analysis of cohort studies. Lipids in Health and Disease, 18. https://doi.org/10.1186/s12944-019-1035-2

Zong, G., Li, Y., Wanders, A. J., Alssema, M., Zock, P. L., Willett, W. C., Hu, F. B., & Sun, Q. (2016). Intake of individual saturated fatty acids and risk of coronary heart disease in US men and women: Two prospective longitudinal cohort studies. The BMJ, 355, i5796. https://doi.org/10.1136/bmj.i5796

DAIRY

~

Julia Hilbrands, MS, MPH, RD
and Deborah Kennedy, PhD
with Jasna Wright
&
The Expert Chef Panel

"I am thankful for laughter, except when milk comes out of my nose."
Quote by Woody Allen

DAIRY FOODS ARE MILK-BASED foods, most commonly from cow's milk, and include foods such as fluid milk, yogurt, and cheese, among others. Dairy foods are consumed in countries across the globe and are a major source of nutrition in many countries. Milk-producing mammals have been domesticated by humans for thousands of years. Initially, this was done as part of nomadic subsistence farming. Protecting and feeding the animals while moving from area to area was part of a symbiotic relationship between the herders and the animals. Later in history, dairy animals were kept for multiple purposes, including milking as well as working animals, and finally, as meat at the end of their lives. Milking by hand turned to machine milking over time with the industrialization of the milk supply. Cows were then bred more specifically for dairy instead of beef. The development of refrigeration and better road transportation in the 1950s allowed milk production to become more centralized in countries such as the United States. In the United States, a dairy cow produced about 5,300 pounds of milk per year in 1950, while in 2019, the average American Holstein cow produced over 23,000 pounds of milk per year (O'Hagan, 2019).

Children are the largest group of milk consumers in the United States, and the nutrients provided in milk are critical for proper growth and bone development (Singh et al., 2015). A recent study by Torres-Gonzalez and colleagues that analyzed data from 2001–2010 found that 80% of children aged 2 to 8 years were milk drinkers, and this proportion dropped to 57% among children aged 9 to 18 years, 42% among adults aged 19 to 70 years, and 60% among adults aged 70+ years (Torres-Gonzalez et al., 2020). Similar findings were reported by Singh et al. (2015), who found that older adults drink more milk than younger adults in every geographic region around the world. This may be a response to the advice given regarding calcium needs and the prevention of osteoporosis.

Global calcium intake is only about half of the recommended 1000 mg to 1300 mg per day suggested by the U.S. National Institutes of Health (NIH), indicating a need for a higher intake of calcium-rich foods such as milk products (National Institutes of Health Office of Dietary Supplements). The study by Singh et al. also found that higher-income countries drink more than twice the amount of milk compared to lower-income countries. Furthermore, countries with high rates of lactose intolerance tend to have lower dairy consumption. Most of the countries with the highest dairy consumption in the world are found in Europe, while the lowest dairy-consuming countries are found in Asia and Africa.

SECTION 1:

DEFINITION AND CHARACTERISTICS OF DAIRY

TYPES OF DAIRY AND DAIRY PRODUCTS

Milk Source

Most of this chapter will focus on milk and milk products derived from cows unless otherwise noted. However, milk and milk products from other animals have been a staple in many cuisines for years and are becoming more common in the Western world. Table 1 outlines the characteristics of milk from various mammal sources.

Table 1: Milk from Various Mammals and Its Defining Characteristics

Source of Milk	Characteristics
Cow's milk	• 3 % to 4% fat (before processing), 3.5% protein, 5% lactose
Buffalo milk	• About twice the fat content of cow's milk • High casein content that facilitates good cheesemaking
Camel milk	• Similar composition to cow's milk but slightly saltier • Can contain 3 times as much vitamin C as cow's milk. This is important for people living in arid and semi-arid areas who have limited access to fruits and vegetables • Also rich in unsaturated fatty acids and B vitamins

Source of Milk	Characteristics
Sheep milk	• Higher fat and protein content than cow's or goat milk, but not as much fat as buffalo or yak milk • Higher lactose content than cow's milk • Good for cheesemaking due to the high solid content
Goat milk	• Similar composition to cow's milk • Often used for cheesemaking
Yak milk	• Slightly sweet taste and smell • High fat and protein content similar to buffalo milk
Equine milk	• Horse and donkey milk is relatively low in fat and protein, similar to human milk • Typically consumed in a fermented form

Source: (Food and Agriculture Organization, 2021)

Liquid Milk

According to the FDA, milk is "the lacteal secretion, practically free from colostrum, obtained by the complete milking of one or more healthy cows" (Code of Federal Regulations Title 21, 2021). Milk is one of the most common beverages consumed worldwide. It comes in several "varieties," if you will, from whole to reduced-fat to skim. The only difference in these types of milk is the fat content — the protein and vitamin/mineral content of all milk varieties are the same. Whole milk contains about 3.5% fat by weight, which is the closest way it comes out of the cow. Fat percentage is reduced from there (see Table 2).

Milk Processing

When processing milk, all fat is removed before the milk is bottled and then re-added (at various percentages) during bottling. The cream is removed via a cream separator that uses centrifugation to separate the fat/cream from the rest of the milk components. This process is called **standardization**.

Milk often goes through the process of **pasteurization**, where it is quickly heated to kill any potential disease-causing pathogens, which reduces the transmission of diseases such as brucellosis and tuberculosis (Willett & Ludwig, 2020). Typically, raw milk is heated until it reaches 161 °F/72 °C, held at that temperature for at least 15 seconds, and then is quickly cooled back down to 39 °F/4 °C, which is the optimal storage temperature for milk. Pasteurization does not have a significant impact on the nutritional value of milk, though it does destroy the very small amount of vitamin C (<10% of the RDA) that is present in raw milk.

Some milk is ultra-pasteurized, and it is often called Ultra High Temperature (UHT) milk, and the U.S. government states, "such product shall have been thermally processed at or above 280 °F/ 138 °C for at least two seconds, either before or after packaging, so as to produce a product which has an extended shelf life." UHT milk typically has a shelf life of six to nine months. Once opened, it becomes perishable and must be stored in the refrigerator. The long shelf life of unopened UHT milk is due to the destruction of microbes in the milk and the deactivation of enzymes that can spoil milk. The high-temperature processing caramelizes the sugars naturally present in the milk, which changes the flavor of the milk slightly.

Since UHT milk can be shipped without refrigeration, it may be slightly better for the environment. UHT milk has slightly less choline than fresh milk, and the quality of the protein in UHT milk may degrade over time, resulting in up to 12% less protein after storage for six months (alKanhal et al., 2001; Manzi et al., 2013). However, UHT milk is the primary type of milk sold in many parts of Europe due to its extended shelf life and ease of transport, and studies have not seen any adverse health outcomes or poor growth trends as a result of UHT milk consumption. UHT milk can be a good source of nutrition for many, as it is safe, convenient, and reasonably priced.

Once the fat is added back to milk after pasteurization, it must go through a **homogenization** process. Otherwise, the fat will continue to separate and rise to the top of the milk. Milk is homogenized by pumping it through very small openings under very high pressure to reduce the size of the fat globules. If the fat globules are small enough, they will stay evenly dispersed throughout the milk and create a uniform, creamy product.

Fortification

Milk is a significant dietary source of **vitamin D,** but this vitamin is not naturally present in dairy products and thus must be added during processing. Vitamin D is crucial for calcium absorption and proper bone mineralization, along with many other important functions. Regulations for vitamin D fortification in the United States are set at the federal level and state that when vitamin D is added to milk, it should be at a level not less than 400 International units (IU) per quart (Code of Federal Regulations Title 21, 2021).

Another vitamin that might be added to milk and dairy products is vitamin A. This vitamin is important for eye health, and while it is a fat-soluble vitamin that is naturally present in milk, some of it is lost during the processing of low-fat milks. According to the FDA, vitamin A should be added in an amount not less than 2000 IU per quart (Code of Federal Regulations Title 21, 2021). Interestingly, vitamin fortification of dairy products is not mandatory in the United States, but it is mandated in Canada and some European countries.

Specialty Milk

Lactose-free Milk

Lactose is a sugar naturally found in milk and many other dairy foods, such as yogurt and ice cream. Lactose-free milk is made by taking cow's milk and either enzymatically breaking down the lactose naturally present or filtering it out. Lactose-free milk can be a good option for those with lactase enzyme deficiency. Lactose-free milk is comparable to regular milk in nutritional content in terms of calcium, protein, vitamin D, B vitamins, and fat. In the case of lactose-free milk, where the lactose has been broken down into its two simple sugars, some people notice that this type of lactose-free milk tastes slightly sweeter, however, the sugar content/ carbohydrate content of the milk is the same (National Dairy Council, 2022). Lactose is found in the fluid part of the milk, so when the fluid is mostly removed to make cheese, much of the lactose is also removed, making hard cheeses naturally low in lactose.

Ultra-filtered Milk

Some companies have a patented process where they take real cow's milk and separate it into its five basic parts: water, vitamins and minerals, lactose, protein and butterfat. They then recombine those parts in different percentages to make beverages that contain more protein and less sugar.

Image: A2 Milk

A2 milk is a variety of cow's milk that is very low in the beta form of casein proteins (called A1) and has mostly the A2 form of casein (New Zealand Commerce Commission, 2003). This variety of cow's milk was introduced to the market by the A2 Milk Company and is mostly sold in New Zealand, Australia, China, and the United States. Milk from mammals other than cows (humans, sheep, goats, donkeys, yaks, camels, buffalo, etc.) also has the predominant A2 form of casein (Jung et al., 2017). A2 milk is produced by selecting cows that produce milk with A2 beta-casein using a genetic test developed by the A2 Milk Company (Woodford, 2009). The A2 Milk Company claims that A1 proteins are harmful, however, there has been a lack of scientific evidence that links A1 proteins to any adverse health effects. The European Food Safety Authority reviewed the scientific literature regarding health effects and A1 proteins and found no relationship between drinking milk containing A1 casein and any disease (De Noni et al., 2009).

Raw Milk

According to the CDC, raw milk can harbor dangerous bacteria. Raw milk has not undergone pasteurization to kill bacteria (which comes from contamination with animal feces, human handling, cow diseases, unsanitary conditions in milk processing, etc.), and so harmful bacteria such as brucella, campylobacter, cryptosporidium, E. coli, listeria, and salmonella can be present. Raw milk does contain enzymes that would be denatured if pasteurized, but there is no evidence that these enzymes are important in human health. Pasteurization does reduce some nutrients available in milk, however, those nutrients that are affected, such as vitamin C, are not nutrients of significance in milk. For more information about raw milk, you can visit: https://www.cdc.gov/foodsafety/rawmilk/raw-milk-questions-and-answers.html.

Fermented and Cultured Milks

There are many dairy products that are made by adding certain microorganisms to milk to create a fermented or cultured product. Adding microorganisms increases the acidity of the milk product. Common fermented dairy products that often appear in a Western diet include yogurt, buttermilk, and sour cream. Other fermented dairy products found around the globe include koumiss, dahi, labneh, ergo, tarag, kurut and kefir.

Yogurt

Versions of yogurt have been around for centuries, dating as far back as 10,000 to 5,000 BCE when nomadic people began to domesticate animals. Herdsman in the Middle East would use bags made of animal guts to transport milk and noticed that the intestinal enzymes that were present caused the milk to sour and curdle but also helped to preserve the milk. Fast forward to the 20th century and the first yogurt factory was opened in 1932 in France. Interestingly, yogurt was first sold in pharmacies because its health benefits drew so much interest (What Is Yogurt?). Historically, fermenting milk into yogurt was a good way to preserve milk and prevent further growth of pathogens.

Today, yogurt is made by adding the microorganisms Lactobacillus delbrueckii subsp. bulgaricus and Streptococcus thermophilus to pasteurized and homogenized milk to create a thick, cultured dairy product. These microorganisms convert lactose to lactic acid, which gives plain yogurt a tangy or slightly sour taste. After this fermentation process, flavoring agents like fruits, sugar, or other ingredients may be added. Greek yogurt has become common in recent decades — Greek yogurt is yogurt that has been strained multiple times after fermentation to remove some liquid and create a product with a smooth mouthfeel and a higher protein content.

Kefir

Image: Kefir

Kefir has been consumed for thousands of years and its name in Slavic means well-being. Kefir is produced by kefir grains, that are made up of acetic- and lactic-acid-producing bacteria, and yeast within a polysaccharide and protein mix. Kefir can be a good option for individuals who are lactose intolerant because during the fermentation process, 30% of the lactose is broken down.

Kefir is rich in amino acids, vitamins, minerals, and antioxidant compounds, and the probiotics present in kefir have probiotic potential. It has both antifungal and antibacterial properties and, in animal studies, has mostly been associated with improved digestion, decreasing cholesterol levels, control of plasma glucose levels, anti-carcinogenic activity, anti-allergenic activity, and more (Rosa et al., 2017). More studies are needed on humans as the results of human trials often conflict with results from animal studies, with the exception of kefir improving diabetic markers (Bourrie et al., 2020).

Buttermilk

Traditionally, buttermilk was the liquid that was left behind after making butter, and this liquid included milk protein and a small amount of fat. Prior to pasteurization, this liquid also contained small amounts of bacteria, and when the liquid was left out at room temperature the bacteria would produce a cultured milk product that was thick and had an acidic or sour taste.

Now, buttermilk is made by adding cultures of Lactococcus lactis or Lactobacillus bulgaricus plus Leuconostoc citrovorum to pasteurized and homogenized milk. When these bacteria ferment the lactose present in milk, they produce lactic acid, which creates an acidic environment. This acidity lends to a sour taste, but it also creates a thicker liquid as milk proteins precipitate or coagulate in acidic environments. Buttermilk is often used as a raising agent in baked goods.

Sour Cream

Sour cream is made in a similar manner to buttermilk, except that lactic acid bacteria are added to pasteurized cream rather than milk. This results in a cultured dairy product with a higher fat content of at least 18% milkfat. Commercial sour creams may also contain some thickening or gelling agents such as sodium citrate, guar gum, carrageenan, or locust bean gum.

Cheeses

Cheese is produced through the coagulation of casein, one of the proteins in milk. Cheese can be soft, hard, semi-hard, hard-ripened, or unripened. There are hundreds of varieties of cheeses worldwide, and the different characteristics are derived from the various types of milk, microorganisms, processes, and added ingredients used.

During cheesemaking, coagulation is achieved by either adding an acid or an enzyme called rennet to liquid milk. Common acid cheeses include cream cheese and queso fresco, while most other types of cheese, such as cheddar and Swiss, make use of rennet. Rennet cheeses also require bacterial cultures for production, making them a fermented food. Lactic acid bacteria are used as the starter culture for cheeses, but there are a wide variety of these cultures available, each of them providing a slightly different flavor and texture to the cheese. For example, Lactobacillus casei and Lactobacillus plantarum are used to make cheddar cheese, while Propionibacterium freudenreichil can be credited for the eye formation in Swiss cheese (Cheese Production).

The wide variety of flavors and textures found in cheeses is not due to different bacterial cultures alone. Differences in temperature, processing time, target pH for each step, the use of salting or brining, and aging time all play a role in the final cheese product. Additionally, cheesemakers may add ingredients like spices, herbs, peppers, or horseradish to create a unique flavor, and the type of milk used (cow, goat, sheep, buffalo, etc.) also contributes to flavor. Additionally, yeasts or molds can be used to provide unique colors and flavors.

Butter and Ghee

Unhomogenized milk and cream contain butterfat in microscopic globules. The globules have phospholipid membranes that keep the fat in milk dispersed rather than clumping together. When cream is agitated, the membranes are damaged and the fats join together and separate from the rest of the cream. Churning creates small butter grains floating in the water-based part of the cream, which is called buttermilk. The buttermilk is drained and rinsed off, and then the fat grains are pressed and kneaded together. Commercially produced butter is about 80% butterfat and 15% water; whereas traditional handmade butter was likely 65% fat and 30% water. Rendering butter removes the water and milk solids, which produces clarified butter, also known as ghee. Ghee is almost entirely butterfat.

Evaporated Milk

This milk product is made by removing about 60% of the milk's water. Once the milk is pasteurized, it's piped into an evaporator, where it's concentrated. It is a heat-sterilized product with an extended shelf life and is often used in baking.

Condensed Milk

Condensed milk is a type of evaporated milk that has been sweetened with sugar (unsweetened condensed milk is simply evaporated milk). Sugar is added before the milk is canned. Sweetened condensed milk is very thick and sweet — in fact, it contains 45% sugar, so it works well as a dessert ingredient. It has a shelf life of about two years.

Dry Milk or Milk Powder

Dry milk is made by removing water from pasteurized milk using a heat treatment followed by evaporation and spray drying to form a powder. This drying process helps to extend the shelf life considerably. Dry milk can be reconstituted into a liquid product by mixing it with water.

Cream

Cream is the higher-fat layer that rises to the top of liquid milk before it is homogenized. Heavy cream contains >36% milkfat, and the fat content can also be lowered to create products like light cream or half and half. Due to its high fat content, cream is also used as the foundation for several dairy desserts.

Ice Cream

This beloved dairy dessert is a mixture of dairy ingredients and ingredients for sweetening and flavoring, such as fruits, nuts, and chocolate. Stabilizers and emulsifiers are often included to promote proper texture and enhance the eating experience. Ice cream must contain at least 10% milkfat before the addition of bulky ingredients and weigh a minimum of 4.5 pounds to the gallon.

Frozen Custard

Similar to ice cream, frozen custard must contain a minimum of 10% milkfat and at least 1.4% egg yolk solids.

Sherbets

As another frozen dairy dessert, sherbets have a milkfat content of between 1% and 2% and a higher sweetener content than ice cream. Sherbets must weigh a minimum of 6 pounds to the gallon.

Gelato

Gelato is characterized by an intense flavor and contains sweeteners, milk, cream, egg yolks, and flavoring.

Table 2: A Description of Milk Products and Their Fat Content

Product	Description/Details	Fat Content
Liquid milk	The most widely consumed, processed, and marketed dairy product worldwide.	
• Whole milk		3.5% fat (8 g/cup)
• Reduced-fat (2%) milk		2% fat (5 g/cup)
• Low-fat (1%) milk		1% fat (2.5 g/cup)
• Skim milk		No more than 0.2% fat
Fermented milks		
• Yogurts	Produced by bacterially fermenting milk. Kefir is a fermented drink made from milk.	0.4% to 3.3% fat
Cheeses	Made by coagulating the milk protein casein. Contains the protein and fat of milk, but most of the liquid and lactose are removed.	20% to 40% fat (average is 30% fat)
Butter and ghee	Butter is created by agitating cream and allowing the fat portion to separate from the liquid. Ghee is clarified butter, which removes more of the water portion.	80% for butter, close to 100% for ghee
Condensed milk	Milk with part of the water removed; sugar is usually added to sweeten it; often used in baking.	8% fat
Evaporated milk	Fresh milk that has been heated to evaporate about 60% of the water; often u Whole grains promote health, while ultra-processed grains do not sed in baking, in soups, and in sauces.	No less than 6.5% fat

Product	Description/Details	Fat Content
Dry milk or milk powder	Milk that has been evaporated until all of the liquid is removed; this extends the shelf life considerably and does not require refrigeration.	A variety of milk powder options are available: whole milk powder, skim milk powder etc. The fat percentages are the same as for fluid milk.
Cream		
• Half and half	A mixture of whole milk and cream.	10.5% to 18% milkfat
• Light cream (or coffee cream)		19% to 30% milkfat (most commonly around 20%)
• Light whipping cream	Cream must contain at least 30% milkfat to produce whipped cream. Whipping cream will double in volume when whipped.	30% to 36% milkfat
• Heavy cream (or heavy whipping cream)	Can retain its whipped state longer than light whipping cream.	> 36% milkfat
Whey products	Whey is a by-product of making cheese; it is often added to foods and used as a protein supplement.	0.3% fat
Ice cream	Made from milk or cream with added sugar and flavors; served as a frozen dessert.	14% to 25% fat; minimum 10% fat

Source: (International Dairy Foods Association, 2022)

SECTION 3:
RECOMMENDATIONS FOR INTAKE

INFANTS AND TODDLERS

Infants should not consume cow's milk before 12 months of age as the higher protein and mineral content are hard for their young kidneys and digestive system to process. Human milk is the ideal form of nutrition from birth to six months of age, and if human milk is unavailable, an iron-fortified FDA-approved infant formula is recommended. After six months of age, infants can have small amounts of yogurt and cheese as part of their solid food intake.

After 12 months of age, toddlers can be offered plain whole cow's milk as their primary beverage. Whole cow's milk helps to meet their calcium, potassium, vitamin D, protein, and fat needs. Flavored milks should be avoided in this age group as they contain unnecessary added sugars. The U.S. Dietary Guidelines recommend that toddlers age 12 to 23 months who are no longer receiving human milk or infant formula consume 1 2/3 to 2 cups of dairy per day (U.S. Department of Agriculture and U.S. Department of Health and Human Services, 2020).

Plant-based milk alternatives should not be used in the first year of life to replace human milk or formula. In the second year of life, unsweetened versions of these beverages may be given in small amounts, but most have significantly less protein than cow's milk and, if used as a dairy replacement, can impact a child's growth and development. Additionally, some plant-based milk alternatives are not fortified with calcium and/or vitamin D. Fortified soy milk is the only milk alternative that can be considered a dairy equivalent as it has a nutrient content that is similar to cow's milk (Centers for Disease Control and Prevention, 2021).

CHILDREN AND ADOLESCENTS

Dairy products continue to be an important source of nutrition through childhood and adolescence. These life stages are characterized by many transitions and the formation of dietary patterns. Children and adolescents themselves, as well as other caregivers and elders, exert a great influence on eating habits. Institutions such as schools or daycares may play a large role in what foods and dairy products are available, and other influences such as peer pressure emerge.

As children age, the recommended daily servings of dairy increase to support nutritional needs and higher calcium intake that is needed during these stages of rapid growth. The U.S. Dietary Guidelines recommend that children ages two to eight years consume 2 to 2.3 cups of dairy products each day, and children between the ages of nine and 18 years should increase to 3 cups of dairy products each day (U.S. Department of Agriculture and U.S. Department of Health and Human Services, 2020). For children and adolescents who cannot tolerate dairy, fortified soy alternatives can also provide the protein and micronutrients needed during these life stages.

Throughout childhood and adolescence, the types of dairy foods consumed change. Liquid milk consumption tends to decline, and more dairy is consumed via cheese, often in the form of processed mixed dishes such as sandwiches, pizza, or pasta.

ADULTS

The recommendation to consume 3 cup-equivalents of dairy or dairy products per day continues into adulthood (U.S. Department of Agriculture and U.S. Department of Health and Human Services, 2020). Even though linear growth is finished by early adulthood, the need for adequate calcium and vitamin D to support bone health continues, and milk and dairy products can be a significant source of these nutrients in the diet. Consumption of dairy foods may also lower the risk of CVD and type 2 diabetes in adults, and it's also been shown that overall dairy consumption increases lean body mass and reduces weight gain (Mozaffarian, 2019).

SENIORS

It is recommended that older adults continue to consume 3 cup-equivalents of dairy or dairy products as they age (U.S. Department of Agriculture and U.S. Department of Health and Human Services, 2020). In older adulthood, adequate dairy consumption is important for bone health and retention of lean muscle mass (Hanach et al., 2019; Iuliano et al., 2021).

Table 3: Recommended Dairy Intake Throughout the Lifespan

Age Group	Recommendations
0 to 11 months	Human milk or iron-fortified infant formula only
12 to 23 months	1 2/3 to 2 cup-equivalents
2 to 8 years	2 to 2.3 cup-equivalents
9 to 13 years	3 cup-equivalents
14 to 18 years	3 cup-equivalents
19 to 59 years	3 cup-equivalents
60⁺ years	3 cup-equivalents

Source: (U.S. Department of Agriculture and U.S. Department of Health and Human Services, 2020)

HOW ARE AMERICANS DOING?

According to the Dietary Guidelines for Americans, about **90% of the U.S. population does not meet dairy recommendations** (U.S. Department of Agriculture and U.S. Department of Health and Human Services, 2020). Infants and toddlers typically meet or exceed recommendations, but average daily intake declines from there.

A study by Hess et al. (2020) found that when Americans aged two years and over who met recommendations for dairy intake were compared to those who did not meet dairy recommendations, nutritional intake was generally better among those consuming more dairy (Hess et al., 2020). People meeting the dairy recommendations were more likely to have adequate intakes of calcium, magnesium, phosphorus, riboflavin, vitamin A, vitamin B_{12}, zinc, choline, and potassium regardless of age, sex, or ethnicity when compared to those eating less than the recommended number of dairy servings. Those consuming the recommended amount of dairy were also more likely to exceed the recommendations for sodium and saturated fat intake but ate less added sugars.

While very few Americans meet the recommendations for dairy intake, patterns of dairy consumption are changing. In 1975, the average American consumed 539 pounds of dairy in a year, whereas in 2020, the average American consumed 655 pounds of dairy in a year (International Dairy Foods Association, 2021). There was a three-pound increase in dairy consumption per person between 2019 to 2020 alone. This increase in dairy consumption in recent years is due to an increase in ice cream, butter, yogurt, and cheese consumption, while intake of liquid milk has been declining. The low-carb/high-fat diet fad, as well as the COVID-19 pandemic, may play a role in these trends in food consumption.

Infants and Toddlers

Children three years old and under tend to be the only age group consuming the recommended number of dairy servings in the U.S. (Dietary Guidelines Advisory Committee, 2020).

Children and Adolescents

Approximately one-quarter of children and adolescents up to age 18 consumed the recommended number of cup equivalents of dairy foods, according to NHANES study data from 2013 to 2016 (Hess et al., 2020). Being younger, male, non-Hispanic, white, and more physically active was associated with a greater likelihood of consuming the recommended number of dairy servings. Among children, milk allergy was cited as one of the primary reasons for avoiding dairy foods. Fortified soy beverages and similar plant-based milk alternatives are suitable options for these individuals (Donovan, 2017; Savage et al., 2016).

Adults

Adults aged 20 years and older were found to consume only 1.5 cup equivalents of dairy foods per day — about half of the recommended number of servings (Dietary Guidelines Advisory Committee, 2020). Among adults 19 years and older in the NHANES data 2013–2016, being male, non-Hispanic, white, and more physically active were associated with an increased likelihood of consuming the recommended number of cup equivalents of dairy foods. Only about 13% of adults met the recommended number of servings per day of dairy foods (Hess et al., 2020).

Seniors

According to NHANES data from 2013 to 2016, only about 13% of adults and seniors consumed 3 cup equivalents per day of dairy foods. White males who were more active were more likely to consume adequate servings of dairy (Hess et al., 2020). Dairy foods are particularly important in this age group due to their contribution to calcium, potassium, vitamin B_{12} and protein, which are important nutrients for the maintenance of bone density, muscle mass, and overall health.

SECTION 4:
IMPORTANT NUTRIENTS IN DAIRY PRODUCTS

FAT

Fats (also referred to as lipids) are one of the key constituents of milk and dairy products. Fat provides energy and is also an important carrier of fat-soluble vitamins (vitamins A, D, E, and K). Fat also provides unique sensory characteristics to milk products, such as creaminess, hardness, spreadability, and flavor (Alothman et al., 2019; Gómez-Cortés et al., 2018). Fat content is one of the most variable nutrients among milk and other dairy products. Within milk alone, fat content can range from almost 8 g per cup serving in whole milk to only minuscule amounts in skim milk (see Table 2). Among dairy products such as heavy cream, ice cream, and cheese, the fat content can be as high as 86 g, 14 g, and 37 g per cup, respectively.

As shown in Table 4, there are several types of fats in dairy products, and they are all metabolized a bit differently and confer slightly different health benefits. While the American Heart Association recommends limiting saturated fats to 5% to 6% of total caloric intake in order to reduce heart disease risk, it does not appear the consumption of saturated fat from dairy products specifically is atherogenic (Fernandez & Calle, 2010). Short-chain and medium-chain fatty acids (types of PUFAs) are important in the regulation of cell metabolism and have beneficial effects on gut microbiota (Gómez-Cortés et al., 2018; Schönfeld & Wojtczak, 2016). Linoleic acid, another type of PUFA, is capable of inhibiting carcinogenesis (Gómez-Cortés et al., 2018). Milk derived from pasture-fed cows specifically can be a source of a small amount of beneficial PUFAs and omega-3 fatty acids (Gómez-Cortés et al., 2018).

Table 4: Fat Content in One 8oz Serving of Various Types of Cows' Milk

	Total Fat (g)	Saturated Fat (g)	MUFA (g)	PUFA (g)	Trans(g)
Whole Milk	7.97	4.63	1.71	0.27	0.28
2% (Reduced Fat) Milk	4.66	2.72	0.98	0.14	0.17
1% (Low fat) milk	2.34	1.40	0.52	0.08	0.09
Skim milk	0.12	0.12	0.04	0.02	0

Source: (USDA, 2018)

PROTEIN

Milk and dairy products are an excellent source of high-quality protein. One 8 oz serving of milk contains 8 grams of protein, regardless of the fat content, and one 5 oz serving of Greek yogurt can contain up to 16 grams of protein (USDA, 2018). Dairy products are complete proteins, meaning they contain all nine essential amino acids that human beings require in their diets. Protein from milk and dairy products is highly digestible and bioavailable, so the body is able to efficiently absorb close to 100% of the protein consumed from dairy sources (Mathai et al., 2017; Timon et al., 2020). Specifically, dairy is a good source of the branched-chain amino acids leucine, isoleucine, and valine, which are especially bioavailable (G. D. Miller et al., 2006; Willett & Ludwig, 2020). In addition, milk protein and several of its post-digestive peptides have been shown to be antimicrobial, antiviral, antifungal, antioxidant, antihypertensive, antimicrobial, antithrombotic, opioid and immunomodulatory (Mills et al., 2011). Milk proteins are also important in the absorption and transport of other nutrients.

The protein found in milk can be classified into two major groups: caseins and whey. Casein is considered an insoluble protein and comprises approximately 80% of the protein in cow's milk, while the remaining 20% is whey protein, a soluble protein (Marangoni et al., 2019; Pereira, 2014). There are several different types of whey protein, all of which play important roles in the body (Alothman et al., 2019). Lactoferrin, lactoperoxidase, and lysozyme act as antimicrobial agents, and lactoglobulins and lactalbumin may have tumor-suppressing activity (Jenssen & Hancock, 2009; Parodi, 2007; Pereira, 2014). Lactoglobulin is also a carrier for retinol, a vitamin A derivative, and it has been shown to have antioxidant and fatty acid-binding capabilities (Mills et al., 2011). Lactoferrin is an important component in iron absorption and may also have anticarcinogenic effects (González-Chávez et al., 2009).

Caseins are considered the solid protein in liquid dairy and make up the primary component of cheese. Caseins have a high capacity to bind minerals, especially calcium and phosphorus and are important in the digestion and transport of these minerals (Holt et al., 2013). It's also thought that caseins have an effect on intestinal motility and may play a role in regulating food intake (Pereira, 2014).

Health Benefits of Casein and Whey

Casein makes up the majority of cow's milk protein, accounting for about 80%, while whey makes up the remaining 20%. The leucine present in cow's milk proteins helps to prevent muscle wasting in conditions where protein breakdown is more prevalent and also helps stimulate muscle protein synthesis. The high content of sulfur-containing amino acids (cysteine and methionine) in whey protein is important for the synthesis of glutathione, a peptide with antioxidant, anticarcinogenic, and immunostimulatory properties. Casein also appears to have anticancer effects, particularly against colon cancer risk. Furthermore, casein appears to have oral health benefits by decreasing plaque-promoting enzymes.

Protein, in general, has a satiating effect, and studies have shown that whey protein specifically helps induce satiety signals, which may help with weight regulation. Casein may also help with cardiovascular health by reducing blood cholesterol. Supplementation studies have found reductions in blood LDL with the addition of casein. For more information on the health benefits of milk and milk proteins, see Section 6.

Sources: (Anderson & Moore, 2004; Bendtsen et al., 2013; Chin-Dusting et al., 2006; Hoffman & Falvo, 2004; Johansson & Lif Holgerson, 2011; Luhovyy et al., 2007; MacDonald et al., 1994; Meinertz et al., 1989; G. D. Miller et al., 2006; Onwulata & Huth, 2008; Parodi, 2007; Yalçin, 2006)

CALCIUM

Milk and dairy products are one of the main sources of calcium in a Western diet, and cow's milk contains around 300 mg of calcium per 8 oz serving. However, despite the high calcium content of milk, almost 30% of adult men and 60% of adult women in the United States do not consume enough calcium each day (U.S. Department of Agriculture and U.S. Department of Health and Human Services, 2020). The RDA for calcium is 1,000 mg per day for adults 19–50 years old, as shown in Table 5 below. Most plant-based dairy alternatives are fortified with calcium, but research shows that the calcium in these beverages may not be as bioavailable as the calcium in cow's milk due to oxalic acids and phytic acids in plant-based milk alternatives reducing calcium absorption (Golden et al., 2014). Approximately 66% of the calcium in cow's milk is bound to casein (protein), while the remainder is found in the serum (liquid) portion of milk (Akkerman et al., 2019).

It has been long understood that calcium is important for bone health, and there is research to suggest that calcium from milk products — along with other nutrients like protein and phosphorus — can delay bone loss, prevent osteoporosis, and reduce frailty later in life (Bonjour et al., 2013; R. P. Heaney, 2007; Lana et al., 2015). In addition to supporting bone health, calcium is important for many other body functions.

Calcium is the most abundant mineral in the human body. It is needed for the regulation of blood pH, proper muscle and nerve function, and the release of several hormones. Hypocalcemia is rare since calcium homeostasis is so tightly regulated in the body. Hypocalcemia usually results from illness, vitamin D or magnesium deficiencies, impaired parathyroid hormones, impaired bone resorption of calcium, or medicine use. When signs and symptoms of calcium deficiency do occur, they affect multiple areas of the body since serum calcium is involved in the function of most organs. Low serum calcium can cause neuromuscular irritability, perioral numbness, tingling in hands and feet, muscle spasms, renal calcification, depression, bipolar disorder, cataracts, heart failure, and seizures (Fong & Khan, 2012; Pepe et al., 2020). Calcium consumption may also play a role in longer-term health outcomes, including risk reduction of cardiovascular disease, preeclampsia, cancer, and in weight regulation, as discussed further below in Section 6.

Calcium requirements vary from 200 mg to 1,200 mg per day throughout the life cycle, with increased needs in females ages 51 to 70 years, and in all individuals over 70 years due to decreased absorption. Recommendations for pregnancy and lactation are the same as others in that age group.

Table 5: Recommended Dietary Allowances (RDAs) for Calcium

Age	Male	Female	Pregnant	Lactating
0–6 months*	200 mg	200 mg		
7–12 months*	260 mg	260 mg		
1–3 years	700 mg	700 mg		
4–8 years	1,000 mg	1,000 mg		
9–13 years	1,300 mg	1,300 mg		
14–18 years	1,300 mg	1,300 mg	1,300 mg	1,300 mg
19–50 years	1,000 mg	1,000 mg	1,000 mg	1,000 mg
51–70 years	1,000 mg	1,200 mg		
70+ years	1,200 mg	1,200 mg		

*Adequate Intake (AI)
Source: (Institute of Medicine, 2010)

VITAMIN A

Full-fat cow's milk can be a good source of vitamin A and beta-carotene, but because vitamin A is a fat-soluble vitamin, some of the content is lost when fat is reduced in milk (see Table 6) (Schuster et al., 2018). However, vitamin A is frequently added back to milk during processing at a level of at least 2,000 IU per quart (International Dairy Foods Association, 2022). Vitamin A is important for promoting good eyesight, particularly in low light. Vitamin A is an essential component of rhodopsin, a protein that absorbs light in the retinal receptors. Vitamin A also supports normal differentiation and functioning of the conjunctival membranes and the cornea of the eye (A. Ross, 2006; C. Ross, 2010; Solomons, 2006). In addition, vitamin A is involved in immune function, reproduction, and the function of several organs, such as the heart, lungs, and kidneys.

VITAMIN D

Vitamin D is not naturally found in many foods, including dairy, but much of the dairy in the American diet is fortified with vitamin D (USDA, 2018). This is because vitamin D is necessary for the absorption of calcium and is a nutrient that is low in the American diet. Vitamin D is also important for maintaining calcium and phosphorus concentrations to allow bone mineralization as well as for cell differentiation and growth, regulation of phosphorus, immune health, reduction of inflammation, blood pressure regulation, and blood sugar regulation (Institute of Medicine, 2010; Jones, 2014; Norman, 2012).In addition to food sources, vitamin D can also be produced endogenously by the skin through sun exposure, but this process can be limited by many factors, such as the time of year, age, and geographic latitude.

Recommendations for vitamin D range from 200 IU to 800 IU throughout the lifespan, with increased needs for those over the age of 70 years (National Institute of Health, Office of Dietary Supplements, 2020b). The active form of vitamin D in the body is 25(OH)D. One 8-oz glass of cow's milk provides approximately 120 International Units of Vitamin D.

PHOSPHOROUS

Phosphorus is an important nutrient for bone health and kidney function, and the phosphorus found in dairy products may help delay sarcopenia and osteoporosis later in life (Bonjour et al., 2013). Cow's milk provides around 250 mg of phosphorus per one-cup serving. Phosphorus is also a component of cell membrane structure and of ATP, the body's main energy source. Additionally, phosphorus plays an important role in regulating gene transcription, activating enzymes, maintaining normal pH in extracellular fluid, and in intracellular energy storage (R. Heaney, 2012).

POTASSIUM

Cow's milk is a significant source of potassium, providing 390 mg per serving. Potassium is a nutrient of public health concern for the general U.S. population, as low intakes have been associated with health concerns (U.S. Department of Agriculture and U.S. Department of Health and Human Services, 2020). Potassium is present in all body tissues and is needed for normal cell functioning due to its role in maintaining intracellular fluid volume and transmembrane electrochemical gradients. Sodium is the main regulator of extracellular fluid volume, and as such, potassium and sodium have a strong relationship (Institute of Medicine, 2005; Stone et al., 2016). In recent years, higher sodium intakes in Western countries have played a role in high blood pressure, which has impacts on cardiovascular health and the risk of stroke. Inadequate potassium intakes equally play a role in hypertension, heart health, and risk of stroke. Consuming a diet with adequate potassium, such as the DASH diet and Mediterranean diet, has been shown to reduce systolic blood pressure (Champagne, 2006).

VITAMIN B$_{12}$

Vitamin B$_{12}$, also known as cobalamin, is a water-soluble vitamin that is formed from the mineral "cobalt." The main functions include red blood cell production, nerve cell development, central nervous system function, conversion of homocysteine to methionine (which decreases the risk of coronary artery disease, peripheral vascular disease, and stroke), and a co-factor for DNA production and metabolism (Carmel, 2014; Institute of Medicine, 1998; National Institute of Health, Office of Dietary Supplements, 2020a). Vitamin B$_{12}$ is naturally found in all animal-source foods such as meat, fish, eggs, and milk products.

Milk is an excellent source of vitamin B$_{12}$, with three times higher bioavailability in dairy than in meat, fish, and poultry (Tucker et al., 2000; Vogiatzoglou et al., 2009). Recommendations for this vitamin range from 0.4 µg to 2.4 µg with increased needs being seen during pregnancy and breastfeeding. One 8-oz glass of milk provides 1.29 µg of vitamin B$_{12}$.

RIBOFLAVIN

Riboflavin, also known as vitamin B$_2$, is a water-soluble vitamin found in foods such as milk, eggs, organ meats, lean meats, green vegetables and fortified grains. Riboflavin is an essential component of two important coenzymes, flavin mononucleotide and flavin adenine dinucleotide. These coenzymes are involved in energy production, cellular function, growth, development and metabolism of fats, drugs, and steroids. Riboflavin is also needed to maintain normal homocysteine levels in the blood (Institute of Medicine, 1998; Rivlin, 2010).

NIACIN

Niacin, also known as vitamin B_3, is found in a variety of foods and is also added to enriched and fortified foods in the United States and Canada. Milk naturally contains a small amount of niacin, though poultry, fish, brown rice, nuts, and enriched cereals contain far more niacin than milk. Niacin is generally well absorbed and highly bioavailable from foods and supplements. Niacin is needed in over 400 enzymes to catalyze reactions in all tissues of the body. Niacin is also needed to create ATP (the body's primary energy form) from carbohydrates, proteins, and fats, as well as in cholesterol and fatty acid synthesis and in cellular antioxidant functioning (Bourgeois & Moss, 2010; Penberthy & Kirkland, 2012).

PANTOTHENIC ACID

Pantothenic acid, also known as vitamin B_5, is found in a wide variety of foods. Almost all plant and animal-source foods contain some amount of pantothenic acid, with milk and yogurt being good sources. This water-soluble vitamin is required for the synthesis of coenzyme A (CoA) and acyl carrier protein. CoA is needed for fatty acid synthesis and degradation, transfer of acetyl and acyl groups, and many other body processes. Acyl carrier protein is needed in fatty acid synthesis (Institute of Medicine, 1998; J. Miller & Rucker, 2012; Sweetman, 2010).

Table 6: Vitamin and Mineral Content of 8 oz of 2% (Reduced fat) Milk

Nutrient	Per 8 oz serving	RDA for Adults (% of RDA per 8 oz serving)
Calcium	309 mg	1,000 mg (31%)
Vitamin A (RAE)	203 µg	900 µg (23%)
Vitamin D	111 IU	600 IU (19%)
Vitamin B12	1.35 µg	2.4 µg (56%)
Riboflavin	0.336 mg	Women: 1.1 mg (31%) Men: 1.3 mg (26%)
Niacin	0.274 mg	Women: 14 mg (2%) Men: 16 mg (2%)
Phosphorus	252 mg	700 mg (36%)
Pantothenic Acid	0.956 mg	5 mg (19%)
Potassium	390 mg	Women: 2600 mg (15%) Men: 3400 mg (11%)

Source: (USDA, 2018)

SECTION 5:
DAIRY AND THE MICROBIOME

The gut microbiome is complex and only beginning to be understood. It impacts many facets of health including gastrointestinal health, weight regulation, mental health and immune function among others. Much of the influence of dairy products on the gut microbiome is by way of probiotics, or beneficial bacteria.

The dairy industry is the largest sector where probiotics are used. A number of dairy products are available with added probiotics, including sour/fermented milk, yogurt, cheese, butter/cream, ice cream, and infant formula. These probiotics are used as a starter culture or in combination with another traditional starter. Adding probiotics to dairy foods gives both sensory changes to the foods (improved taste, aroma, texture, etc.) as well as health-promoting properties. Yogurt and fermented milk, such as kefir, are some of the most well-known and widely consumed foods with probiotics. In the past, fermented foods were valued due to their increased shelf life, food safety, and sensory aspects. However, the scientific community is increasingly discovering that the fermentation process enhances nutritional and functional properties in foods by creating bioactive compounds and by adding live microorganisms to the diet (Marco et al., 2017).

Probiotics have four main mechanisms of action: improving the gut barrier, interfering with pathogens, immunomodulation, and producing neurotransmitters (Sánchez et al., 2017). Some probiotic strains are effective in treating antibiotic-associated diarrhea (Hempel et al., 2012), while others have been found to be helpful in managing inflammatory bowel disease (Jakubczyk et al., 2020), and due to the gut-brain axis, probiotics have also been found to play a role in mental health. A number of randomized controlled trials have found that probiotic supplementation can help reduce depression and anxiety symptoms (Akkasheh et al., 2016; Kazemi et al., 2019; Slykerman et al., 2017). A systematic review and meta-analysis by Companys et al. found that fermented milk consumption was associated with a 4% reduction in the risk of stroke, ischemic heart disease, and cardiovascular mortality (Companys et al., 2020). Yogurt intake was associated with a 27% reduction in risk of type 2 diabetes and a 20% reduction in risk of metabolic syndrome.

A recent systematic review of the links between dairy food intake and gut microbiota found eight randomized controlled trials of good quality on this subject (Aslam et al., 2020). Seven of the studies examined the effect of type of dairy (milk, yogurt, kefir) and dairy proteins (whey and casein) on the gut microbiota, while one study looked at the effects of quantity of dairy intake on the microbiota. Three studies showed that milk, yogurt, and kefir increase beneficial strains of Lactobacillus and Bifidobacterium in the gut. One study found that yogurt lowered a pathogenic strain of Bacteroides fragilis. The reviewers concluded that milk and fermented milk products such as kefir and yogurt likely help change the gut microbiota in a beneficial manner. Further studies are needed to understand this potential.

SECTION 6:
DAIRY INTAKE AND HEALTH OUTCOMES

METABOLIC SYNDROME

Metabolic syndrome (MetS) comprises a constellation of conditions, including high blood pressure, high blood sugar, excess body fat around the waist, and abnormal blood cholesterol levels. These conditions together increase one's risk of heart disease, stroke, and diabetes. The consumption of dairy products such as milk and yogurt may help to improve these conditions and reduce the risk of chronic disease (Astrup, 2014; Mena-Sánchez et al., 2019). In a recent study of over 15,000 Brazilian adults aged 35 to 74 years, total and full-fat dairy food intakes were inversely associated with MetS (Drehmer et al., 2016). Similarly, a recent meta-analysis of cohort studies found a 15% lower risk of MetS for each one serving per day increment of dairy consumption (Kim & Je, 2016).

Dairy intake may also aid in weight management. Intake of yogurt was found to be inversely associated with weight gain over a four-year time period in both women and men (Mozaffarian et al., 2011), and in an 11.2-year cohort study, the risk of becoming overweight or obese was lower among women in the highest quintile of dairy intake (Rautiainen et al., 2016).

CARDIOVASCULAR DISEASE

For years, the Dietary Guidelines for Americans and the American Heart Association have recommended the consumption of low-fat and fat-free dairy products so as to minimize saturated fat intake and thus reduce the risk of cardiovascular disease (Arnett Donna K. et al., 2019; U.S. Department of Agriculture and U.S. Department of Health and Human Services, 2020). After all, milk and dairy products can be a major source of saturated fatty acids, which have been linked to an increased risk of CVD, CHD, and stroke.

On the contrary, numerous cohort studies and meta-analyses have found that dairy intake is inversely related to cardiovascular disease risk (Astrup et al., 2016; Drouin-Chartier et al., 2016; Fontecha et al., 2019; Gómez-Cortés et al., 2018; Lovegrove & Hobbs, 2016; Siri-Tarino et al., 2015; Soedamah-Muthu et al., 2011).

Data from the PURE study (Prospective Urban Rural Epidemiology) illustrates this relationship well. The PURE study is a large multinational cohort study that includes dietary intakes of over 136,000 individuals between the ages of 35 and 70 from 21 different countries in five different contents over a nine-year follow-up period (Dehghan et al., 2018). After nine years of follow-up, researchers observed that those with a higher intake of total dairy (>2 servings/day) had a lower risk of major CVD, CV mortality, and stroke than those with no dairy intake. More specifically, a higher intake of milk and yogurt was associated with lower CVD risk, while cheese intake showed no association. The authors concluded that dairy consumption was associated with a lower risk of mortality and major CVD events.

Fats

Many researchers have found that there is no clear evidence that dairy food consumption of any fat level is associated with a higher risk of CVD, and recommendations to reduce dairy food consumption should be made with caution (German et al., 2009).

A review by German and colleagues found that milk fat has been shown to increase plasma HDL-C levels, and most saturated fats in milk have no impact on LDL-C levels (German et al., 2009). A cohort study in Sweden observed that among women, milk fat biomarkers were significantly higher among controls than among those who experienced a myocardial infarction (Warensjö et al., 2010). This relationship was also seen in men, though it did not reach statistical significance. Another finding of this study was that the intake of cheese and fermented milk products was inversely related to the incidence of myocardial infarction.

Some may question the consumption of cheese in particular, as it contains a high amount of saturated fat. In response to this thought, Raziani and colleagues (Raziani et al., 2016) recently conducted a randomized control trial where they had 139 subjects with two or more MetS risk factors, and they divided these subjects into three groups: a regular fat cheese group, a reduced-fat cheese group, and a no cheese group (iso-caloric, higher in carbohydrates). After 12 weeks of follow-up, levels of LDL-C were not significantly different between any of the groups, and HDL-C levels were higher in the cheese groups compared to the no-cheese groups. In addition, insulin, blood glucose, blood pressure, and waist circumference did not differ between groups. Their conclusion: a high daily intake of regular cheese does not significantly alter LDL-C levels or other MetS risk factors.

So why is it that saturated fat from dairy products appears to have no or even a beneficial impact on CVD risk, while saturated fat from other sources is harmful? It is thought that when saturated fats are consumed as part of the whole food matrix, like those in milk, cheese, and yogurt, their detrimental effects may be counteracted (Astrup et al., 2019; Gijsbers et al., 2016; Unger et al., 2019). The specific types of fatty acids (15:0 and 17:0) in dairy products may also be beneficial to cardiovascular health, though more research is needed in that area (de Souza et al., 2015; Liang et al., 2018; Yu & Hu, 2018). As reviewed previously, the saturated fat in dairy is also accompanied by numerous other beneficial nutrients, including calcium, magnesium, phosphorus, potassium, and probiotics (if fermented), and the provision of these nutrients in dairy may ameliorate the impact of saturated fat on CVD risk as well (Astrup, 2014; Soerensen et al., 2014).

TYPE 2 DIABETES

There is also a modest inverse relationship between the consumption of dairy and the risk of type 2 diabetes (Aune et al., 2013; Gijsbers et al., 2016; Gómez-Cortés et al., 2018; Schwing-shackl et al., 2017; Tong et al., 2011). It's suggested that the biggest benefit comes with a dairy intake of three servings per day, and this reduces type 2 diabetes risk by 2% to 15% (Mitri et al., 2019). A recent review found that among 12 meta-analyses, most reported an inverse associa-tion between the incidence of type 2 diabetes and dairy consumption, and this risk decreases incrementally as consumption of total dairy products and low-fat dairy products increases (Alvarez-Bueno et al., 2019).

This relationship may be strongest when looking at cheese and yogurt specifically. For example, Chen and colleagues conducted a meta-analysis using data from three cohorts: the Health Professionals Follow-Up Study (41,436 men), the Nurses' Health Study (67,138 women), and the Nurses' Health Study II (85,884 women) (M. Chen et al., 2014). While they found that neither low-fat nor high-fat dairy intake was associated with type 2 Diabetes risk, yogurt intake was consistently associated with a reduced risk. Specifically, the pooled data from all three cohorts showed that **each serving of yogurt/day resulted in a 17% decrease in type 2 diabetes risk**. Turning our attention to cheese, a study of almost 27,000 Swedish adults observed a decreased risk of type 2 diabetes among those with higher consumption of cheese, cream, butter, and high-fat fermented dairy (Ericson et al., 2015).

The mechanism(s) behind these associations still remains unclear, though it has been ob-served that a high consumption of dairy products improves insulin sensitivity and reduces circulating insulin levels (Mitri et al., 2019). For example, Stancliffe and colleagues conducted a study where they randomized 48 adults with MetS to receive either an adequate dairy (3.5 daily servings) or low-dairy (0.5 daily servings) diet for 12 weeks (Stancliffe et al., 2011). The adequate dairy group showed a significant reduction in plasma insulin levels after just one week, and these reduced levels were maintained throughout the study. Additionally, despite no change in body weight between groups, fat mass was significantly reduced in the adequate dairy group compared to the low dairy group. This may suggest the possibility of dairy in restricting body fat accumulation (Wennersberg et al., 2009). Rideout and colleagues produced similar findings of improved insulin resistance and plasma insulin levels when comparing a high intake of low-fat dairy products (four servings/day) with a low intake (one to two servings/day) over a six-month period (Rideout et al., 2013). The specific long-chain fatty acids in dairy products (15:0 and 17:0) may have a role in insulin action as they have been positively associated with lower glucose levels as well as higher systemic and hepatic insulin sensitivity, though more research is needed in this area (Kratz et al., 2014).

CANCER

The relationship between dairy consumption and cancer risk is less clear than it is for cardiovascular disease and type 2 diabetes, but there is some evidence that consuming dairy products decreases the risk of some cancers, particularly colorectal cancer, bladder cancer, and esophageal cancer (Schwingshackl et al., 2018; Zhang et al., 2019). In a recent systematic review, there was consistent evidence of a decrease in colorectal cancer risk with higher consumption of total dairy products and milk (Barrubés et al., 2019). Interestingly in this study, no significant associations were observed between colorectal cancer risk and intake of low-fat dairy products, whole milk, fermented dairy products or cultured milk. In contrast, other studies have found a significant risk reduction associated with cheese and yogurt intake (Zhang et al., 2019). Yogurt consumption has also been associated with a decreased risk of bladder cancer when comparing those in moderate and high intake categories with non-consumers (Acham et al., 2020; Bermejo et al., 2019). According to the World Cancer Research Fund, the cancer-protecting effects of milk can be attributed to its high calcium content as well as lactic acid-producing bacteria (World Cancer Research Fund/American Institute for Cancer Research, 2018). The other beneficial components of milk, such as lactoferrin, vitamin D, and short-chain fatty acids, may also have protective benefits.

The influence of dairy on breast cancer risk has also been studied, though this relationship is much less clear. Garcia and colleagues recently conducted a systematic review of the association between breast cancer and dairy product consumption (García et al., 2020). Of the 18 studies that met their inclusion criteria, 11 studies showed that dairy consumption was inversely associated with breast cancer, two studies showed a positive association, and five studies found a non-significant association. A 2019 study by Chen and colleagues found that data does not support a strong association between the consumption of dairy and breast cancer risk, even when comparing low-fat/skim milk, whole milk, and yogurt separately (L. Chen et al., 2019). The World Cancer Research Fund states in their most recent report that there is limited evidence that consuming dairy products may decrease the risk of breast cancer (World Cancer Research Fund/American Institute for Cancer Research, 2018).

BONE HEALTH

Bone, just like muscle tissue, is constantly being remodeled. During early life, adequate intakes of calcium and vitamin D, along with an overall adequate diet, are essential for bone deposition and for adequate growth and development. In later life, decreasing estrogen levels in women during and after menopause leads to increased bone resorption that outpaces bone formation. For this reason, postmenopausal women are at higher risk of osteoporosis due to lower bone mass density and bone quality. Osteoporosis increases the risk of fracture, especially to the hip, vertebrae, and forearms (Institute of Medicine, 2010; Song, 2017). Calcium plays an important role in bone health. However, observational evidence is mixed on the link between calcium intake and measures of bone strength in older adults.

The 2001–2006 NHANES data on adults aged 60 and older (55% women) found an association between higher dietary calcium intake and higher lumbar spine bone mass density in women only (Yao et al., 2021). In contrast, a randomized controlled trial in Australia in women over 65 years with an average intake of 886 mg per day of dietary calcium found no association between calcium intake and bone mass density (Bristow et al., 2019). A two-year randomized controlled trial in 500 healthy postmenopausal women found that consuming 500 ml (16 oz) per day of enriched skimmed milk (900 mg calcium and 600 IU vitamin D) increased bone mass density at the femoral neck (Reyes-Garcia et al., 2018). The U.S. Preventive Services Task Force (USPSTF) concluded from the body of research on calcium and vitamin D supplementation studies and studies examining the effects of dairy consumption that daily doses of less than 1,000 mg of calcium and 400 IU of vitamin D are insufficient to prevent fractures in postmenopausal women and there is inadequate evidence using higher doses to examine the potential benefits in this population (US Preventive Services Task Force et al., 2018).

While further studies are needed to better understand the role of calcium, vitamin D, and milk products in preventing fractures among older adults, some recent studies may help clarify this relationship. For example, a recent randomized controlled trial found that improving calcium and protein intake by using dairy foods reduced the risk of falls and fractures among over 7,000 institutionalized older adults (Iuliano et al., 2021).

GASTROINTESTINAL HEALTH

Dairy foods have a complex impact on the gastrointestinal (GI) tract. While people with lactose intolerance experience unpleasant and uncomfortable effects from consuming dairy foods that have lactose, milk products can also have beneficial effects on GI health. (For more information on lactose intolerance, see the section below on this topic.) A recent systematic review by Aslam et al. found that consuming milk, yogurt, and kefir increased beneficial bacteria strains and decreased harmful strains, having an overall positive effect on the gut microbiome (Aslam et al., 2020). Fermented milk products such as yogurt and kefir also contain probiotics, which improve the gut barrier and interfere with potential pathogens, thereby improving GI health (Sánchez et al., 2017).

There have been reports that in individuals for whom cow's milk causes GI distress, sheep milk or goats' milk may be better tolerated. There are a few nutritional differences that may account for this. While all animal milk contains casein, cow's milk contains a combination of A1 beta-casein and A2 beta-casein, while sheep and goats' milk contains primarily just A2 beta-casein with little to no of the A1 variety (Turkmen, 2017). When A1 beta-casein is digested, it leads to the production of a compound called beta-casomorphine-7, which is associated with intestinal inflammation and various digestive issues in some people (Jianqin et al., 2016). The issues could be avoided by drinking sheep or goat's milk that has very little A1 beta-casein. Another quality of these milks is that they have smaller fat globules and a lower lactose content which may also aid in digestibility. However, research in this area is still in its infancy, and there is currently no evidence to support the idea that sheep or goat milk is more healthful or more easily digestible for most individuals.

WEIGHT

Dairy products can aid in weight management due in part to the satiating effect of their protein content. The protein content of milk aids in satiety since protein takes longer to digest than simple carbohydrates. Furthermore, higher-fat dairy products are particularly satiating since fat digests even more slowly than protein. Milk proteins have been found to be more satiating than other protein sources (Anderson & Moore, 2004; McGregor & Poppitt, 2013). Whey protein found in milk induces satiety signals and contributes to short-term and longer-term food intake regulation (Bendtsen et al., 2013; Luhovyy et al., 2007). One study found that 45 g of whey protein resulted in better satiety and more reduced food intake at a subsequent meal when compared to egg albumin and soy protein (Anderson et al., 2004). Another study found that 48 g of whey protein resulted in further reduced food intake at a buffet meal more than a similar intake of casein (Hall et al., 2003). A study examining the impact of whey on the satiety hormone glucagon-like-peptide-1 found that a high-protein breakfast (58% energy from protein) using dairy foods enriched with whey isolate raised glucagon-like-peptide-1 levels over the following three hours more than a breakfast with unenriched yogurt (Blom et al., 2006).

A study by Baer et al. found that 23 weeks of consuming supplemental protein in the form of whey or soy vs. the same amount of calories in the form of carbohydrates resulted in lower body weight and body fat in the two protein groups (Baer et al., 2011). Waist circumference was smaller in the whey protein group compared to the other two groups, and fasting ghrelin was also lower in the whey group compared to the soy and carbohydrate groups. In rat studies, similar findings have been shown. Feeding insulin-resistant obese rats whey protein is associated with decreased calorie intake, decreased body fat, and improvements in insulin sensitivity compared to feeding them protein from red meat (Belobrajdic et al., 2004).

In general, there have been mixed findings regarding dairy product intake and lower body weight from observational and clinical trials with humans. An observational study found that higher intakes of calcium from dairy were associated with less being overweight in children in eight European countries (Nappo et al., 2019). In contrast, a Portuguese study found no association between dairy foods and weight among teens and young adults aged 13 to 21 (Marabujo et al., 2018). A systematic review and meta-analysis of 41 randomized controlled trials found that high dairy food intake had no impact on weight or body fat but did see an impact on body fat when high dairy intake was combined with an energy-restricted diet (Booth et al., 2015). In contrast, a recent intervention study among overweight/obese postmenopausal women found a greater degree of weight loss and fat loss among women consuming either low-fat dairy foods (four to five servings/day) or calcium and vitamin D supplements as compared to the placebo group (Ilich et al., 2019).

IMMUNITY

Several animal studies have shown that milk proteins, particularly whey protein, can positively influence immune responses. Mice that were fed with whey protein had higher mucosal antibody responses to ovalbumin and cholera toxin compared to mice on a standard diet (Low et al., 2001). Another study found that mice fed undenatured whey protein had higher T helper cells and a higher ratio of helper to suppressor cells compared to those on a casein diet (Bounous et al., 1993). Mice that were fed whey have also been observed to have an increase in white blood cells, lymphocyte counts, and IFN-gamma in spleen cells compared to mice that were fed casein and soy protein (Ford et al., 2001). Several in vitro studies have also found that whey protein improves markers of immunity, including cytokine secretion, lymphocytes, and leukocytes (Cross & Gill, 1999; Wang et al., 2000; Zimecki & Kruzel, 2000). Some in vitro and rodent studies have also shown the immunomodulatory effects of casein (Hata et al., 1998; Li & Mine, 2004; Otani et al., 2000; Pessi et al., 2001; Requena et al., 2009).

Beyond animal studies, there is also some evidence that points to an immunomodulating effect of cow's milk in humans. There is strong evidence that consumption of cow's milk early in life is associated with a lower prevalence of allergies, respiratory tract infections, and asthma (Perdijk et al., 2018). It has also been shown that children who grow up on a farm have a lower prevalence of these conditions than children who do not (von Mutius & Vercelli, 2010). However, more studies are needed to understand the immune effects of consuming dairy in humans.

INFLAMMATION

There have been an increasing number of studies on the topic of dairy and inflammation in the past few years, indicating a growing interest in this area. A recent systematic review of 16 clinical trials found that consuming milk products did not show a pro-inflammatory effect in healthy subjects or in subjects with metabolic abnormalities such as type 2 diabetes or MetS (Ulven et al., 2019). In fact, the majority of the studies saw a significant anti-inflammatory effect in both groups.

It is well-known that high-fat meals increase the postprandial concentration of proinflammatory cytokines (IL-6 and TNF-alpha) and the acute-phase protein CRP, and it appears that full-fat milk products (cheese and butter) have this same impact on inflammatory responses following their immediate consumption (Emerson et al., 2017; Pacheco et al., 2008; Payette et al., 2009; Poppitt et al., 2008). However, in the longer term, consuming dairy foods high in saturated and total fat as part of an overall balanced eating pattern does not appear to promote inflammation, as none of the studies included in the systematic review by Ulven et al. reported an increase in circulating inflammatory markers between the dairy and control groups (Ulven et al., 2019). In other studies, consuming kefir and yogurt actually reduced inflammatory markers TNF-alpha and CRP (O'Brien et al., 2015; Pei et al., 2017).

SECTION 7:
WHEN TO LIMIT DAIRY

LACTOSE INTOLERANCE

Lactose is a disaccharide found in milk and dairy foods. The enzyme lactase is needed to break lactose down into galactose and glucose before these sugars can be absorbed in the small intestine. There are two types of lactase deficiency: primary lactase deficiency and secondary lactase deficiency. Primary deficiency is the most common type, where a person makes less lactase. It is most common in adults but can also occur in children. Secondary deficiency can be temporary and is a lactase deficiency brought on by a medical condition such as acute illness or diarrhea. Lactose intolerance is not an allergy (see cow's milk protein allergy below for more information). When lactose remains undigested and enters the large intestine, bacteria break the lactose down and cause symptoms such as bloating, gas, cramping, nausea, and diarrhea. Lactose intolerance can be diagnosed with a blood test following consumption of a lactose-containing drink. If a person's blood sugar does not rise after the drink, they may be lactose-intolerant. Alternatively, a hydrogen breath test can be done. After consuming a high-lactose drink, a high level of hydrogen present in a person's breath can indicate lactose intolerance. A stool acidity test can also indicate lactose intolerance. If someone is not digesting lactose, their stool will contain lactic acid, glucose, and fatty acids. Lactose intolerance can also be diagnosed via biopsies of the small intestine taken during an endoscopy. It's important not to self-diagnose lactose intolerance as symptoms could be indicative of other gastrointestinal conditions, such as irritable bowel disease or Celiac disease.

Lactose intolerance is very common worldwide, though the true prevalence of lactose intolerance is unknown as it is not often tested for and many individuals self-diagnose (Bailey et al., 2013). As shown in Table 7, there are differences in prevalence between ethnic groups, likely due to genetic factors. However, scientific findings indicate that the prevalence of true lactose intolerance may be overestimated as there are many other physiologic conditions that can appear similar to lactose intolerance (McBean & Miller, 1998).

To manage lactose intolerance, lactase pills or drops can be taken when a person eats or drinks foods containing lactose. Alternatively, a person can choose to consume only dairy foods with lower levels of lactose, such as hard cheese and small amounts of yogurt. Lactose-free milk is also available in most grocery stores. Having milk products at the same time as other foods may help to lessen symptoms among some people, and data suggests that adults with lactose intolerance may tolerate up to 8 oz of milk with meals (McBean & Miller, 1998). Keeping a food and symptom diary may also help to identify the quantities of lactose-containing foods that can be tolerated. Dairy alternatives such as soy milk and other fortified beverages may also be a good option.

Individuals with lactose intolerance consume less than the recommended levels of dairy foods, and it is known that avoiding dairy may lead to nutrient deficiencies and an increased risk of several chronic diseases (Bailey et al., 2013; Suchy et al., 2010). In most cases, individuals don't need to avoid dairy entirely, and when working with individuals with lactose intolerance, it is important to ensure they are still consuming a nutritionally adequate diet.

Table 7: Estimated Prevalence of Lactose Intolerance Among Various Ethnic Groups

Ethnic Group	Prevalence
Northern Europeans	2% to 15%
American Whites	6% to 22%
Central Europeans	9% to 23%
Indians, Northern	20% to 30%
Indians, Southern	60% to 70%
Hispanics	50% to 80%
Ashkenazi Jews	60% to 80%
Blacks	60% to 80%
American Indians/First Nations	80% to 100%
Other Asians	95% to 100%

Source: (Harrington & Mayberry, 2008)

MILK ALLERGY

Cow's milk allergy happens when the body's immune system reacts to proteins found in milk — casein and whey. Milk allergy is most common in young children, though most outgrow the allergy by the age of five. Symptoms of milk allergy can be immediate or delayed. Immediate symptoms may include itchy rash, hives, redness, swelling, itchy eyes, runny nose, coughing, vomiting, or, in rare cases swallowing and breathing difficulties. Delayed symptoms may include diarrhea, constipation, reflux, vomiting, mucus/blood in stools, nausea, abdominal pain, gas, and bloating.

Immediate reactions are usually mediated by Immunoglobulin E (IgE), which triggers histamine to be released and involves symptoms in the skin and gut. This is in contrast to delayed reactions which are usually mediated by non-IgE immune reactions and may involve IgG or IgA. Non-IgE-mediated allergy symptoms typically occur in the gut but may also occur in the skin. IgE-mediated milk allergy can be diagnosed with a skin prick test, while non-IgE-mediated milk allergy can be diagnosed with a blood test. In both cases, milk allergy is managed by avoiding all foods containing milk and milk products. However, as most people do outgrow milk allergy and milk allergy is unusual in adults, reinvestigating tolerance over time (with the help of a health professional such as an allergist or dietitian) may be worthwhile. Some individuals with a milk allergy may be able to tolerate milk baked into products, though this should be discussed with an allergist before attempting.

CONSTIPATION

Randomized controlled trials show that in some children, non-IgE mediated cow's milk protein allergy may be a cause of chronic constipation. In children with chronic constipation, some show improvement in constipation with an oligoantigenic diet (a diet that excludes cow's milk, soy milk, and eggs) (Borrelli et al., 2009; Iacono et al., 2006). Observational studies have shown that among children aged 4 months to 3 years, short duration of breastfeeding and high cow's milk intake increases the risk of constipation (Andiran et al., 2003; Carroccio et al., 2013; Dehghani et al., 2012; Irastorza et al., 2010; Simeone et al., 2008). The body of evidence in this area is small, however, and further studies may be warranted.

SECTION 8:

ENVIRONMENTAL CONSIDERATIONS OF DAIRY

DAIRY AND CLIMATE CHANGE

Agriculture is a significant contributor to greenhouse gas (GHG) emissions worldwide, and recent studies show that the dairy sector's GHG emissions increased by 18% between 2005 and 2015 (FAO & GDP, 2018). Across the globe, all cattle are estimated to produce about 11% of all human-induced GHG emissions. Within the U.S., this figure is a bit lower at 3.4 %, and dairy cattle alone are responsible for about 1.3% of all human-induced GHG emissions (Rotz, 2018). These emissions come from the maintenance of crop and pasture land, manure storage, and the enteric fermentation from the animals themselves. A dairy cow is estimated to produce more than 330 kg of methane annually, a GHG that is 25% more potent than carbon dioxide. However, while total emissions have increased, dairy farming is becoming more efficient, resulting in declining emissions and impact per unit of production (FAO & GDP, 2018).

Water use is another topic of concern in dairy farming. Milk itself is about 87% water, so milking cows need to drink several gallons of water each day in order to sustain production. Additional water is needed to dispose of manure, clean milking equipment, and water pastures, and it's estimated that 30 to 50 gallons of water are needed per dairy cow per day (Brugger, 2007). This water use is especially concerning given that a majority of large dairy farms in the U.S. are in dry states like New Mexico, Texas, and California, where water use is a growing concern.

**Figure 2: The Amount of CO$_2$ Equivalents To
Create One Kilogram of Product**

It takes 21 pounds of whole milk to make one pound of butter.

DAIRY AND POLLUTION

The majority of milk and dairy products on the market today come from huge dairy farms, or "mega-dairies," that house thousands of cows at a time (Chrisman, 2020). These operations often contribute significantly to land, water, and air pollution. A considerable challenge at these mega-dairies is disposing of manure, as a 2,000-cow farm can generate up to a quarter of a million pounds of manure daily (US Environmental Protection Agency). Manure is high in nitrogen and phosphorus, and while these nutrients are important fertilizers in proper amounts, they are at toxic levels in manure. In these large farms, manure is often scraped or washed into large pits or lagoons, which then release large amounts of methane into the air and are prone to leaks into ground or surface water (Flaherty & Cativiela, 2017). On large dry lots, manure may also turn into dust that is inhaled by the cows, the farmworkers, and the local community alike. In fact, cities in the San Joaquin Valley which is in the heart of California's dairy country, have some of the highest rates of particulate air pollution in the U.S. (Charles, 2016).

However, not all dairy farming is automatically equated to pollution. Smaller herds grazing on pasture deposit much of their waste directly into the land in amounts that break down naturally and are beneficial to the soil. The "wear and tear" of cows on a pasture is also beneficial for the land — the impact of hooves and fertilization helps to build a healthful soil structure and stimulates deeper root growth which, in turn, helps control erosion and make the soil able to retain more water, lessening the effects of droughts and reducing flooding (USDA Natural Resources Conservation Service, Grazing Lands Technology Institute, 1996). While pastured cows still enterically produce methane, well-managed grasslands are able to sequester tons of GHGs and play a vital role in healthful ecosystems (Voth & Gilker, 2017).

DAIRY AND ANIMAL WELFARE

The treatment of animals in large dairy operations is also a growing concern. Many animals on these farms are kept in crowded lots with little vegetation or shade to escape the elements and are given no room to lie down. Cows that are not let out to pasture are fed a diet primarily of grain which can lead to acidosis, a digestive condition that can cause many different health problems for the cow. Cows on mega-dairies also have a shortened life expectancy. While dairy cattle can live to age 15 or 20 in a well-managed herd and can effectively produce milk for 12 to 15 years, cows on mega-dairies often remain in the herd for only about five years until their productivity begins to decline and they are sold to slaughter (Chrisman, 2020).

GROWTH HORMONE AND ANTIBIOTIC USE

Recombinant bovine somatotropin (rBST), previously called bovine growth hormone, is a synthetic hormone sometimes used in dairy cattle to increase milk production. It was approved by the FDA in 1993 and is now found in less than one in five dairy cows (American Cancer Society, 2014; US Food and Drug Administration, 2021). The U.S. does not require companies to label the use of rBST in dairy products, but the use of rBST has been banned in Canada and the European Union. The use of rBST was approved by the FDA because it was not deemed a health risk to humans. It is a large protein that is degraded by digestive enzymes in the stomach and small intestine, and the hormone itself shows no biological activity in humans. Of greater concern is that milk from cows treated with rBST often has higher levels of IGF-1, a hormone that helps cells grow and may influence the development of cancer, especially prostate, breast, and colorectal cancer. However, the exact nature of this association remains unclear, and many studies have found weak or no relationship between the two factors, and the American Cancer Society states they have no formal position regarding rBST (American Cancer Society, 2014).

A related topic is the use of antibiotics in dairy cows. On one hand, the use of antibiotics over the past several decades has resulted in more healthful and more productive animals. However, with the widespread use of antibiotics, there is concern about the development of antibiotic-resistant bacteria, both in food-producing animals and strains that could transfer to humans. While there have been isolated reports of antibacterial resistance among food-producing animals, there are not any studies that report the emergence and establishment of antibiotic-resistant microbes among dairy cows or humans (Oliver et al., 2011). Antimicrobial resistance among dairy pathogens, particularly those found in milk, likely poses little risk to humans if milk is pasteurized.

ORGANIC AND GRASS-FED DAIRY

Choosing organic and/or grass-fed dairy products from small, local farms may help to avoid some of the environmental concerns mentioned above. Additionally, grass-fed milk has been found to have nearly twice the amount of beneficial unsaturated fats as conventional milk (Benbrook et al., 2018). However, the total amount of these fats in grass-fed milk is still significantly lower than in other good sources such as fatty fish or vegetable oils.

If you are looking for the terms "organic" or "grass-fed" on the labels of dairy products, it's important to know what exactly they refer to. The term "USDA Organic" is regulated by the federal government, and the rules state that cows cannot be given growth hormones or antibiotics, all feed must be certified organic and cannot contain any animal by-products, and the animals cannot be continuously confined (AMS, 2018). Of note, an organic cow can still receive a diet primarily consisting of grain as long as the grain is organic.

The term "grass-fed," on the other hand, is not federally regulated. Some farmers with grass-fed animals keep their cows on pasture all of the time, while others supplement the cow's diet with some grain, usually to boost milk production. However, one distinction is that dairy from cows eating nothing but grass (and hay in the winter) can be labeled "100% grass-fed."

SECTION 9:

DAIRY AND MEDICATIONS

There are certain medications that should not be taken with dairy products due to the potential for calcium to interfere with the absorption of the medications. This can result in the medication being less effective. It is always best to check with a pharmacist or clinician to make sure which nutrients or foods may interact with any new medication.

Table 8: Medications That Are Affected by Dairy*

Class of Medication	Medication	Time Frame to Avoid Interactions
Antibiotics	Tetracycline – tetracycline, minocycline, and doxycycline	Avoid dairy one hour before and 2 hours after taking this medication
	Fluoroquinolone – ciprofloxacin, levofloxacin, and moxifloxacin	Avoid dairy 2 hours before and 2 hours after taking this medication

Class of Medication	Medication	Time Frame to Avoid Interactions
Bisphosphonates	Risedronate, alendronate, and ibandronate	Wait one hour after the medication to consume dairy
Iron Supplements	Ferrous sulfate, and ferrous gluconate	Wait at least 2 hours after taking an iron supplement before having any dairy
Thyroid Medications	Levothyroxine, Armor thyroid, and liothyronine	Wait 4 hours after taking medication to consume dairy
Anti-influenza	Xofluza	
Laxative	Bisacodyl (Dulcolax)	Avoid within an hour of dairy consumption

(https://www.goodrx.com/well-being/diet-nutrition/medications-and-dairy-products)
and (Christianson & Salling, 2020) *This is not a complete list.

SECTION 10:

CLINICAL AND CULINARY RECOMMENDATIONS AND COMPETENCIES

Messaging from the Menus of Change Annual Report 2020

REIMAGINE DAIRY IN A SUPPORTING ROLE

Clinical recommendations and competencies are the foundation from which culinary competencies were created. The goal for the culinary medicine practitioner is to help clients and patients develop the skills necessary to meet the clinical recommendations by teaching skill-based learning outlined in the culinary competencies.

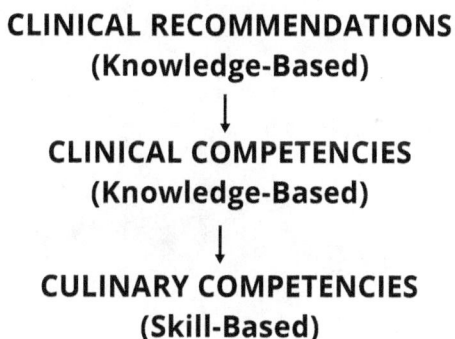

CLINICAL RECOMMENDATIONS
(Knowledge-Based)
↓
CLINICAL COMPETENCIES
(Knowledge-Based)
↓
CULINARY COMPETENCIES
(Skill-Based)

CLINICAL RECOMMENDATIONS

1. 3 cup-equivalents of dairy or dairy products per day for adults (U.S. Department of Agriculture and U.S. Department of Health and Human Services, 2020).
2. Consume dairy, "including fat-free and low-fat milk, yogurt, and cheese, and/or lactose-free versions and fortified soy beverages and yogurt as alternatives" (U.S. Department of Agriculture and U.S. Department of Health and Human Services, 2020).

CLINICAL COMPETENCIES

1. List the nutrients for which dairy supplies a "good source"
2. Explain which cohorts are at risk of not meeting their daily dairy requirement of dairy
3. Relate the importance of consuming dairy for overall health
4. Discuss the conditions that require limiting or avoiding dairy in one's diet
5. List medications that react with dairy

CULINARY COMPETENCIES FOR DAIRY
SHOPPING AND STORING COMPETENCIES

1. Identify the sugar content in a serving of yogurt
   a. Demonstrate how to read the Nutrition Facts panel
   b. Demonstrate how to find the added sugar content in a serving of yogurt
2. Describe the various steps in processing milk
3. Identify protein content in a serving of yogurt
4. Identify low-fat sources of dairy
5. Identify the most healthful milk option
6. Identify the most healthful cheese option
7. Demonstrate proper storage of dairy products

Stocking the Kitchen

1. Stock a variety of milks
2. Stock yogurt
3. Stock a variety of cheeses

COOKING/PREPARING COMPETENCIES

1. Prepare a healthful white sauce
2. Prepare a yogurt sauce
3. Prepare homemade yogurt (optional)

4. Thicken sauces using healthful ingredients
5. Prepare a dairy-based breakfast
6. Prepare a dairy-based dessert

FLAVOR DEVELOPMENT COMPETENCIES

1. Describe how to use cheese to increase the flavor profile of a dish
2. Demonstrate how to use dairy products to improve the texture and flavor profile of a dish

SERVING COMPETENCIES

1. Model-consuming dairy products
2. Demonstrate proper serving sizes of dairy products
3. Explain a dairy-equivalent
4. Serve healthful dairy-based desserts
5. Serve the appropriate number of dairy servings per day

SAFETY COMPETENCIES

1. Transport dairy products safely
2. Identify rancid dairy products
3. Identify dairy products that can increase the risk of foodborne illness

SECTION 11:
AT THE STORE

MILK

There are many milk alternatives available in stores, and decoding certain terms is necessary. The following are important terms to understand when shopping for milk that were discussed earlier in this chapter — homogenization, standardization, fortification, raw, and A2 milk. They also vary in the percentage of fat each contains (Table 9). They are listed here from the lowest to highest amount of fat — skim, 1%, 2%, full fat, half and half, and whipping cream.

Lactose-free or Minimal Lactose Foods

For some individuals, they cannot digest the sugar — lactose — in milk products. Some manufacturers will add the enzyme that digests lactose (lactase) to the milk to remove the lactose so that individuals can consume it without unwanted side effects. Lactose-free milk has the same nutrient profile (with the exception of the sugar lactose) as regular milk.

Chocolate Milk

> 48% of Americans have no idea where chocolate milk comes from, and 7% think that it comes from brown cows.

Do the benefits of consuming chocolate milk (calcium, for example) outweigh the risks of the added sugar that is present in chocolate milk? Let the math answer that question. If a child drinks just one 8-ounce glass of chocolate milk a day, which equals 10 to 15 grams of added sugar, that would equal 890 teaspoons (19 cups) to 1246 teaspoons (26 cups) of added sugar per year.

Organic Milk

For milk to be labeled organic, the cows must (Milk Safety | Dairy Health Benefits):
- Be exclusively given feed grown without the use of pesticides or commercial fertilizers.
- Be given access to a pasture periodically.
- Not be given supplemental hormones to promote growth.
- Not be given certain medications to treat illness. Cows are allowed to be given antibiotics but only in the case of an emergency.
- The USDA's Guidelines for Organic Certification of Dairy Livestock lays out the specifics. (https://www.ams.usda.gov/sites/default/files/media/Dairy%20-%20Guidelines.pdf)

Fortified

Fortified milk is more common in the United States than unfortified milk, although there is no law requiring fortification. Many states, however, require a standard value for certain nutrients present in milk, like calcium, iron, and protein. Common nutrients that are added are vitamins A (vitamin A palmitate) and D (vitamin D_3), plus others may also be added, like zinc, iron, and folic acid.

Fat Content

Do you choose whole-fat or low-fat dairy at the store? The answer depends on what your total diet looks like and your overall health. The fats present in whole-fat dairy products are a combination of mostly saturated fats and some mono-unsaturated fats. The recommendation for saturated fat intake is to consume no more than 10% of calories, which would equal 20 grams in a 2,000-calorie diet. If your overall diet is relatively low in saturated fat (low in animal products), then there is room for some whole-fat dairy products. Table 9 lists the amount of saturated fat in dairy products. If other saturated fats — animal meat products — are consumed, they should be accounted for in the daily consumption of saturated fats.

Table 9: Saturated Fat and Sodium in Whole-Fat Dairy Products

Whole Fat Dairy Product	Saturated Fat* (grams)	Sodium* (mg)
8 ounces: Whole fat milk	4.6	94
Reduced fat (2% milk)	2.7	95
Low fat Milk (1%)	1.4	95
Skim milk (fat-free)	0.1	100
Yogurt 1 cup	4.77**	104
Cheese hard		
Cheddar 1 slice (21 grams)	4	135
American 1 slice (20.6 grams)	3.7	342
Swiss 1 ounce (28.35 grams)	4.4	439
Gruyere 1 ounce (28.35 grams)	5.4	202
Parmesan 1 ounce (28.35 grams)	4.2	335
Asiago (30 grams)	6	360
Manchego 1 ounce (28 grams)	8	210
Romano 1 ounce (28.35 grams)	4.9	405
Goat cheese hard 1 ounce (28.35 grams)	7	120
Cheese soft		
Brie 1 ounce (28.35 grams)	5	178
Feta (28.35 grams)	3.8	323
Camembert 1 ounce (28.35 grams)	4.3	239
Queso fresco ¼ cup (30.5 grams)	4	229
Blue cheese 1 ounce (28.35 grams)	5.3	326
Mozzarella 1 ounce (28.35 grams)	3.9	138
Cottage cheese ½ cup (105 grams)	3.6	331
Cream cheese 1 tablespoon (14.5 grams)	2.9	46
Goat cheese soft 1 ounce (28.35 grams)	4	130
Ricotta ½ cup	7.3	125

*U.S. Department of Agriculture, Agricultural Research Service. FoodData Central, 2019. fdc.nal.usda.gov.
** Depending on the brand it can vary widely from 7 to 14 grams for one cup (look at the label).

The Nutrition Source from Harvard (https://nutritionsource.hsph.harvard.edu/dairy/) summarizes the evidence on whether or not to consume whole-fat or low-fat dairy products. One of the most important factors to consider is what type of food replaces the calories from fat when one consumes low-fat dairy. If those calories are replaced with whole grains, nuts, and healthful oils, great. If, however, they are replaced with refined grains and sugar, then that is not a more healthful option.

YOGURT

Fermentation is another issue to consider when purchasing and consuming dairy products as that process leads to a product lower in lactose (great for those that are lactose intolerant) and a product that provides healthful bacteria to the gastrointestinal tract, which brings with it a host of health benefits.

Putting it Into Practice: How to Choose a Healthful Yogurt

You are likely bombarded with over 30 different yogurts to choose from when you go to the store. Which one is the most healthful? Let's break it down into simple steps.

Type: Greek yogurt has more protein than regular yogurt. Chobani, Fage, and Skyr are some of the popular high-protein Greek options. If you are going to buy non-Greek yogurt, the lower-fat, plain varieties typically offer the highest protein content.

Added sugars: Find how many grams of added sugar there are per serving? What is the percent daily value? Aim for an unsweetened yogurt or one with minimal added sugar. Be careful, as some yogurts use artificial sweeteners like sucralose (Splenda), acesulfame potassium, and aspartame; of note, stevia and monk fruit are not artificial sweeteners.

Fat content: It depends on the individual situation (see above for more specifics). Choose low-fat or nonfat dairy when fewer calories and saturated fat are desired.

Flavor: Typically, flavored yogurt has a high amount of added sugar. Plain yogurt has 0 grams of added sugar, but some people don't like the taste. If going for a flavored yogurt, compare the nutrition facts label of different brands to find the one with the least amount of added sugar.

Ingredients list: This is another area where you can compare between two brands. Some brands add additives, colors, or other unnecessary ingredients. The fewer the ingredients, the better!

For help, check out What's New in The Yogurt Aisle (https://www.cspinet.org/article/whats-new-yogurt-aisle) by The Center for Science in the Public Interest.

CHEESE

A lot of people like cheese, and who can blame them? It is savory and creamy, and when melted, who can resist its gooey deliciousness? Since cheese is high in saturated fat, it is important to watch the amount of it consumed. If there was little to no saturated fat consumed that day (little to no animal products), then there is room for cheese. Refer to Table 9 for the amount of saturated fat in a serving of cheese and compare that with the daily allotment (13 grams in a 2,000-calorie diet). It is also important to watch the sodium content in processed cheese.

There are many factors to consider when selecting cheese, such as the number of calories, lactose content, and amount of saturated fat and sodium. Depending on what the greatest need is, consider the following:

- If lactose intolerance is an issue, select hard cheeses as they are lower in lactose as most of the whey is squeezed out when making it. Cheeses with low lactose levels are — cheddar, parmesan, and Swiss.
- For lower-calorie options, consider cheese made with skim or low-fat milk, be sure to look at the sodium content though, as it may be higher to make up for the loss of fat.
- If sodium is an issue, choose lower-sodium cheeses.

> Culinary Techniques—shred or grate cheese to get the illusion of a larger portion of cheese. Choose stronger smelling cheese that boosts the flavor profile, so less is needed.

BUTTER VERSUS MARGARINE

Defining Margarine

Figure 3: The Timeline of Margarine

In 1866 Napoleon III offered money for the development of an inexpensive food-fat, and three years later, a French chemist invented margarine by flavoring beef tallow with milk (McGee, 2004). It certainly was not a healthful product, but it was cheap. It was mass-produced in the United States by 1880, and between the 1970s and mid-1990s, low-fat spreads went from a market share of 5% to more than 74%. Figure 3 lays out the timeline for margarine (Dostalova, 2003).

Table 10: Comparing Butter and Margarine

	Butter	Margarine
CO_2 emissions (grams per Kg product)	23,794	1,350
Type of fat	High in saturated fat, which increases total and LDL cholesterol.	Some are low in saturated fat and high in unsaturated fat. Some are high in stearic acid.
Hydrogenated oil	Minimal partially hydrogenated trans fat and it is found naturally in butter (0.5g per tablespoon).	No trans fat, but does have fully hydrogenated oils created by force, which leads to stearic acid, a saturated fat.
Percentage of fat	70 to 80%	70 to 80%
Fortified/Enriched	If the milk had vitamin D added, so would the butter.	Some have plant sterols added.

Because both butter and margarine contain saturated fats, neither is really "better" than the other. Both should be used sparingly, and poly and mono-unsaturated oils should replace them as often as they can. The Presidential Advisory from the American Heart Association is very clear that replacing saturated fat with unsaturated fat — especially polyunsaturated fat — will lower the incidence of cardiovascular disease (Sacks et al., 2017).

Oils high in **polyunsaturated fats** include canola, corn, peanut, safflower (high linoleic), sunflower (high linoleic) and soybean oils. Canola, safflower (high oleic), sunflower (high oleic) and olive oils are high in **mono-unsaturated** fat.

From a culinary perspective, many recipes can still achieve good taste and texture by replacing some, if not all, of the butter/margarine with vegetable oil. Other spreads for toast and sandwiches can include heart-healthful options such as peanut butter and other nut/seed butters, avocado, and hummus. Low- and reduced-fat margarines do not work well for baking or cooking as they contain stabilizers that can scorch pans. In baking, the increase in water content affects the liquid-solid balance, and the extra starch, gum, and protein prevent melting.

In summary, the choice between butter or margarine will largely be based on an individual's taste preference. Some margarines have functional ingredients added, such as plant sterols, and others are dairy/lactose-free and vegan, which allows those with intolerances, allergies, and plant-based diets to use these options. For cardiovascular and overall health, both butter and margarine should be used in smaller quantities and heart-healthful fats such as polyunsaturated and monounsaturated fats should be promoted.

SECTION 12:
DAIRY AND SAFETY

Milk is highly perishable and should be kept from direct exposure to oxygen and strong light. Sunlight or fluorescent lights can cause a reaction between riboflavin and methionine, which contains sulfur (McGee, 2004). In addition, even with pasteurization, millions of bacteria are present.

It is very important to refrigerate milk and limit its exposure to oxygen at room temperature. The odor when milk turns rancid is very distinctive and should be the first clue to discard the milk. Other safety tips for dairy products are listed below.

1. Milk should be kept at or below 40 °F/4 °C. Pasteurized milk has a shelf life of 10 to 21 days, and ultra-pasteurized milk (UPM) has a shelf life of 30 to 90 days. Once opened, the UPM can last 7 to 10 days.
2. When shopping, pick up dairy products last (check that they are cold) in order to increase the chance that they remain cool enough until you get them home. If travel time is more than 30 minutes, add frozen items or an ice pack to the bag to keep them cool.
3. Look for the "sell by" date and don't buy products if they are after this date.
4. Don't leave dairy products out at room temperature for more than two hours.
5. Don't return unused milk or cream to their original container.
6. Butter that has been opened needs to be kept in the refrigerator for one to two months.
7. Soft cheeses tend to be made with unpasteurized milk, so it is best to avoid in vulnerable populations — those who are immune-compromised, children, and pregnant women, for example.

The Food Keeper App — https://www.foodsafety.gov/keep-food-safe/foodkeeper-app — has a lot more information on food and beverage storage.

SECTION 13:

IN THE KITCHEN

ON THE TONGUE

The flavor of milk is subtle and has been described as "milky, acidic, vanilla-like, caramel-like, aldehydic, fruity, beany, buttery, meaty, and vegetative" (Zhu & Xiao, 2017). It has a sweet-like flavor due to the sugar lactose, which is 60% less sweet than sucrose, and a slightly salty taste due to the minerals in milk (Helstad, 2019). Milk also has a pleasant mouthfeel due to fat globules and colloidal protein (Forss, 1969).

The flavor of fresh milk is influenced by the animal's feed. The flavor and color (a yellow hue) of milk from grass-fed cows differs from grain-fed cows due to the higher amount of unsaturated fats and the transfer of carotenoids, phenols, and other molecules in the grass to the milk (Faccia, 2020; Manzocchi et al., 2021).

The flavor of milk can change due to heat with the low temperature of pasteurization, adding a slightly sulfur and green-leaf note (McGee, 2004). This is due to breaking down enzymes and bacteria and destroying the more delicate aromas. At high heat — above 170 °F/76 °C — a world of other flavors develops. One can sense notes of almonds, vanilla, and cultured butter in addition to an eggy smell. With prolonged boiling, a butterscotch flavor develops due to the Maillard reaction.

THE ROLE OF DAIRY IN THE KITCHEN

1. Milk has a great ability to foam. Skim milk foams the best due to the higher protein content but has less flavor than higher-fat milk.
2. Milk moistens baked goods as well as adds protein, color, flavor, and an overall richness.
3. Milk can be a thickened agent along with starch. The salts present in milk promote protein coagulation.
4. Yogurt's acidity and calcium content act as a natural tenderizer.
5. Yogurt adds moisture and tang to baked goods.
6. Freezing milk will result in the clumping of the fat and protein particles and is not a good idea.

Culinary Tip: Wet the bottom of a pan before adding milk to prevent scorching when heated.

YOGURT
Making Yogurt

Image: Making Yogurt

Yogurt has many flavor assets — it is savory, creamy, and acidic. Because of that, yogurt can accompany a variety of dishes, from the spicy (to cool it down) to the savory, where it is used as a marinade due to its acidity, and to the sweet, where it is added on top of desserts. It can add creaminess without saturated fats to meat dishes, dry dishes (grains, waffles, latkes), spread on pitas and flatbreads, mixed into dressings and used as a dip for raw vegetables. The options are almost endless.

Making yogurt is super easy. There are three steps to making your own yogurt — heating, which unwinds the curd proteins and removes unwanted bacteria, cooling the milk to a temperature where healthful bacteria can thrive, and then fermenting the warm milk with bacteria (McGee, 2004).

Image: How to Make Yogurt

Yogurt-Based Sauces
Tzatziki Sauce

Image: Tzatziki Sauce

Ingredients**

- 1 small grated without seeds English cucumber
- 1 cup Greek yogurt
- 1 tablespoon lemon juice + 1 teaspoon zest
- 1 clove minced garlic
- ½ teaspoon salt
- 1 tablespoon dill chopped
- 1 tablespoon chopped mint leaves
- Black pepper to taste

Instructions

1. Prepare the cucumber: Peel the cucumber if it has a thick skin. Remove any seeds and grate. Squeeze any water out by placing the grated cucumber in a clean kitchen towel and wring out the water
2. Add all ingredients, stir, and allow the sauce to marinate for at least 2 hours to improve the flavor

Thickening Sauces

- Yogurt can be used to thicken sauces as long as the heat is only moderate. The sauce will curdle if it reaches boiling. Yogurt adds thickness — as opposed to thickening the liquid — as the casein proteins are already coagulated. Tips to using yogurt as a thickener:
  - Remove the watery whey before adding yogurt as a thickener
  - Add yogurt toward the end of cooking when the dish is cooling, not simmering
  - Beware when using yogurt in an acidic sauce (tomatoes, for example), as that will cause it to curdle. To prevent this, lower the heat and use full-fat yogurt (the fat prevents casein proteins from combining)
  - Do not beat the yogurt in sauces vigorously; fold or gently stir instead

Making a White Sauce – Béchamel

Image: White Sauce/Bechamel

A béchamel sauce is a classic French white sauce that is used to make lasagna, creamed chicken, the gravy in a pot pie and much more. There are three basic ingredients plus optional added flavors — salt and nutmeg. Cheese can also be added to make a cheese sauce.

- To make a classic béchamel the ratio of butter: flour: milk is 1 tablespoon: 1 tablespoon: 1 cup.
- To make a béchamel with skim milk, an extra tablespoon of flour is needed for every cup of milk.
- For a low-fat version made with olive oil and low-fat milk, The New York Times has a great recipe using 2 tablespoons flour, 2 tablespoons olive oil, and 2 cups 1% (low-fat) milk. (Olive Oil Béchamel Recipe).

The key to making this white sauce is to melt the fat (butter or oil) and combine with the flour. Let it cook for several minutes, which will reduce the taste of the flour. Then add the milk slowly, heat on medium (stirring occasionally) until thickened, and add cheese or spices if desired.

Milk and Heat

When cooking with dairy, it is important to not heat the milk too high (do not boil unless directed) as this will lead to curdling. Curdling occurs because the whey protein unfolds (denatures) and binds with the casein creating clumps of protein. To undo this, place in a blender.

Desserts or Breakfast

Yogurt Parfaits

Image: Yogurt Parfaits

Layer in a glass or bowl yogurt, granola, and fruit. This makes a great breakfast, snack, or dessert item.

Cottage Cheese and Fruit

Image: Cottage Cheese and Fruit

Add fresh fruit to cottage cheese for a quick and sweet/savory breakfast, lunch, or snack. Yum!

Cheese and Fruit Plate

Image: Cheese and Fruit Plate

Fresh figs, grapes, pears, and apples pair very well with a touch of cheese. Add the ingredients to a plate with nuts for a delicious snack or dessert. For a pop of eye appeal, drizzle a bit of honey on top.

SECTION 14:
SERVING DAIRY

Table 3 lays out the number of dairy or dairy equivalents recommended per day (3 cups a day for those nine years of age and older), and Table 11 defines a dairy equivalent. Refer to previous sections to decide which type of dairy products to serve. Because of the health value of probiotics, it makes sense to have yogurt as one of the dairy servings per day. That leaves one or two cups of milk to consume at mealtime or between meals as part of a snack.

Tale 11: Dairy Equivalents

	Amount That Counts as 1 Cup in The Dairy Group
Milk	1 cup milk 1 half-pint container milk ½ cup evaporated milk 1 cup calcium-fortified soy milk 1 half-pint container calcium-fortified soy milk
Yogurt	1 cup yogurt (dairy or fortified soy)

	Amount That Counts as 1 Cup in The Dairy Group
Cheese	1 ½ ounces hard cheese (cheddar, mozzarella, swiss, parmesan)
	⅓ cup shredded cheese
	1 ounce processed cheese (American)
	½ cup ricotta cheese
	2 cups cottage cheese
	2 ounces queso fresco
	2 slices queso blanco

Copied from https://www.myplate.gov/eat-healthy/dairy

The Culinary Institute of America Menus of Change recommends "reimaging dairy in a supporting role" (CIA & Harvard TH Chan, 2020). For example, instead of making a cheesy white sauce for pasta, create an olive oil herb blend and top with grated cheese; replace butter with oil; and use yogurt without added sugar.

SUMMARY

Milk products have been a staple in the diets of many cultures around the world and continue to be an important nutritional source for people today. Dairy foods are high in essential nutrients, including protein, fats, calcium, magnesium, potassium, vitamin B_{12} and riboflavin, among others. The micronutrients in milk products are highly bioavailable. Milk in the U.S. is also fortified with vitamin D, making it one of the few food sources of this important nutrient. Fermented milk and yogurt also provide additional benefits through their effects on the microbiome.

Despite initial concern over the potential impact of the saturated fat content of dairy foods, studies show that those who consume higher quantities of dairy products tend to have lower rates of cardiovascular disease, type 2 diabetes, and cancer. This may be in part due to the food matrix effect or the structure of the specific fats found in dairy foods, as well as other beneficial nutrients such as calcium, potassium, magnesium, and phosphorus present in milk products. Milk products are an excellent source of highly bioavailable calcium, which is important for bone health and the prevention of osteoporosis. Americans generally consume far less than the recommended number of servings of dairy foods, and more emphasis on the inclusion of dairy as part of a healthy eating pattern may be warranted.

For those who cannot tolerate dairy or, for various other reasons, prefer plant-based milks, the next section summarizes these beverages and their by-products.

APPENDIX A: USDA Dairy Recommendations Over Time

Date	Recommendation	Food Guide
1930s	2 cups of milk	H.K. Stiebeling
1940s	2 cups or more of milk and milk products	Basic Seven Foundation Diet
1956 to 1970s	Milk group – 2 cups or more	Basic Seven Foundation Diet
1979	Milk-cheese group – 2 (1 cup, 1 ½ oz cheese)	Hassle-Free Foundation Diet
1984	Milk, yogurt, cheese – 2 to 3	Food Guide Pyramid Diet
2005	Consume 3 cups per day of fat-free or low-fat milk or equivalent milk products. Avoid raw (unpasteurized) milk or any products made from unpasteurized milk.	2005 - 2010 DGA
2010	Increase intake of fat-free or low-fat milk and milk products, such as milk, yogurt, cheese, or fortified soy beverages. Choose foods that provide more potassium, dietary fiber, calcium, and vitamin D, which are nutrients of concern in American diets. These foods include vegetables, fruits, whole grains, and milk and milk products.	2010 - 2015 DGA
2015	A healthy eating pattern includes – Fat-free or low-fat dairy, including milk, yogurt, cheese, and/or fortified soy beverages	2015-2020 DGA
2020	Core elements that make up a healthy dietary pattern include – Dairy, including fat-free or low-fat milk, yogurt, and cheese, and/or lactose-free versions and fortified soy beverages and yogurt as alternatives. All fluid, dry, or evaporated milk, including lactose-free and lactose-reduced products and fortified soy beverages (soy milk), buttermilk, yogurt, kefir, frozen yogurt, dairy desserts, and cheeses. Most choices should be fat-free or low-fat. Cream, sour cream, and cream cheese are not included due to their low calcium content.	2020-2025 DGA

https://www.ers.usda.gov/webdocs/publications/42215/5831_aib750b_1_.pdf
https://www.ncbi.nlm.nih.gov/books/NBK469839/

PLANT-BASED MILK ALTERNATIVES

~

Joi Lenczowski MD, Dana Henderson MS RD CDCES,
Caroline Rosseler MS RD, and Deborah Koehn MD, FACP, BC-ADM, ABCL

Image: Plant Based Milk

HUMANS HAVE CONSUMED THE milk of buffalo, camels, sheep, goats, horses and yaks for thousands of years. While cow's milk remains the most produced and consumed milk beverage worldwide, production and consumption of plant-based milk alternatives are steadily rising. Milk sales in the United States decreased from 55,003 million pounds sold in 2010 to 47,672 million pounds sold in 2018, accounting for a $1.1 billion sales decline in 2018 alone (Dairy Farmers of America). Conversely, plant-based milk alternative sales grew by 9% in 2018, accounting for a growth of $1.6 billion in sales (Singh et al., 2015).

Plant-based milk alternatives are fluids resulting from the size reduction of plant materials extracted in water and homogenized. Although there are numerous types of plant-based milk alternatives, they can be categorized into five main groups based on their plant origin (Sethi et al., 2016):

1. **Cereal-based**: oat milk, rice milk, corn milk, spelt milk
2. **Legume-based**: soy milk, peanut milk, lupin milk, pea milk
3. **Nut-based**: almond milk, coconut milk, hazelnut milk, pistachio milk, walnut milk
4. **Seed-based**: sesame milk, flax milk, hemp milk, sunflower milk
5. **Pseudo-cereal-based**: quinoa milk, teff milk, amaranth milk

Among these groups, plant-based milk alternatives vary in their production methods, nutritional content, market presence, and sensory qualities. The Food and Drug Administration (FDA) does not have a standard of identity for these beverages, so be sure to read the list of ingredients and nutrition facts panel. For example, soy milk is the oldest plant-based milk alternative on the market and has been touted for its isoflavones' protective effects against cancer, cardiovascular disease, and osteoporosis. However, many consumers were deterred by its beany flavor, resulting in more modern production methods, including vacuum treatment at high temperatures to strip the more volatile compounds. Alternatively, newer plant-based milk alternatives, such as quinoa, hemp, and sunflower, have limited market presence and research on their nutritional benefits. Production methods of these products continue to evolve with consumer preference, ranging from blending varieties of milk for texture to fortifying products to meet consumers' health needs.

SECTION 1:

REASONS CONSUMERS SWITCH TO PLANT-BASED MILK ALTERNATIVES

Specific preferences aside, there are medical — including **allergies and intolerance** — and **ethical reasons** consumers are switching to plant-based beverages. Cow's milk allergy is one of the most common food allergies during the first year of life, with developed countries' prevalence ranging from 0.5% to 3% (Flom & Sicherer, 2019). Lactose intolerance is far more common. Lactose malabsorption, a precondition for lactose intolerance, may be as high as 68% worldwide (Misselwitz et al., 2019). Lactose intolerance varies among populations (see Table 7), with rates ranging as low as 5% in British populations to almost 100% in some Asian countries (Lomer et al., 2008).

As there is tremendous variability in the nutrient profiles among different plant-based milk alternatives, individuals may also choose one of these beverages to better support their **specific dietary concerns**. For example, individuals with diabetes may prefer the lower carbohydrate content of almond milk (4 g) compared to cow's milk (12 g) or oat milk (24 g).

Fat and thus calorie content is also extremely variable among plant-based milk alternatives, so those trying to lose weight or reduce their saturated fat consumption may opt for a lower-fat variety, while those trying to gain weight may opt for a higher-fat variety. Many popular varieties, such as almond and cashew milk, only contain 1 g of fat and 40 to 60 kilocalories per cup while coconut milk can contain up to 42 g of fat and 424 kilocalories per cup.

Most plant-based milk alternatives are low in protein, ranging between 1 gram to 4 grams of protein per cup compared to the 8 grams in cow's milk. However, those looking for a higher protein variety may opt for soy (8 grams) or pea milk (8 grams). Micronutrient content varies widely between milks due to manufacturing differences including processing and fortification (see section 2).

Consumers may also switch to plant-based beverages due to ethical reasons regarding animal welfare and environmental impact. Controversial practices of dairying include artificial insemination, removal of calves from their mother hours after birth, and the killing of male calves, and consumers concerned by these practices may shift their shopping habits. Additionally, many plant-based beverage consumers are attracted to the smaller ecological footprint of nondairy milk; one glass of dairy milks results in almost three times the greenhouse gas emissions, land use, and water use of any nondairy milks (Poore & Nemecek, 2018).

With the rise of plant-based milk alternatives, consumers are often confused by the labeling of plant-based beverages as "milks." They thus may not understand the nutritional differences between dairy milk and plant-based milk alternatives. A recent Consumer Reports found that more than half of people who buy plant-based milk alternatives believe these beverages are more healthful than cow's milk (Meltzer Warren, 2019). According to the FDA definition, milk is defined as "the lacteal secretion, practically free from colostrum, obtained by the complete milking of one or more healthy cows." The FDA has not set a standard of identity for plant-based milk alternatives, and in the past few years, bills — including the Dairy Pride Act — have been introduced upon the continued insistence of dairy farmers to limit the use of the word "milk" to animal-produced beverage. While this and other bills may protect the interest of dairy farmers and their product(s), it may also be of benefit to consumers as it will make the nutritional differences between cow's milk and plant-based milk alternatives more explicit and may lead consumers to make a more informed beverage choice.

SECTION 2:
COMPARISON OF NUTRIENTS

The focus of this section is on the nutrients present in cow's milk that are also found in alternate sources. This is important to note as when replacing, for example, dairy products in the Mediterranean diet with plant-based milk alternatives. One cannot assume the health benefits are the same due to the specific nutrient profile of dairy milk and food matrix effects. The major nutrients that this section will highlight are calcium, vitamin D, protein, vitamin B_{12} and saturated fat. Table 12 and Table 13 is a comparison of nutrients in cow's milk versus plant-based milk alternatives.

With the exception of soy milk, other plant-based milks are not to be considered as part of the dairy group and therefore do not count toward the daily dairy recommendation (U.S. Department of Agriculture and U.S. Department of Health and Human Services, 2020).

Many plant-based milk alternatives are fortified with important nutrients — both macro and micronutrients — that are either lost during processing or not present in adequate amounts in the first place. Note that some fortified nutrients may be more or less bioavailable than their naturally occurring counterparts found in cow's milk and also that many micronutrients are not measured in plant-based dairy alternatives, so they are unable to be compared (R. P. Heaney et al., 2005). In addition, many retailers are now producing plant-based dairy alternative blends by blending at least two plant-based products together to maximize nutrient offerings.

Table 12: Macronutrient Composition of Cow's Milk and Plant-based Milk Alternatives per 8 oz serving

Type	Product Name	Energy (kcal)	Protein (g)	Fat (g)	Saturated Fat (g)	Carbo-hydrate (g)	Fiber (g)	Sugars (g)	Added Sugars (g)
Cow's milk	2% Cow's milk	122	8.2	4.7	2.7	12	0	12	0
Almond	Silk Original	60	1	2.5	0	8	0	7	7
	Almond Breeze Original	60	1	2.5	0	8	<1	7	7
Cashew	Pacific Foods Original	80	1	4.5	0.5	8	N/A	6	5
Coconut	So Delicious Original (diluted beverage)	70	0	4.5	4	9	1	7	7
	Thai Kitchen (canned)	360	0	36	30	3	0	3	N/A
Combination	Silk Original Protein (Pea, Almond and Cashew)	130	10	8	0.5	3	<1	2	2
Flax	Good Karma Original	50	0	2.5	N/A	7	0	7	7
Hemp	Living Harvest/ Tempt Original	101	2	7	0.5	8	0	6	N/A
Oat	Oatly Original	120	3	5	0.5	16	1.9	7	N/A

Type	Product Name	Energy (kcal)	Protein (g)	Fat (g)	Saturated Fat (g)	Carbo-hydrate (g)	Fiber (g)	Sugars (g)	Added Sugars (g)
	Planet Oat Original	90	2	1.5	2	19	2	4	4
Pea	Ripple Unsweetened Original	80	8	4.5	0.5	<1	<1	0	0
Rice	Rice Dream Original	130	0	2.5	0	27	v	12	12
Soy	Silk Original	110	8	4.5	0.5	9	2	6	5

Sources: (DREAM Plant Based, 2022; Planet Oat, 2022; Ripple Foods, 2022; Silk, 2022; So Delicious Dairy Free, 2022; USDA, 2018)

Table 13: Micronutrient Composition of Cow's Milk and Plant-based Milk Alternatives per 8 oz serving

Type	Product Name	Calcium (mg)	Vit D (IU)	Iron (mg)	Potassium (mg)	Sodium (mg)	Vit B_{12} (mcg)	Vit A (IU)
Cow's Milk	2% Cow's milk	309	111	0	390	95.6	1.4	677
Almond	Silk Original	450	100	0.5	0	150	N/A	500
	Almond Breeze Original	450	200	0.7	170	150	N/A	500
Cashew	Pacific Foods Original	44	N/A	N/A	N/A	95	N/A	N/A
Coconut	So Delicious Original (diluted beverage)	130	100	0.3	40	10	3	140
		0	N/A	1.1	N/A	N/A	N/A	0
Combination	Silk Original (Pea, Almond and Cashew)	450	100	1.7	80	230	N/A	N/A
Flax	Good Karma Original	N/A	N/A	N/A	N/A	80	N/A	N/A
Hemp	Living Harvest/ Tempt Original	300	101	1	N/A	110	1.5	499
Oat	Oatly Original	350	N/A	0.3	389	101	1.2	N/A
	Planet Oat Original	350	160	0.3	400	120	0.2	600

Type	Product Name	Calcium (mg)	Vit D (IU)	Iron (mg)	Potassium (mg)	Sodium (mg)	Vit B$_{12}$ (mcg)	Vit A (IU)
Pea	Ripple Unsweetened Original	440	240	0	405	125	2.5	367
Rice	Rice Dream Original	20	0	0.5	30	95	N/A	N/A
Soy	Silk Original	450	120	1.3	380	90	3	500

Sources: (DREAM Plant Based, 2022; Planet Oat, 2022; Ripple Foods, 2022; Silk, 2022; So Delicious Dairy Free, 2022; USDA, 2018)

Calcium

As previously discussed, calcium is the most abundant mineral in the body whose functions include supporting bone health, regulating blood pH, and regulating muscle and nerve function. The calcium content in 8 oz cow's milk is about 30% of the daily value or about 300 mg, but calcium does not naturally occur in adequate amounts in plant-based milk alternatives. Thus, most plant-based milk alternatives are fortified with calcium in the form of calcium carbonate, often to a level even higher than in cow's milk. However, the simple addition of calcium does not mean nutritional equivalence (Singhal et al., 2017). Calcium in cow's milk is highly bioavailable due in part to the presence of lactose and casein that aid in intestinal absorption. The calcium in plant-based milk alternatives does not have the help of lactose and casein, and additional compounds like phytic acid that are present in many plant-based products may further impede absorption, making the calcium in plant-based milks less bioavailable.

Table 14: Amount of Calcium in Dairy and Plant-Based Milk

Type of "Milk"	Amount*
Cow	300 mg
Almond	22 to 495 mg
Soy	0 to 385 mg
Rice	22 to 330 mg
Coconut	to 495 mg

*Higher amounts reflect the amount of calcium being added to the product
Source: (Vanga & Raghavan, 2018a)

Vitamin D

Recall that vitamin D is not found in many foods but is required for the proper absorption and function of calcium as well as for cell differentiation and growth, regulation of phosphorous, immune health, blood pressure regulation and blood sugar regulation.

The FDA ruled in 2016 that plant-based milk beverages may be fortified with up to 205 IU of vitamin D per serving, which could make them better sources of vitamin D than cow's milk. The new nutrition label requires that the amount of vitamin D is to be listed, so consumers will be better able to meet and track their vitamin D intake from plant-based milk alternatives (Harrar, S, 2016).

There are two different forms of vitamin D, though only one is typically used for fortification. The vitamin D in fortified cow's milk is vitamin D_3, the type of vitamin D derived from animals, and is also the type commonly found in plant-based dairy alternatives (Armas et al., 2004; Singhal et al., 2017). The other form, vitamin D_2, is derived from plants and is a good option for supplementation for strict vegetarians or vegans. Additional differences in vitamins D_3 and D_2 are listed in Table 15.

Table 15: Types of Vitamin D

Vitamin D_3	Vitamin D_2
Cholecalciferol	Ergocalciferol
From animal sources	From plant sources
More expensive	Cheaper
Better at raising serum levels of 25(OH)D when a bolus dose (large dose) was given	Raises serum levels of 25(OH)D to the same degree when given as a daily supplement

Source: (Tripkovic et al., 2012)

Protein

Protein is an important macronutrient whose functions include muscle and connective tissue development, enzyme production, and antibody development, among others. Amino acids act as the building block of proteins, and the amino acids present in a protein food can make the food either a complete or an incomplete protein. Complete proteins are those which contain all nine essential amino acids, which must be consumed from the diet, and offer the most bioavailable form of protein from a singular source. Complete proteins are found in animal products, such as cow's milk, as well as the plant-based proteins **soy, amaranth, and quinoa**. Incomplete proteins are proteins that offer some of the essential amino acids, but not all nine. Incomplete proteins are also typically less bioavailable than complete proteins.

In contrast to cow's milk which provides about 8 grams of protein per 8 oz serving, many of the plant-based dairy alternatives on the shelves are low in protein (as low as 1 gram per 8 oz serving) with inadequate information on the types of amino acids present. One exception is soy and pea milk beverages which offer about 8 grams of protein per 8 oz (Parrish, 2018; Singhal et al., 2017). Some plant-based dairy alternatives are fortified with pea protein to increase protein content, however, pea protein is not considered a complete protein.

When thinking about sources of protein, it's also important to consider the quality of protein from those sources. The digestible indispensable amino acids score (DIAAS) is one measure of protein digestibility and degree of absorption. Using this method, dairy proteins can be considered "excellent/high" quality sources of protein with DIAAS >100, soy protein qualifies as a "good" source of protein with DIAAS between 75 and 100, and pea protein is a lower quality protein with DIASS <75 (Mathai et al., 2017). If an individual is relying on a plant-based milk alternative as a significant source of protein in their diet, it's important to recognize the difference in protein quality and be sure there are other sources of quality protein in the diet if needed.

Vitamin B$_{12}$

Recall that vitamin B$_{12}$ is a water-soluble vitamin that is involved in many processes in the body including red blood cell production, nerve cell development, DNA production and metabolism. It is found naturally only in animal source foods, but milk alternatives may be fortified with B$_{12}$, up to 3.01 µg per 8 oz serving, more than double the amount found in cow's milk however the details regarding the source of fortification and bioavailability are not available in the current research (Parrish, 2018; Singhal et al., 2017). Plant-based milk alternatives can be an important source of vitamin B$_{12}$ for strict vegetarians and vegans who consume little to no natural sources of this vitamin.

Saturated Fat

Saturated fat is a type of fat typically associated with animal products, though it is also found in foods or products containing coconut or palm oil. A diet high in saturated fats is associated with unfavorable health outcomes, such as cardiovascular disease and metabolic syndrome, while research has shown that replacing saturated fats in the diet with unsaturated fats shows more favorable outcomes for health (De Lorgeril et al., 1996; Nordmann et al., 2011).

The USDA recommends less than 10% of calories from saturated fats in the 2020-2025 Dietary Guidelines for Americans (U.S. Department of Agriculture and U.S. Department of Health and Human Services, 2020). Many milk alternatives contain only a small amount of unsaturated fat and are free of saturated fat. One exception to this is coconut milk as it does contain some saturated fat (Parrish, 2018).

Iodine

Iodine is a mineral that is essential for hormone synthesis, and milk is often one of the main dietary sources of iodine. Plant-based milk alternatives tend to have a low iodine concentration and the fortification of iodine in these beverages is inconsistent. Individuals who avoid dairy products and opt instead for milk alternatives may be at risk of iodine deficiency (Eveleigh et al., 2022). In fact, a recent study that examined data from the U.K. National Diet and Nutrition Study found that iodine intake and markers of iodine status were lower in exclusive consumers of plant-based milk alternatives than in cows' milk consumers, and as a group the exclusive consumers of plant-based milk alternatives were classified as iodine deficient by the World Health Organization criterion (Dineva et al., 2021).

SECTION 3:
EMULSIFIERS IN PLANT-BASED MILK ALTERNATIVES

Plant-based milk alternatives can have many different types of additives, the most common of which is an emulsifier. Since plant-based beverages are often a mixture of oil and water, a hydrocolloid — a substance that has both a hydrophobic and hydrophilic component — helps to keep the composition smooth and silky.

Interestingly, emulsifiers can originate from animals (gelatin), plants (guar gum, pectin), aquatic plants (seaweeds), microbes (xanthan gum and gellan gum) and/or be synthetically produced such as lecithin. They have a long cultural history, with Asian countries using seaweed, the Americas using fruit pectin, and Mediterranean countries using locust bean gum. In Table 16, emulsifiers that are used within the plant-based beverages are listed. See Appendix A for common plant-based milk alternatives for the type of emulsifier used in each.

Table 16: Safety of Emulsifiers Used in Plant-Based Milk Alternatives

Emulsifier	Source	Safety
Carrageenan	Seaweed	Non-carcinogenic, tumorigenic, genotoxic or reproductively toxic. It is a safe food additive and is released into the feces unchanged [a].
Sodium Alginate	Seaweed	It has been proven to be a safe additive. Caution with infants and young children [b]

Emulsifier	Source	Safety
Xanthan Gum	Fermented Polysaccharide	Unlikely to be absorbed by the intestinal tract and is partially fermented by the intestinal microbiota in the large intestine. No carcinogenicity effects were seen at the highest doses. Since Xanthan gum is not absorbed by the intestines it can result in abdominal discomfort at higher doses as it acts as a bulk laxative [c].
Gellan Gum	Fermented polysaccharide	At this time, no known genotoxicity, carcinogenic toxicity or reproductive toxicity has been identified in the use of gellan gum [d].
Lecithin (a.k.a. phosphatidylcholine)	Soybean, egg yolk, sunflower oil, or rape seed oil	At this time, no genotoxicity or carcinogenicity has been identified; however, some animal studies have generated concern about choline's impact on neurodevelopment. Consequently, recommendations at this time include limiting exposure to large doses of lecithin during gestation, lactation, and post-weaning period. In addition, sensitive individuals should avoid this additive as some hypersensitivity can occur to residual soy and egg proteins in the extracted lecithin [e].
Guar Gum	Seed gums	No adverse effects were reported in sub-chronic and carcinogenicity studies at the highest dose tested; no concern with respect to the genotoxicity. No adequate assessment has been done in infants and young children [f].

a (McKim et al, 2019), b (EFSA Panel, 2017d), c (EFSA Panel, 2017c), d (EFSA Panel, 2018), e (EFSA Panel, 2017b), f (EFSA Panel, 2017a)

In general, most added emulsifiers used in plant-based milk alternatives are safe for adults without any concern for toxicity, though the data is lacking for infants and young children. Lecithin may be harmful for individuals, fetuses and infants who are hypersensitive to egg. Since emulsifiers are complex polysaccharides that pass through the gut without being absorbed or minimally modified by the gut bacteria, they can act as a stool bulking agent. There is potential that these stool bulking emulsifiers can lower cholesterol and blood sugar but at the same time increase stool frequency and flatulence.

SECTION 4:

HEALTH BENEFITS OF PLANT-BASED MILK ALTERNATIVES

There is minimal direct research on the health benefits of plant-based milk alternatives. Extrapolation from data derived from health benefits of the basic source of the milk, e.g., soybeans, almonds, or such, may not be justified, as the primary source is modified in commercial production. This modification results in both loss of primary components and addition of supplements. However, there are still some important things to note.

Soy milk and health

Diabetes

Currently, no consensus is available on the impact of soy milk on overall health. Multiple studies have shown a decreased incidence of type 2 diabetes mellitus (T2DM) with ingestion of soy products, primarily tofu. However, studies directly investigating soy milk have reported conflicting results, with both increased risk and decreased risk of T2DM. Nguyen et al noted that a higher dietary intake of soy-foods and isoflavones lowers the risk of T2DM, and this decreased risk was also noted with increased soy milk ingestion (Nguyen et al., 2017). A similar inverse association between soy milk ingestion and T2DM was reported in a sub-analysis of the Shanghai Women's Health Study (Villegas et al., 2008).

However, a study based on data from the Singapore Chinese Health Study (SCHS), a population-based, prospective investigation, found that while consumption of unsweetened non-fried whole soy proteins decreased the risk of T2DM, ingestion of sweetened soymilk beverages was associated with an increased risk of T2DM. In this study, however, 17 grams of added sugar were present per serving of soy milk, complicating the interpretation of the data (Mueller et al., 2012). It is possible that unsweetened soy milk decreases the risk for T2DM, but current research is not conclusive.

Lipid Levels

Research studies are conflicted in their results on the impact of soy milk on lipid profiles. A randomized controlled trial with 31 participants comparing two different commercially available soy milks versus low-fat dairy milk concluded that a 25 g dose of daily soy protein from soy milk led to a modest 5% lowering of LDL-C relative to dairy milk among adults with elevated LDL-C. The effect did not differ by type of soy milk and neither did soy milk significantly affect other lipid variables, insulin, or glucose (Gardner et al., 2007). In contrast, a single-blind randomized trial with 32 postmenopausal women comparing vanilla soymilk and reduced-fat dairy milk showed no significant difference in total, HDL, or LDL cholesterol or triglyceride levels with ingestion of three daily servings of soy milk, (21 g soy protein) (Beavers et al., 2010).

Oat Milk and Health

Oat milk ingestion has been associated with small decreases in total cholesterol and LDL cholesterol when used as a replacement for cow's milk. Two randomized clinical trials of oat milk versus soy milk, rice milk, or cow's milk (<70 participants each) showed a 4% to 9% decrease in total and LDL cholesterol levels with ingestion of oat milk. The high content of beta-glucans in oat milk may be responsible for the decreased plasma cholesterol and LDL cholesterol concentrations, however, the effect could also be due to a replacement of saturated fat by unsaturated fat. Oat milk can be recommended as an alternative to other milk drinks for patients who would benefit from reduced LDL cholesterol values (Onning et al., 1998, 1999).

Almond Milk and Health

Despite the considerable literature on the health benefits of almonds, such as improved glycemic control, there is currently no literature systematically investigating the impact of almond milk on health.

SECTION 5:

POTENTIAL RISK OF CONSUMING PLANT-BASED MILK ALTERNATIVES

Arsenic in Rice Milk

Recently there has been concern about arsenic in rice and rice products as one's lifetime exposure to arsenic can increase their risk for bladder and lung cancer. The attributable risk from rice and rice products to bladder and lung cancer remains small at 39 cases per million people (compared to 90,000 total cases of bladder and lung cancer per million people over a lifetime). Risk increases though with increased daily servings of rice and rice products (U.S. Food and Drug Administration, 2016).

Regulations in the European Union and the U.S. state that arsenic levels in drinking water should not exceed 10 micrograms/L (Meharg et al., 2008). However, there have been reports that have found arsenic levels in rice milk that exceed these limits. For example, Meharg and colleagues found a mean arsenic level of 22 micrograms/L among 15 rice milks with a range of 10.2 to 33.3 micrograms/L, and Shannon & Rodriguez found an average arsenic concentration of 7.1 micrograms/L with a range of 2.7 to 17.9 micrograms/L among 15 rice milk samples (Meharg et al., 2008; Shannon & Rodriguez, 2014). The decision whether or not to recommend rice milk in a person's diet should be weighed against the consumption of other rice and rice products in the individual's diet.

Effect of Plant-Based Milk Alternatives on Dentition

Risk of cavity formation due to ingestion of plant-based milk alternatives has been studied in in-vitro models of biofilm formation. Based on these investigations, unsweetened almond milk has the lowest potential to contribute to dental caries, while soy milk has the highest potential. Almond milk sweetened with sucrose does have an increased risk of contributing to dental cavities. Thus, for patients who are lactose-intolerant or suffer from milk allergy, unsweetened almond milk is a better alternative than soy-based products with respect to dental health (Lee et al., 2018).

Pros and Cons of Plant Based Milk

Image: Pros and Cons of Plant Based Milk

In summary, some plant-based milk alternatives can provide a nutrient profile similar to cow's milk (not identical) as long as the following is met:
- Make sure the plant-based milk has vitamin B_{12} added (1.29 µg), or find an alternate source of B_{12} in the diet, especially for vegetarians
- Calcium is added to provide at least 300 mg — preferably in the form of calcium carbonate
- Vitamin D is added to provide 120 IU — vitamin D_3, which is sourced from animals is better absorbed than D_2 — for vegetarians make sure there are other sources as well
- If protein is a concern, choose soy milk, pea protein milk, or a milk blend with added pea protein that contains at least 5 to 6 grams of protein per 8 oz serving.

SECTION 6:

INFANTS, CHILDREN, AND PLANT-BASED MILK ALTERNATIVES

Breast milk or an iron-fortified infant formula should be an infant's sole food source during the first four to six months of life. After one year, the USDA recommends infants over one year of age consume two to three servings of whole cow's milk per day for a nutritionally complete diet. This suggested amount makes up roughly 25% to 30% of total energy needs of those one to three years and provides numerous macro- and micronutrients, including protein, fat, calcium, phosphorus and vitamin B_{12} (Drewnowski, 2011; Fox et al., 2006; Grimes et al., 2017; Groetch & Nowak-Wegrzyn, 2013). Over the past several years, more parents have been opting for plant-based milk alternatives due to allergies, intolerances, cultural traditions or health beliefs. A plant-based milk alternative should provide a similar nutrient profile as cow's milk, or attention is needed to make sure these nutrients are provided elsewhere in the child's diet. Severe nutrient deficiencies have been reported in young infants and children using plant-based milks without proper nutritional guidance (Le Louer et al., 2014).

The North American Society for Pediatric Gastroenterology, Hepatology, and Nutrition (NASPGHAN) claims that **soy milk and soy formula may be a suitable substitute** for the majority of infants and young children. However, parents opting for almond, rice, coconut, hemp, flaxseed and cashew milks should be advised that these products have inadequate nutrient profiles to meet the nutritional needs for protein, calcium, and vitamin D. While these products can be included safely as a component of the diet, families with children where cow's milk is medically contraindicated or not culturally appropriate should receive special counseling from clinicians or registered dietitians to determine alternative dietary sources of protein, calcium, iron, vitamin B_{12} and vitamin D (Merritt et al., 2020).

SECTION 7:

THE ELDERLY AND PLANT-BASED MILK ALTERNATIVES

Similar to the way plant-based milk alternatives should be approached with caution for infants and young children, they may also be problematic for the elderly. Older individuals have limited appetites and consume fewer calories, so the foods they do consume must be nutrient-dense in order for their nutrient needs to be met. In this population especially, poor nutrition could induce frailty and speed the progression of chronic disease.

It is well established that adequate calcium and protein intake in the elderly can delay sarcopenia and bone loss (Lana et al., 2015). Dairy products are good sources of these important nutrients, but it's unclear if the same benefits could be gained from fortified plant-based milk alternatives, especially if the bioavailability of the protein, vitamin, and mineral content of these beverages is in question. Some researchers have suggested that increasing plant-based foods, including plant-based milk alternatives, and reducing animal-based products could have unintended consequences on the protein intake of older adults and put them at risk of nutrient deficiencies (Houchins et al., 2017; Scholz-Ahrens et al., 2020). Like with infants and children, if older adults wish to consume a plant-based milk alternative or are required to do so for medical reasons, it is important to be sure that they are consuming sufficient amounts of protein, vitamins, and minerals elsewhere in their diet.

SECTION 8:

ENVIRONMENTAL CONSIDERATIONS OF PLANT-BASED MILK ALTERNATIVES

It is well established that the production of dairy products from cow's milk has a significant environmental impact, but plant-based milk alternatives also come with an environmental impact of their own. One thing to keep in mind is that different producers and manufacturers may have different processing methods that impact the beverage's environmental impact, so even plant-based milk alternatives from the same plant source may not be equivalent.

The first environmental issue that comes to mind regarding plant-based milk alternatives is **water usage**. Almond milk especially has a high water footprint, and a recent study calculated that it takes 3.2 gallons of water to grow a single almond (Fulton et al., 2019). This becomes especially problematic considering that about 80% of the world's almonds are grown in California, an area with ongoing concerns regarding their water supply (USDA Foreign Agricultural Service). Of all the plant-based milk alternatives, oats generally use the least water and soy and pea are a close second. Hemp farming requires more water than these three but still less than almond (Mekonnen & Hoekstra, 2010).

Land use is another environmental factor to consider. Soybeans require a lot of land compared to other plants like almonds or rice (Poore & Nemecek, 2018). On the other hand, soybeans and peas are nitrogen-fixing plants, so they naturally add nitrogen back into the soil, eliminating the need for nitrogen-containing fertilizers.

GHG emissions associated with plant-based milk alternatives are certainly lower than cow's milk. Soy and pea protein milks have comparable GHG emissions, and a study by the brand Oatly found that oat milk production results in 80% lower GHG emissions and uses 60% lower energy than cow's milk (Climate Footprint).

While plant-based milk alternatives have a lower impact on the environment overall, the issue is more complex as cow's milk contains several key nutrients that prove to be challenging to replace (Vanga & Raghavan, 2018b). In a recent modeling study by Cifelli and colleagues, a nutritionally optimal diet that eliminates dairy foods requires a greater volume of food and more calories and still falls short of several key nutrients (Cifelli et al., 2020). Additionally, an optimal dietary pattern that incorporates plant-based milk alternatives may cost up to six times as much as a diet that follows the USDA pattern that incorporates dairy. While a diet that removes dairy may lead to lower GHG emissions, careful consideration needs to be given to nutritional adequacy.

SECTION 9:

CLINICAL AND CULINARY RECOMMENDATIONS AND COMPETENCIES

1. Identify the plant-based milk alternative for the infant and young child.
2. Compare and contrast "good sources" of nutrients in dairy versus plant-based milk.
3. List the advantages and disadvantages of replacing dairy with various plant-based milks.
4. Choose a plant-based milk based on the nutrient(s) needed.
5. Make a plant-based milk (optional).

SECTION 10:

AT THE STORE

Steps to Choosing a Plant-Based Milk Alternative

- There is no one-size-fits-all when selecting plant-based milk alternatives at the store as it depends on what purpose the beverage needs to serve. For example, reasons can include that you want it to be:

- **Similar to dairy in its overall nutrient profile**. For various reasons described previously, individuals switch to a plant-based milk alternative and many do so not realizing that dairy comes with its unique nutrient profile. Reasons may include it being:
  - A substitute when following the Mediterranean diet. In this case, data is not sufficient enough to say the benefits of following a Mediterranean diet would be the same if for example soy milk was substituted for dairy.
  - A dairy substitute for children after weaning. As described above, NASPGHAN suggests substituting soy milk for dairy for infants and young children.
  - Lactose intolerant. These individuals can consume Lactaid and other dairy products with little or no amount of lactose. This is described in the Dairy – In the Store section.
  - A dairy allergy.
  - An overall substitute for vegetarians or flexitarians.
- **A good source of protein**. In this case, look for an equivalent of 8 grams of protein in an 8-ounce (1 cup) serving on the Nutrition Facts Label. Choose from soy, amaranth, and quinoa, which are complete sources of protein.
- **A good source of calcium, vitamin D, and/or vitamin B_{12}**. In this case look for 300 mg calcium, 120 IU of vitamin D, and/or 1.29 µg of vitamin B_{12} per 8-ounce (1 cup) serving on the Nutrition Facts Label. Note 20% DV of vitamin B_{12} = 0.48 µg and in order to get 1.29 µg per serving the DV would need to be 54%.
- **A substitute for dairy in recipes** — see Section 11.

SECTION 11:

IN THE KITCHEN

Plant-Based Milk

Image: Making Nut Milk

Making homemade nut milks is quite simple but does require some planning. They will not contain fortified amounts of calcium, vitamin D, protein or B_{12}, so making sure that these nutrients are consumed from somewhere else in the diet is important.

Cashew Milk

- For drinking 2% like-milk:
    - Soak 1 cup raw cashews overnight and then purée in a food processor with 4 cups of water.
    - Add additional flavorings (optional): maple syrup, dates, honey, vanilla, and purée .
    - Place in a nut-bag or cheese cloth and strain the milk from the nut residue. The nut residue can be baked and added to granola or cookie batter.
- For cashew milk that you are going to use in a soup where you need a creamier whole-like milk
    - Soak 1 cup raw cashews overnight and then purée in a food processor with 2 cups of room temperature water.

Consumers may choose plant-based milk alternatives based on their cooking properties. Soy milk is the most common replacement in recipes calling for cow's milk due to its similar protein content. Its protein content adds structure for baking and its stability at high temperatures enables its use in savory dishes. In comparison, sweeter and lower-protein milk varieties such as almond milk are better for desserts and smoothies. For creamier dishes, many opt for coconut milk due to its higher fat content and thus creamy texture.

Plant-Based Yogurt in Three Easy Steps

- **Step 1:** Select a plant-based milk — 14 ounce can of coconut milk or 1 ¾ cup soy or cashew milk. The milk with higher fat content makes a creamy yogurt whereas the milk with lower fat content — almond and rice — makes a thin pourable mixture.
- **Step 2:** Add 4 probiotic capsules (or 1 teaspoon), mix together, add to a clean glass jar (do not use metal), top with cheesecloth and a rubber band. Make sure the probiotics are 'live' and contain L. acidophilus or S. thermophilus.
- **Step 3:** Allow to ferment for 24 to 48 hours in a warm space (oven with light on but no heat).

*Note: to make a Greek yogurt, place the prepared yogurt in a cheesecloth over a bowl and let the liquid seep out. Keep an eye on it as you don't want to turn into cheese (or do you?).

SUMMARY

Plant-based milk alternatives are plentiful, and some can offer a similar nutrient profile as dairy milk. However, only soy fortified beverages can count toward a dairy serving. Specifically, for the nutrients calcium, vitamin D, protein and vitamin B_{12} many plant-based milk alternatives are fortified to help them offer just as much, if not more than dairy milk, though the bioavailability of these nutrients is not yet known (Parrish, 2018). Most plant-based milk alternatives also offer a beverage choice that is lower in saturated fat than full-fat or reduced-fat dairy milk, with the exception of coconut milk (Parrish, 2018). There is a need for further research on the micronutrient composition of these dairy alternatives, as well as the types of nutrients they are being fortified with, and the bioavailability of these nutrients to better determine the impact that they have on a person's health.

Plant-based beverages can not only be incorporated into a healthful eating pattern but also promote a healthful environment. It is important for clients and clinicians alike to understand that the type of plant-based dairy alternative they are choosing will differ in terms of fortification of nutrients and the presence of emulsifiers.

APPENDIX A: Plant-Based Milk Alternatives and Emulsifiers

		Xanthan Gum	Gellan Gum	Guar Gum	Sunflower Lecithin	Locust Bean	Carrageenan	None
Pacific								
	Almond Original	x	x					
	Cashew Original	x	x	x				
	Hemp Original	x	x					
	Coconut Original	x	x	x				
	Oat Original		x					
	Hazelnut	x	x		x	x		
	Soy							x
West Soy								x
Almond Breeze								
	Almond Original		x		x			
Silk								
	Soy		x					
	Almond		x		x	x		
	Cashew		x		x	x		
	Oat		x		x	x		
	Coconut		x		x	x		
Simple Truth								
	Soy						x	
	Almond	x	x		x			
	Oat		x					
	Coconut	x	x	x			x	
Ripple								
	Original		x	x	x			
Whole foods								
	365 soy		x			x		
	365 Almond		x			x		

		Xanthan Gum	Gellan Gum	Guar Gum	Sunflower Lecithin	Locust Bean	Carrageenan	None
	365 Coconut		x			x		
	Cosmic Cashew							x
	Oatley							x
Walmart								
	Soy		x					
	Almond				x		x	
	Planet Oat		x					

REFERENCES

Acham, M., Wesselius, A., van Osch, F. H. M., Yu, E. Y.-W., van den Brandt, P. A., White, E., Adami, H.-O., Weiderpass, E., Brinkman, M., Giles, G. G., Milne, R. L., & Zeegers, M. P. (2020). Intake of milk and other dairy products and the risk of bladder cancer: A pooled analysis of 13 cohort studies. European Journal of Clinical Nutrition, 74(1), 28–35. https://doi.org/10.1038/s41430-019-0453-6

Akkasheh, G., Kashani-Poor, Z., Tajabadi-Ebrahimi, M., Jafari, P., Akbari, H., Taghizadeh, M., Memarzadeh, M. R., Asemi, Z., & Esmaillzadeh, A. (2016). Clinical and metabolic response to probiotic administration in patients with major depressive disorder: A randomized, double-blind, placebo-controlled trial. Nutrition (Burbank, Los Angeles County, Calif.), 32(3), 315–320. https://doi.org/10.1016/j.nut.2015.09.003

Akkerman, M., Larsen, L. B., Sørensen, J., & Poulsen, N. A. (2019). Natural variations of citrate and calcium in milk and their effects on milk processing properties. Journal of Dairy Science, 102(8), 6830–6841. https://doi.org/10.3168/jds.2018-16195

alKanhal, H. A., al-Othman, A. A., & Hewedi, F. M. (2001). Changes in protein nutritional quality in fresh and recombined ultra high temperature treated milk during storage. International Journal of Food Sciences and Nutrition, 52(6), 509–514.

Alothman, M., Hogan, S. A., Hennessy, D., Dillon, P., Kilcawley, K. N., O'Donovan, M., Tobin, J., Fenelon, M. A., & O'Callaghan, T. F. (2019). The "Grass-Fed" Milk Story: Understanding the Impact of Pasture Feeding on the Composition and Quality of Bovine Milk. Foods (Basel, Switzerland), 8(8), E350. https://doi.org/10.3390/foods8080350

Alvarez-Bueno, C., Cavero-Redondo, I., Martinez-Vizcaino, V., Sotos-Prieto, M., Ruiz, J. R., & Gil, A. (2019). Effects of Milk and Dairy Product Consumption on Type 2 Diabetes: Overview of Systematic Reviews and Meta-Analyses. Advances in Nutrition (Bethesda, Md.), 10(suppl_2), S154–S163. https://doi.org/10.1093/advances/nmy107

American Cancer Society. (2014, September 10). Recombinant Bovine Growth Hormone. https://www.cancer.org/cancer/cancer-causes/recombinant-bovine-growth-hormone.html

AMS. (2018). Guidelines for Organic Certification of Dairy Livestock. USDA. https://www.ams.usda.gov/sites/default/files/media/Dairy%20-%20Guidelines.pdf

Anderson, G. H., & Moore, S. E. (2004). Dietary proteins in the regulation of food intake and body weight in humans. The Journal of Nutrition, 134(4), 974S-9S. https://doi.org/10.1093/jn/134.4.974S

Anderson, G. H., Tecimer, S. N., Shah, D., & Zafar, T. A. (2004). Protein source, quantity, and time of consumption determine the effect of proteins on short-term food intake in young men. The Journal of Nutrition, 134(11), 3011–3015. https://doi.org/10.1093/jn/134.11.3011

Andiran, F., Dayi, S., & Mete, E. (2003). Cows milk consumption in constipation and anal fissure in infants and young children. Journal of Paediatrics and Child Health, 39(5), 329–331. https://doi.org/10.1046/j.1440-1754.2003.00152.x

Armas, L. A. G., Hollis, B. W., & Heaney, R. P. (2004). Vitamin D2 is much less effective than vitamin D3 in humans. The Journal of Clinical Endocrinology and Metabolism, 89(11), 5387–5391. https://doi.org/10.1210/jc.2004-0360

Arnett Donna K., Blumenthal Roger S., Albert Michelle A., Buroker Andrew B., Goldberger Zachary D., Hahn Ellen J., Himmelfarb Cheryl Dennison, Khera Amit, Lloyd-Jones Donald, McEvoy J. William, Michos Erin D., Miedema Michael D., Muñoz Daniel, Smith Sidney C., Virani Salim S., Williams Kim A., Yeboah Joseph, & Ziaeian Boback. (2019). 2019 ACC/AHA Guideline on the Primary Prevention of Cardiovascular Disease: A Report of the American College of Cardiology/American Heart Association Task Force on Clinical Practice Guidelines. Circulation, 140(11), e596–e646. https://doi.org/10.1161/CIR.0000000000000678

Aslam, H., Marx, W., Rocks, T., Loughman, A., Chandrasekaran, V., Ruusunen, A., Dawson, S. L., West, M., Mullarkey, E., Pasco, J. A., & Jacka, F. N. (2020). The effects of dairy and dairy derivatives on the gut microbiota: A systematic literature review. Gut Microbes, 12(1), 1799533. https://doi.org/10.1080/19490976.2020.1799533

Astrup, A. (2014). Yogurt and dairy product consumption to prevent cardiometabolic diseases: Epidemiologic and experimental studies. The American Journal of Clinical Nutrition, 99(5 Suppl), 1235S-42S. https://doi.org/10.3945/ajcn.113.073015

Astrup, A., Geiker, N. R. W., & Magkos, F. (2019). Effects of Full-Fat and Fermented Dairy Products on Cardiometabolic Disease: Food Is More Than the Sum of Its Parts. Advances in Nutrition (Bethesda, Md.), 10(5), 924S-930S. https://doi.org/10.1093/advances/nmz069

Astrup, A., Rice Bradley, B. H., Brenna, J. T., Delplanque, B., Ferry, M., & Torres-Gonzalez, M. (2016). Regular-Fat Dairy and Human Health: A Synopsis of Symposia Presented in Europe and North America (2014-2015). Nutrients, 8(8), E463. https://doi.org/10.3390/nu8080463

Aune, D., Norat, T., Romundstad, P., & Vatten, L. J. (2013). Dairy products and the risk of type 2 diabetes: A systematic review and dose-response meta-analysis of cohort studies. The American Journal of Clinical Nutrition, 98(4), 1066–1083. https://doi.org/10.3945/ajcn.113.059030

Baer, D. J., Stote, K. S., Paul, D. R., Harris, G. K., Rumpler, W. V., & Clevidence, B. A. (2011). Whey protein but not soy protein supplementation alters body weight and composition in free-living overweight and obese adults. The Journal of Nutrition, 141(8), 1489–1494. https://doi.org/10.3945/jn.111.139840

Bailey, R. K., Fileti, C. P., Keith, J., Tropez-Sims, S., Price, W., & Allison-Ottey, S. D. (2013). Lactose intolerance and health disparities among African Americans and Hispanic Americans: An updated consensus statement. Journal of the National Medical Association, 105(2), 112–127. https://doi.org/10.1016/s0027-9684(15)30113-9

Barrubés, L., Babio, N., Becerra-Tomás, N., Rosique-Esteban, N., & Salas-Salvadó, J. (2019). Association Between Dairy Product Consumption and Colorectal Cancer Risk in Adults: A Systematic Review and Meta-Analysis of Epidemiologic Studies. Advances in Nutrition (Bethesda, Md.), 10(suppl_2), S190–S211. https://doi.org/10.1093/advances/nmy114

Beavers, K. M., Serra, M. C., Beavers, D. P., Hudson, G. M., & Willoughby, D. S. (2010). The lipid-lowering effects of 4 weeks of daily soymilk or dairy milk ingestion in a postmenopausal female population. Journal of Medicinal Food, 13(3), 650–656. https://doi.org/10.1089/jmf.2009.0171

Belobrajdic, D. P., McIntosh, G. H., & Owens, J. A. (2004). A high-whey-protein diet reduces body weight gain and alters insulin sensitivity relative to red meat in wistar rats. The Journal of Nutrition, 134(6), 1454–1458. https://doi.org/10.1093/jn/134.6.1454

Benbrook, C. M., Davis, D. R., Heins, B. J., Latif, M. A., Leifert, C., Peterman, L., Butler, G., Faergeman, O., Abel-Caines, S., & Baranski, M. (2018). Enhancing the fatty acid profile of milk through forage-based rations, with nutrition modeling of diet outcomes. Food Science & Nutrition, 6(3), 681–700. https://doi.org/10.1002/fsn3.610

Bendtsen, L. Q., Lorenzen, J. K., Bendsen, N. T., Rasmussen, C., & Astrup, A. (2013). Effect of dairy proteins on appetite, energy expenditure, body weight, and composition: A review of the evidence from controlled clinical trials. Advances in Nutrition (Bethesda, Md.), 4(4), 418–438. https://doi.org/10.3945/an.113.003723

Bermejo, L. M., López-Plaza, B., Santurino, C., Cavero-Redondo, I., & Gómez-Candela, C. (2019). Milk and Dairy Product Consumption and Bladder Cancer Risk: A Systematic Review and Meta-Analysis of Observational Studies. Advances in Nutrition (Bethesda, Md.), 10(suppl_2), S224–S238. https://doi.org/10.1093/advances/nmy119

Blom, W. A. M., Lluch, A., Stafleu, A., Vinoy, S., Holst, J. J., Schaafsma, G., & Hendriks, H. F. J. (2006). Effect of a high-protein breakfast on the postprandial ghrelin response. The American Journal of Clinical Nutrition, 83(2), 211–220. https://doi.org/10.1093/ajcn/83.2.211

Bonjour, J.-P., Kraenzlin, M., Levasseur, R., Warren, M., & Whiting, S. (2013). Dairy in adulthood: From foods to nutrient interactions on bone and skeletal muscle health. Journal of the American College of Nutrition, 32(4), 251–263. https://doi.org/10.1080/07315724.2013.816604

Booth, A. O., Huggins, C. E., Wattanapenpaiboon, N., & Nowson, C. A. (2015). Effect of increasing dietary calcium through supplements and dairy food on body weight and body composition: A meta-analysis of randomised controlled trials. The British Journal of Nutrition, 114(7), 1013–1025. https://doi.org/10.1017/S0007114515001518

Borrelli, O., Barbara, G., Di Nardo, G., Cremon, C., Lucarelli, S., Frediani, T., Paganelli, M., De Giorgio, R., Stanghellini, V., & Cucchiara, S. (2009). Neuroimmune interaction and anorectal motility in children with food allergy-related chronic constipation. The American Journal of Gastroenterology, 104(2), 454–463. https://doi.org/10.1038/ajg.2008.109

Bounous, G., Baruchel, S., Falutz, J., & Gold, P. (1993). Whey proteins as a food supplement in HIV-seropositive individuals. Clinical and Investigative Medicine. Medecine Clinique Et Experimentale, 16(3), 204–209.

Bourgeois, C., & Moss, J. (2010). Niacin. In P. Coates, J. Betz, M. Blackman, G. Cragg, M. Levine, J. Moss, & J. White (Eds.), Encyclopedia of Dietary Supplements (2nd ed., pp. 562–569). Informa Healthcare.

Bourrie, B. C. T., Richard, C., & Willing, B. P. (2020). Kefir in the Prevention and Treatment of Obesity and Metabolic Disorders. Current Nutrition Reports, 9(3), 184–192. https://doi.org/10.1007/s13668-020-00315-3

Bristow, S. M., Horne, A. M., Gamble, G. D., Mihov, B., Stewart, A., & Reid, I. R. (2019). Dietary Calcium Intake and Bone Loss Over 6 Years in Osteopenic Postmenopausal Women. The Journal of Clinical Endocrinology and Metabolism, 104(8), 3576–3584. https://doi.org/10.1210/jc.2019-00111

Brugger, M. (2007). Fact Sheet: Water Use on Ohio Dairy Farms. Ohio State Univeristy Extension, 3.

Carmel, R. (2014). Cobalamin (vitamin B12). In A. Ross, B. Caballero, R. Cousins, K. Tucker, & T. Ziegler (Eds.), Modern Nutrition in Health and Disease (11th ed., pp. 369–389). Lippincott Williams & Wilkins.

Carroccio, A., Mansueto, P., Morfino, G., D'Alcamo, A., Di Paola, V., Iacono, G., Soresi, M., Scerrino, G., Maresi, E., Gulotta, G., Rini, G., & Bonventre, S. (2013). Oligo-antigenic diet in the treatment of chronic anal fissures. Evidence for a relationship between food hypersensitivity and anal fissures. The American Journal of Gastroenterology, 108(5), 825–832. https://doi.org/10.1038/ajg.2013.58

Centers for Disease Control and Prevention. (2021, July 23). Fortified Cow's Milk and Milk Alternatives. Centers for Disease Control and Prevention. https://www.cdc.gov/nutrition/infantandtoddlernutrition/foods-and-drinks/cows-milk-and-milk-alternatives.html

Champagne, C. M. (2006). Dietary interventions on blood pressure: The Dietary Approaches to Stop Hypertension (DASH) trials. Nutrition Reviews, 64(2 Pt 2), S53-56. https://doi.org/10.1111/j.1753-4887.2006.tb00234.x

Charles, J. (2016). Menu of State Laws Regarding Odors Produced by Concentrated Animal Feeding Operations. Centers for Disease Control, Office of State, Tribal, Local and Territorial Support, 8.

Cheese Production. (n.d.). Milk Facts. Retrieved January 23, 2022, from http://milkfacts.info/Milk%20Processing/Cheese%20Production.htm

Chen, L., Li, M., & Li, H. (2019). Milk and yogurt intake and breast cancer risk: A meta-analysis. Medicine, 98(12), e14900. https://doi.org/10.1097/MD.0000000000014900

Chen, M., Sun, Q., Giovannucci, E., Mozaffarian, D., Manson, J. E., Willett, W. C., & Hu, F. B. (2014). Dairy consumption and risk of type 2 diabetes: 3 cohorts of US adults and an updated meta-analysis. BMC Medicine, 12, 215. https://doi.org/10.1186/s12916-014-0215-1

Chin-Dusting, J., Shennan, J., Jones, E., Williams, C., Kingwell, B., & Dart, A. (2006). Effect of dietary supplementation with beta-casein A1 or A2 on markers of disease development in individuals at high risk of cardiovascular disease. The British Journal of Nutrition, 95(1), 136–144. https://doi.org/10.1079/bjn20051599

Chrisman, S. (2020). The FoodPrint of Dairy. https://foodprint.org/reports/the-foodprint-of-dairy/

Christianson, E., & Salling, J. (2020). Meded101 Guide to Drug Food Interactions.

CIA, & Harvard TH Chan. (2020). Menus of Change: 2020 Summit & Resources. https://www.ciaprochef.com/MOC/Resources.pdf/

Cifelli, C. J., Auestad, N., & Fulgoni, V. L. (2020). Replacing the nutrients in dairy foods with non-dairy foods will increase cost, energy intake and require large amounts of food: National Health and Nutrition Examination Survey 2011-2014. Public Health Nutrition, 1–12. https://doi.org/10.1017/S1368980020001937

Climate footprint. (n.d.). Oatly. Retrieved February 6, 2022, from https://www.oatly.com/en-us/stuff-we-make/climate-footprint

Code of Federal Regulations Title 21. (2021, October 1). U.S. Food and Drug Administration. https://www.accessdata.fda.gov/scripts/cdrh/cfdocs/cfcfr/CFRSearch.cfm?fr=133.3

Companys, J., Pla-Pagà, L., Calderón-Pérez, L., Llauradó, E., Solà, R., Pedret, A., & Valls, R. M. (2020). Fermented Dairy Products, Probiotic Supplementation, and Cardiometabolic Diseases: A Systematic Review and Meta-analysis. Advances in Nutrition (Bethesda, Md.), 11(4), 834–863. https://doi.org/10.1093/advances/nmaa030

Cross, M. L., & Gill, H. S. (1999). Modulation of immune function by a modified bovine whey protein concentrate. Immunology and Cell Biology, 77(4), 345–350. https://doi.org/10.1046/j.1440-1711.1999.00834.x

Dairy Farmers of America. (n.d.). Retrieved February 6, 2022, from https://www.dfamilk.com/

De Lorgeril, M., Salen, P., Martin, J. L., Mamelle, N., Monjaud, I., Touboul, P., & Delaye, J. (1996). Effect of a mediterranean type of diet on the rate of cardiovascular complications in patients with coronary artery disease. Insights into the cardioprotective effect of certain nutriments. Journal of the American College of Cardiology, 28(5), 1103–1108. https://doi.org/10.1016/S0735-1097(96)00280-X

De Noni, I., FitzGerald, R. J., Korhonen, H. J. T., Le Roux, Y., Livesey, C. T., Thorsdottir, I., Tome, D., & Witkamp, R. (2009). Review of the potential health impact of β-casomorphins and related peptides (pp. 1–107). European Food Safety Authority. https://www.efsa.europa.eu/en/efsajournal/pub/rn-231

de Souza, R. J., Mente, A., Maroleanu, A., Cozma, A. I., Ha, V., Kishibe, T., Uleryk, E., Budylowski, P., Schünemann, H., Beyene, J., & Anand, S. S. (2015). Intake of saturated and trans unsaturated fatty acids and risk of all cause mortality, cardiovascular disease, and type 2 diabetes: Systematic review and meta-analysis of observational studies. BMJ (Clinical Research Ed.), 351, h3978. https://doi.org/10.1136/bmj.h3978

Dehghan, M., Mente, A., Rangarajan, S., Sheridan, P., Mohan, V., Iqbal, R., Gupta, R., Lear, S., Wentzel-Viljoen, E., Avezum, A., Lopez-Jaramillo, P., Mony, P., Varma, R. P., Kumar, R., Chifamba, J., Alhabib, K. F., Mohammadifard, N., Oguz, A., Lanas, F., ... Prospective Urban Rural Epidemiology (PURE) study investigators. (2018). Association of dairy intake with cardiovascular disease and mortality in 21 countries from five continents (PURE): A prospective cohort study. Lancet (London, England), 392(10161), 2288–2297. https://doi.org/10.1016/S0140-6736(18)31812-9

Dehghani, S.-M., Ahmadpour, B., Haghighat, M., Kashef, S., Imanieh, M.-H., & Soleimani, M. (2012). The Role of Cow's Milk Allergy in Pediatric Chronic Constipation: A Randomized Clinical Trial. Iranian Journal of Pediatrics, 22(4), 468–474.

Dietary Guidelines Advisory Committee. (2020). Scientific Report of the 2020 Dietary Guidelines Advisory Committee: Advisory Report to the Secretary of Agriculture and the Secretary of Health and Human Services.

Dineva, M., Rayman, M. P., & Bath, S. C. (2021). Iodine status of consumers of milk-alternative drinks v. cows' milk: Data from the UK National Diet and Nutrition Survey. The British Journal of Nutrition, 126(1), 28–36. https://doi.org/10.1017/S0007114520003876

Donovan, S. M. (2017). In V. A. Stallings & M. P. Oria (Eds.), National Academies of Sciences, Engineering, and Medicine. Finding a Path to Safety in Food Allergy. National Academies Press.

Dostalova, J. (2003). Low Fat Foods: Low Fat Spreads. In Encyclopedia of Food Sciences and Nutrition | ScienceDirect. Academic Press. https://www.sciencedirect.com/referencework/9780122270550/encyclopedia-of-food-sciences-and-nutrition

DREAM Plant Based. (2022). Dream Plant Based. https://www.dreamplantbased.com/

Drehmer, M., Pereira, M. A., Schmidt, M. I., Alvim, S., Lotufo, P. A., Luft, V. C., & Duncan, B. B. (2016). Total and Full-Fat, but Not Low-Fat, Dairy Product Intakes are Inversely Associated with Metabolic Syndrome in Adults. The Journal of Nutrition, 146(1), 81–89. https://doi.org/10.3945/jn.115.220699

Drewnowski, A. (2011). The contribution of milk and milk products to micronutrient density and affordability of the U.S. diet. Journal of the American College of Nutrition, 30(5 Suppl 1), 422S-8S. https://doi.org/10.1080/07315724.2011.10719986

Drouin-Chartier, J.-P., Brassard, D., Tessier-Grenier, M., Côté, J. A., Labonté, M.-È., Desroches, S., Couture, P., & Lamarche, B. (2016). Systematic Review of the Association between Dairy Product Consumption and Risk of Cardiovascular-Related Clinical Outcomes. Advances in Nutrition (Bethesda, Md.), 7(6), 1026–1040. https://doi.org/10.3945/an.115.011403

EFSA Panel. (2017a). Re-evaluation of guar gum (E 412) as a food additive. https://efsa.onlinelibrary.wiley.com/doi/10.2903/j.efsa.2017.4669

EFSA Panel. (2017b). Re-evaluation of lecithins (E322) as a food additive.

EFSA Panel. (2017c). Re-evaluation of Xanthan gum (E415) as a food additive.

EFSA Panel. (2017d). Re-evaluation of alginic acid and its sodium, potassium, ammonium, and calcium salts. https://efsa.onlinelibrary.wiley.com/doi/full/10.2903/j.efsa.2017.5049

EFSA Panel. (2018). Re-evaluation of Gellan Gum (E418) as Food Additive.

Emerson, S. R., Kurti, S. P., Harms, C. A., Haub, M. D., Melgarejo, T., Logan, C., & Rosenkranz, S. K. (2017). Magnitude and Timing of the Postprandial Inflammatory Response to a High-Fat Meal in Healthy Adults: A Systematic Review. Advances in Nutrition (Bethesda, Md.), 8(2), 213–225. https://doi.org/10.3945/an.116.014431

Ericson, U., Hellstrand, S., Brunkwall, L., Schulz, C.-A., Sonestedt, E., Wallström, P., Gullberg, B., Wirfält, E., & Orho-Melander, M. (2015). Food sources of fat may clarify the inconsistent role of dietary fat intake for incidence of type 2 diabetes. The American Journal of Clinical Nutrition, 101(5), 1065–1080. https://doi.org/10.3945/ajcn.114.103010

Eveleigh, E., Coneyworth, L., Zhou, M., Burdett, H., Malla, J., Nguyen, V. H., & Welham, S. (2022). Vegans and vegetarians living in Nottingham (UK) continue to be at risk of iodine deficiency. The British Journal of Nutrition, 1–46. https://doi.org/10.1017/S0007114522000113

Faccia, M. (2020). The Flavor of Dairy Products from Grass-Fed Cows. Foods, 9(9), 1188. https://doi.org/10.3390/foods9091188

FAO & GDP. (2018). Climate change and the global dairy cattle sector: The role of the dairy sector in a low-carbon future. (CC BY-NC-SA-3.0 IGO). FAO. http://www.fao.org/3/CA2929EN/ca2929en.pdf

Fernandez, M. L., & Calle, M. (2010). Revisiting dietary cholesterol recommendations: Does the evidence support a limit of 300 mg/d? Current Atherosclerosis Reports, 12(6), 377–383. https://doi.org/10.1007/s11883-010-0130-7

Flaherty, R., & Cativiela, J. (2017, August 21). California Dairy 101: Overview of dairy farming and manure methane reduction opportunities. Dairy and Livestock Working Group. https://ww2.arb.ca.gov/sites/default/files/classic/cc/dairy/documents/08-21-17/dsg1-dairy-101-presentation.pdf

Flom, J. D., & Sicherer, S. H. (2019). Epidemiology of Cow's Milk Allergy. Nutrients, 11(5), 1051. https://doi.org/10.3390/nu11051051

Fong, J., & Khan, A. (2012). Hypocalcemia: Updates in diagnosis and management for primary care. Canadian Family Physician Medecin De Famille Canadien, 58(2), 158–162.

Fontecha, J., Calvo, M. V., Juarez, M., Gil, A., & Martínez-Vizcaino, V. (2019). Milk and Dairy Product Consumption and Cardiovascular Diseases: An Overview of Systematic Reviews and Meta-Analyses. Advances in Nutrition (Bethesda, Md.), 10(suppl_2), S164–S189. https://doi.org/10.1093/advances/nmy099

Food and Agriculture Organization. (2021). Gateway to Dairy and Dairy Products. http://www.fao.org/dairy-production-products/en/

Ford, J. T., Wong, C. W., & Colditz, I. G. (2001). Effects of dietary protein types on immune responses and levels of infection with Eimeria vermiformis in mice. Immunology and Cell Biology, 79(1), 23–28. https://doi.org/10.1046/j.1440-1711.2001.00788.x

Forss, D. (1969). Flavors of Dairy Products: A Review of Recent Advances | Elsevier Enhanced Reader. Journal of Dairy Science, 52(6), 832–840. https://doi.org/10.3168/jds.S0022-0302(69)86659-2

Fox, M. K., Reidy, K., Novak, T., & Ziegler, P. (2006). Sources of energy and nutrients in the diets of infants and toddlers. Journal of the American Dietetic Association, 106(1 Suppl 1), S28-42. https://doi.org/10.1016/j.jada.2005.09.034

Fulton, J., Norton, M., & Shilling, F. (2019). Water-indexed benefits and impacts of California almonds. Ecological Indicators, 96(1), 711–717.

García, E. V., Sala-Serra, M., Continente-Garcia, X., Serral Cano, G., & Puigpinós-Riera, R. (2020). The association between breast cancer and consumption of dairy products: A systematic review. Nutricion Hospitalaria, 34(3), 589–598. https://doi.org/10.20960/nh.02649

Gardner, C. D., Messina, M., Kiazand, A., Morris, J. L., & Franke, A. A. (2007). Effect of two types of soy milk and dairy milk on plasma lipids in hypercholesterolemic adults: A randomized trial. Journal of the American College of Nutrition, 26(6), 669–677. https://doi.org/10.1080/07315724.2007.10719646

German, J. B., Gibson, R. A., Krauss, R. M., Nestel, P., Lamarche, B., van Staveren, W. A., Steijns, J. M., de Groot, L. C. P. G. M., Lock, A. L., & Destaillats, F. (2009). A reappraisal of the impact of dairy foods and milk fat on cardiovascular disease risk. European Journal of Nutrition, 48(4), 191–203. https://doi.org/10.1007/s00394-009-0002-5

Gijsbers, L., Ding, E. L., Malik, V. S., de Goede, J., Geleijnse, J. M., & Soedamah-Muthu, S. S. (2016). Consumption of dairy foods and diabetes incidence: A dose-response meta-analysis of observational studies. The American Journal of Clinical Nutrition, 103(4), 1111–1124. https://doi.org/10.3945/ajcn.115.123216

Golden, N. H., Abrams, S. A., & Committee on Nutrition. (2014). Optimizing bone health in children and adolescents. Pediatrics, 134(4), e1229-1243. https://doi.org/10.1542/peds.2014-2173

Gómez-Cortés, P., Juárez, M., & de la Fuente, M. A. (2018). Milk fatty acids and potential health benefits: An updated vision. Trends in Food Science & Technology, 81, 1–9. https://doi.org/10.1016/j.tifs.2018.08.014

González-Chávez, S. A., Arévalo-Gallegos, S., & Rascón-Cruz, Q. (2009). Lactoferrin: Structure, function and applications. International Journal of Antimicrobial Agents, 33(4), 301.e1-8. https://doi.org/10.1016/j.ijantimicag.2008.07.020

Grimes, C. A., Szymlek-Gay, E. A., & Nicklas, T. A. (2017). Beverage Consumption among U.S. Children Aged 0-24 Months: National Health and Nutrition Examination Survey (NHANES). Nutrients, 9(3), E264. https://doi.org/10.3390/nu9030264

Groetch, M., & Nowak-Wegrzyn, A. (2013). Practical approach to nutrition and dietary intervention in pediatric food allergy. Pediatric Allergy and Immunology: Official Publication of the European Society of Pediatric Allergy and Immunology, 24(3), 212–221. https://doi.org/10.1111/pai.12035

Hall, W. L., Millward, D. J., Long, S. J., & Morgan, L. M. (2003). Casein and whey exert different effects on plasma amino acid profiles, gastrointestinal hormone secretion and appetite. The British Journal of Nutrition, 89(2), 239–248. https://doi.org/10.1079/BJN2002760

Hanach, N. I., McCullough, F., & Avery, A. (2019). The Impact of Dairy Protein Intake on Muscle Mass, Muscle Strength, and Physical Performance in Middle-Aged to Older Adults with or without Existing Sarcopenia: A Systematic Review and Meta-Analysis. Advances in Nutrition (Bethesda, Md.), 10(1), 59–69. https://doi.org/10.1093/advances/nmy065

Harrar, S. (2016, October 17). Is There Vitamin D in Mil Alternatives? Consumer Reports. https://www.consumerreports.org/vitamins-supplements/vitamin-d-in-milk-alternatives/

Harrington, L. K., & Mayberry, J. F. (2008). A re-appraisal of lactose intolerance. International Journal of Clinical Practice, 62(10), 1541–1546. https://doi.org/10.1111/j.1742-1241.2008.01834.x

Hata, I., Higashiyama, S., & Otani, H. (1998). Identification of a phosphopeptide in bovine alpha s1-casein digest as a factor influencing proliferation and immunoglobulin production in lymphocyte cultures. The Journal of Dairy Research, 65(4), 569–578. https://doi.org/10.1017/s0022029998003136

Heaney, R. (2012). Phosphorus. In J. Erdman, I. MacDonald, & S. Zeisel (Eds.), Present Knowledge in Nutrition (10th ed., pp. 447–458). Wiley-Blackwell.

Heaney, R. P. (2007). Bone health. The American Journal of Clinical Nutrition, 85(1), 300S-303S. https://doi.org/10.1093/ajcn/85.1.300S

Heaney, R. P., Rafferty, K., & Bierman, J. (2005). Not All Calcium-fortified Beverages Are Equal. Nutrition Today, 40(1), 39–44.

Helstad, S. (2019). Corn Sweeteners. In Corn: Chemstry and Technology (3rd ed.). Elsevier. https://www.sciencedirect.com/topics/agricultural-and-biological-sciences/sweetness

Hempel, S., Newberry, S. J., Maher, A. R., Wang, Z., Miles, J. N. V., Shanman, R., Johnsen, B., & Shekelle, P. G. (2012). Probiotics for the prevention and treatment of antibiotic-associated diarrhea: A systematic review and meta-analysis. JAMA, 307(18), 1959–1969. https://doi.org/10.1001/jama.2012.3507

Hess, J. M., Cifelli, C. J., & Fulgoni Iii, V. L. (2020). Energy and Nutrient Intake of Americans according to Meeting Current Dairy Recommendations. Nutrients, 12(10), E3006. https://doi.org/10.3390/nu12103006

Hoffman, J. R., & Falvo, M. J. (2004). Protein—Which is Best? Journal of Sports Science & Medicine, 3(3), 118–130.

Holt, C., Carver, J. A., Ecroyd, H., & Thorn, D. C. (2013). Invited review: Caseins and the casein micelle: their biological functions, structures, and behavior in foods. Journal of Dairy Science, 96(10), 6127–6146. https://doi.org/10.3168/jds.2013-6831

Houchins, J. A., Cifelli, C. J., Demmer, E., & Fulgoni, V. L. (2017). Diet Modeling in Older Americans: The Impact of Increasing Plant-Based Foods or Dairy Products on Protein Intake. The Journal of Nutrition, Health & Aging, 21(6), 673–680. https://doi.org/10.1007/s12603-016-0819-6

Iacono, G., Bonventre, S., Scalici, C., Maresi, E., Di Prima, L., Soresi, M., Di Gesù, G., Noto, D., & Carroccio, A. (2006). Food intolerance and chronic constipation: Manometry and histology study. European Journal of Gastroenterology & Hepatology, 18(2), 143–150. https://doi.org/10.1097/00042737-200602000-00006

Ilich, J. Z., Kelly, O. J., Liu, P.-Y., Shin, H., Kim, Y., Chi, Y., Wickrama, K. K. A. S., & Colic-Baric, I. (2019). Role of Calcium and Low-Fat Dairy Foods in Weight-Loss Outcomes Revisited: Results from the Randomized Trial of Effects on Bone and Body Composition in Overweight/Obese Postmenopausal Women. Nutrients, 11(5), E1157. https://doi.org/10.3390/nu11051157

Institute of Medicine. (1998). Dietary Reference Intakes for Thiamin, Riboflavin, Niacin, Vitamin B6, Folate, Vitamin B12, Pantothenic Acid, Biotin, and Choline. In Dietary Reference Intakes for Thiamin, Riboflavin, Niacin, Vitamin B6, Folate, Vitamin B12, Pantothenic Acid, Biotin, and Choline. National Academies Press (US). https://www.ncbi.nlm.nih.gov/books/NBK114318/

Institute of Medicine. (2005). Dietary Reference Intakes for Water, Potassium, Chloride, and Sulfate. National Academies Press.

Institute of Medicine. (2010). Dietary Reference Intakes for Calcium and Vitamin D. National Academies Press.

International Dairy Foods Association. (2021, September 30). U.S. Dairy Consumption Beats Expectations in 2020 and Continues to Surge Upward Despite Disruption Caused by Pandemic. IDFA. https://www.idfa.org/news/u-s-dairy-consumption-beats-expectations-in-2020-and-continues-to-surge-upward-despite-disruption-caused-by-pandemic

International Dairy Foods Association. (2022). IDFA. https://www.idfa.org/news/international-dairy-foods-association

Irastorza, I., Ibañez, B., Delgado-Sanzonetti, L., Maruri, N., & Vitoria, J. C. (2010). Cow's-milk-free diet as a therapeutic option in childhood chronic constipation. Journal of Pediatric Gastroenterology and Nutrition, 51(2), 171–176. https://doi.org/10.1097/MPG.0b013e3181cd2653

Iuliano, S., Poon, S., Robbins, J., Bui, M., Wang, X., Groot, L. D., Loan, M. V., Zadeh, A. G., Nguyen, T., & Seeman, E. (2021). Effect of dietary sources of calcium and protein on hip fractures and falls in older adults in residential care: Cluster randomised controlled trial. BMJ, 375, n2364. https://doi.org/10.1136/bmj.n2364

Jakubczyk, D., Leszczyńska, K., & Górska, S. (2020). The Effectiveness of Probiotics in the Treatment of Inflammatory Bowel Disease (IBD)-A Critical Review. Nutrients, 12(7), E1973. https://doi.org/10.3390/nu12071973

Jenssen, H., & Hancock, R. E. W. (2009). Antimicrobial properties of lactoferrin. Biochimie, 91(1), 19–29. https://doi.org/10.1016/j.biochi.2008.05.015

Jianqin, S., Leiming, X., Lu, X., Yelland, G. W., Ni, J., & Clarke, A. J. (2016). Effects of milk containing only A2 beta casein versus milk containing both A1 and A2 beta casein proteins on gastrointestinal physiology, symptoms of discomfort, and cognitive behavior of people with self-reported intolerance to traditional cows' milk. Nutrition Journal, 15, 35. https://doi.org/10.1186/s12937-016-0147-z

Johansson, I., & Lif Holgerson, P. (2011). Milk and oral health. Nestle Nutrition Workshop Series. Paediatric Programme, 67, 55–66. https://doi.org/10.1159/000325575

Jones, G. (2014). Vitamin D. In A. Ross, B. Caballero, R. Cousins, K. Tucker, & T. Ziegler (Eds.), Modern Nutrition in Health and Disease (11th ed.). Lippincott Williams & Wilkins.

Jung, T.-H., Hwang, H.-J., Yun, S.-S., Lee, W.-J., Kim, J.-W., Ahn, J.-Y., Jeon, W.-M., & Han, K.-S. (2017). Hypoallergenic and Physicochemical Properties of the A2 β-Casein Fractionof Goat Milk. Korean Journal for Food Science of Animal Resources, 37(6), 940–947. https://doi.org/10.5851/kosfa.2017.37.6.940

Kazemi, A., Noorbala, A. A., Azam, K., Eskandari, M. H., & Djafarian, K. (2019). Effect of probiotic and prebiotic vs placebo on psychological outcomes in patients with major depressive disorder: A randomized clinical trial. Clinical Nutrition (Edinburgh, Scotland), 38(2), 522–528. https://doi.org/10.1016/j.clnu.2018.04.010

Kim, Y., & Je, Y. (2016). Dairy consumption and risk of metabolic syndrome: A meta-analysis. Diabetic Medicine: A Journal of the British Diabetic Association, 33(4), 428–440. https://doi.org/10.1111/dme.12970

Kratz, M., Marcovina, S., Nelson, J. E., Yeh, M. M., Kowdley, K. V., Callahan, H. S., Song, X., Di, C., & Utzschneider, K. M. (2014). Dairy fat intake is associated with glucose tolerance, hepatic and systemic insulin sensitivity, and liver fat but not β-cell function in humans. The American Journal of Clinical Nutrition, 99(6), 1385–1396. https://doi.org/10.3945/ajcn.113.075457

Lana, A., Rodriguez-Artalejo, F., & Lopez-Garcia, E. (2015). Dairy Consumption and Risk of Frailty in Older Adults: A Prospective Cohort Study. Journal of the American Geriatrics Society, 63(9), 1852–1860. https://doi.org/10.1111/jgs.13626

Le Louer, B., Lemale, J., Garcette, K., Orzechowski, C., Chalvon, A., Girardet, J.-P., & Tounian, P. (2014). [Severe nutritional deficiencies in young infants with inappropriate plant milk consumption]. Archives De Pediatrie: Organe Officiel De La Societe Francaise De Pediatrie, 21(5), 483–488. https://doi.org/10.1016/j.arcped.2014.02.027

Lee, J., Fu, Z., Chung, M., Jang, D.-J., & Lee, H.-J. (2018). Role of milk and dairy intake in cognitive function in older adults: A systematic review and meta-analysis. Nutrition Journal, 17(1), 82. https://doi.org/10.1186/s12937-018-0387-1

Li, E. W. Y., & Mine, Y. (2004). Immunoenhancing effects of bovine glycomacropeptide and its derivatives on the proliferative response and phagocytic activities of human macrophagelike cells, U937. Journal of Agricultural and Food Chemistry, 52(9), 2704–2708. https://doi.org/10.1021/jf0355102

Liang, J., Zhou, Q., Kwame Amakye, W., Su, Y., & Zhang, Z. (2018). Biomarkers of dairy fat intake and risk of cardiovascular disease: A systematic review and meta analysis of prospective studies. Critical Reviews in Food Science and Nutrition, 58(7), 1122–1130. https://doi.org/10.1080/10408398.2016.1242114

Lighter Béchamel | Cook's Illustrated. (n.d.). Retrieved February 18, 2022, from http://www.cooksillustrated.com/how_tos/5627-lighter-bechamel

Lomer, M. C. E., Parkes, G. C., & Sanderson, J. D. (2008). Review article: Lactose intolerance in clinical practice--myths and realities. Alimentary Pharmacology & Therapeutics, 27(2), 93–103. https://doi.org/10.1111/j.1365-2036.2007.03557.x

Lovegrove, J. A., & Hobbs, D. A. (2016). New perspectives on dairy and cardiovascular health. The Proceedings of the Nutrition Society, 75(3), 247–258. https://doi.org/10.1017/S002966511600001X

Low, P. P. L., Rutherfurd, K. J., Cross, M. L., & Gill, H. S. (2001). Enhancement of Mucosal Antibody Responses by Dietary Whey Protein Concentrate. Food and Agricultural Immunology, 13(4), 255–264. https://doi.org/10.1080/09540100120094519

Luhovyy, B. L., Akhavan, T., & Anderson, G. H. (2007). Whey proteins in the regulation of food intake and satiety. Journal of the American College of Nutrition, 26(6), 704S-12S. https://doi.org/10.1080/07315724.2007.10719651

MacDonald, R. S., Thornton, W. H., & Marshall, R. T. (1994). A cell culture model to identify biologically active peptides generated by bacterial hydrolysis of casein. Journal of Dairy Science, 77(5), 1167–1175. https://doi.org/10.3168/jds.S0022-0302(94)77054-5

Manzi, P., Di Costanzo, M. G., & Mattera, M. (2013). Updating Nutritional Data and Evaluation of Technological Parameters of Italian Milk. Foods (Basel, Switzerland), 2(2), 254–273. https://doi.org/10.3390/foods2020254

Manzocchi, E., Martin, B., Bord, C., Verdier-Metz, I., Bouchon, M., De Marchi, M., Constant, I., Giller, K., Kreuzer, M., Berard, J., Musci, M., & Coppa, M. (2021). Feeding cows with hay, silage, or fresh herbage on pasture or indoors affects sensory properties and chemical composition of milk and cheese. Journal of Dairy Science, 104(5), 5285–5302. https://doi.org/10.3168/jds.2020-19738

Marabujo, T., Ramos, E., & Lopes, C. (2018). Dairy products and total calcium intake at 13 years of age and its association with obesity at 21 years of age. European Journal of Clinical Nutrition, 72(4), 541–547. https://doi.org/10.1038/s41430-017-0082-x

Marangoni, F., Pellegrino, L., Verduci, E., Ghiselli, A., Bernabei, R., Calvani, R., Cetin, I., Giampietro, M., Perticone, F., Piretta, L., Giacco, R., La Vecchia, C., Brandi, M. L., Ballardini, D., Banderali, G., Bellentani, S., Canzone, G., Cricelli, C., Faggiano, P., ... Poli, A. (2019). Cow's Milk Consumption and Health: A Health Professional's Guide. Journal of the American College of Nutrition, 38(3), 197–208. https://doi.org/10.1080/07315724.2018.1491016

Marco, M. L., Heeney, D., Binda, S., Cifelli, C. J., Cotter, P. D., Foligné, B., Gänzle, M., Kort, R., Pasin, G., Pihlanto, A., Smid, E. J., & Hutkins, R. (2017). Health benefits of fermented foods: Microbiota and beyond. Current Opinion in Biotechnology, 44, 94–102. https://doi.org/10.1016/j.copbio.2016.11.010

Mathai, J. K., Liu, Y., & Stein, H. H. (2017). Values for digestible indispensable amino acid scores (DIAAS) for some dairy and plant proteins may better describe protein quality than values calculated using the concept for protein digestibility-corrected amino acid scores (PDCAAS). The British Journal of Nutrition, 117(4), 490–499. https://doi.org/10.1017/S0007114517000125

McBean, L. D., & Miller, G. D. (1998). Allaying fears and fallacies about lactose intolerance. Journal of the American Dietetic Association, 98(6), 671–676. https://doi.org/10.1016/S0002-8223(98)00152-7

McGee, H. (2004). On Food and Cooking: The Science and Lore of the Kitchen (1st edition). Scribner Books.

McGregor, R. A., & Poppitt, S. D. (2013). Milk protein for improved metabolic health: A review of the evidence. Nutrition & Metabolism, 10(1), 46. https://doi.org/10.1186/1743-7075-10-46

McKim et al. (2019). Clarifying the confusion between poligeenan, degraded carrageenan, and carrageenan: A review of the chemistry, nomenclature, and in vivo toxicology by the oral route. 59(19), 3054–3073.

Meharg, A. A., Deacon, C., Campbell, R. C. J., Carey, A.-M., Williams, P. N., Feldmann, J., & Raab, A. (2008). Inorganic arsenic levels in rice milk exceed EU and US drinking water standards. Journal of Environmental Monitoring: JEM, 10(4), 428–431. https://doi.org/10.1039/b800981c

Meinertz, H., Nilausen, K., & Faergeman, O. (1989). Soy protein and casein in cholesterol-enriched diets: Effects on plasma lipoproteins in normolipidemic subjects. The American Journal of Clinical Nutrition, 50(4), 786–793. https://doi.org/10.1093/ajcn/50.4.786

Mekonnen, M. M., & Hoekstra, A. Y. (2010). The Green, Blue and Grey Water Footprint of Crops and Derived Crop Products, Value of Water Research Report Series No. 47. UNESCO-IHE. https://waterfootprint.org/media/downloads/Report47-WaterFootprintCrops-Vol2.pdf

Meltzer Warren, R. (2019, September 25). Are Plant Milks Good for You? Consumer Reports. https://www.consumerreports.org/plant-milk/are-plant-milks-more-healthful-than-cows-milk/

Mena-Sánchez, G., Becerra-Tomás, N., Babio, N., & Salas-Salvadó, J. (2019). Dairy Product Consumption in the Prevention of Metabolic Syndrome: A Systematic Review and Meta-Analysis of Prospective Cohort Studies. Advances in Nutrition (Bethesda, Md.), 10(suppl_2), S144–S153. https://doi.org/10.1093/advances/nmy083

Merritt, R. J., Fleet, S. E., Fifi, A., Jump, C., Schwartz, S., Sentongo, T., Duro, D., Rudolph, J., Turner, J., & NASPGHAN Committee on Nutrition. (2020). North American Society for Pediatric Gastroenterology, Hepatology, and Nutrition Position Paper: Plant-based Milks. Journal of Pediatric Gastroenterology and Nutrition, 71(2), 276–281. https://doi.org/10.1097/MPG.0000000000002799

Milk Safety | Dairy Health Benefits. (n.d.). The Dairy Alliance. Retrieved April 9, 2022, from https://thedairyalliance.com/dairy-farming/milk-safety/

Miller, G. D., Jarvis, J. K., & McBean, L. D. (2006). Handbook of Dairy Foods and Nutrition (3rd ed.). CRC Press.

Miller, J., & Rucker, R. (2012). Pantothenic acid. In J. Erdman, I. MacDonald, & S. Zeisel (Eds.), Present Knowledge in Nutrition (10th ed., pp. 375–390). Wiley-Blackwell.

Mills, S., Ross, R. P., Hill, C., Fitzgerald, G. F., & Stanton, C. (2011). Milk intelligence: Mining milk for bioactive substances associated with human health. International Dairy Journal, 21(6), 377–401. https://doi.org/10.1016/j.idairyj.2010.12.011

Misselwitz, B., Butter, M., Verbeke, K., & Fox, M. R. (2019). Update on lactose malabsorption and intolerance: Pathogenesis, diagnosis and clinical management. Gut, 68(11), 2080–2091. https://doi.org/10.1136/gutjnl-2019-318404

Mitri, J., Mohd Yusof, B.-N., Maryniuk, M., Schrager, C., Hamdy, O., & Salsberg, V. (2019). Dairy intake and type 2 diabetes risk factors: A narrative review. Diabetes & Metabolic Syndrome, 13(5), 2879–2887. https://doi.org/10.1016/j.dsx.2019.07.064

Mozaffarian, D. (2019). Dairy Foods, Obesity, and Metabolic Health: The Role of the Food Matrix Compared with Single Nutrients. Advances in Nutrition (Bethesda, Md.), 10(5), 917S–923S. https://doi.org/10.1093/advances/nmz053

Mozaffarian, D., Hao, T., Rimm, E. B., Willett, W. C., & Hu, F. B. (2011). Changes in diet and lifestyle and long-term weight gain in women and men. The New England Journal of Medicine, 364(25), 2392–2404. https://doi.org/10.1056/NEJMoa1014296

Mueller, N. T., Odegaard, A. O., Gross, M. D., Koh, W.-P., Yu, M. C., Yuan, J.-M., & Pereira, M. A. (2012). Soy intake and risk of type 2 diabetes in Chinese Singaporeans [corrected]. European Journal of Nutrition, 51(8), 1033–1040. https://doi.org/10.1007/s00394-011-0276-2

Nappo, A., Sparano, S., Intemann, T., Kourides, Y. A., Lissner, L., Molnar, D., Moreno, L. A., Pala, V., Sioen, I., Veidebaum, T., Wolters, M., Siani, A., & Russo, P. (2019). Dietary calcium intake and adiposity in children and adolescents: Cross-sectional and longitudinal results from IDEFICS/I.Family cohort. Nutrition, Metabolism, and Cardiovascular Diseases: NMCD, 29(5), 440–449. https://doi.org/10.1016/j.numecd.2019.01.015

National Dairy Council. (2022). https://www.usdairy.com/about-us/national-dairy-council

National Institute of Health, Office of Dietary Supplements. (2020a, March 20). Vitamin B12 Health Professional Sheet. https://ods.od.nih.gov/factsheets/VitaminB12-HealthProfessional/

National Institute of Health, Office of Dietary Supplements. (2020b, March 24). Vitamin D Health Professional Sheet. https://ods.od.nih.gov/factsheets/VitaminD-HealthProfessional/

National Institutes of Health Office of Dietary Supplements. (n.d.). Vitamin and Mineral Supplement Fact Sheets. Retrieved March 28, 2020, from https://ods.od.nih.gov/factsheets/list-VitaminsMinerals/

New Zealand Commerce Commission. (2003, November 21). Advertising of A2 milk changes following Commerce Commission warning. Commerce Commission. https://comcom.govt.nz/news-and-media/media-releases/archive/advertising-of-a2-milk-changes-following-commerce-commission-warning

Nguyen, C. T., Pham, N. M., Do, V. V., Binns, C. W., Hoang, V. M., Dang, D. A., & Lee, A. H. (2017). Soyfood and isoflavone intake and risk of type 2 diabetes in Vietnamese adults. European Journal of Clinical Nutrition, 71(10), 1186–1192. https://doi.org/10.1038/ejcn.2017.76

Nordmann, A. J., Suter-Zimmermann, K., Bucher, H. C., Shai, I., Tuttle, K. R., Estruch, R., & Briel, M. (2011). Meta-analysis comparing Mediterranean to low-fat diets for modification of cardiovascular risk factors. The American Journal of Medicine, 124(9), 841-851.e2. https://doi.org/10.1016/j.amjmed.2011.04.024

Norman, A. (2012). Vitamin D. In H. Henry, J. Erdman, I. MacDonald, & S. Zeisel (Eds.), Present Knowledge in Nutrition (10th ed.). Wiley-Blackwell.

O'Brien, K. V., Stewart, L. K., Forney, L. A., Aryana, K. J., Prinyawiwatkul, W., & Boeneke, C. A. (2015). The effects of postexercise consumption of a kefir beverage on performance and recovery during intensive endurance training. Journal of Dairy Science, 98(11), 7446–7449. https://doi.org/10.3168/jds.2015-9392

O'Hagan, M. (2019, June 19). From Two Bulls, 9 Million Dairy Cows. Undark Magazine.

Olive Oil Béchamel Recipe. (n.d.). NYT Cooking. Retrieved February 18, 2022, from https://cooking.nytimes.com/recipes/1017372-olive-oil-bechamel

Oliver, S. P., Murinda, S. E., & Jayarao, B. M. (2011). Impact of Antibiotic Use in Adult Dairy Cows on Antimicrobial Resistance of Veterinary and Human Pathogens: A Comprehensive Review. Foodborne Pathogens and Disease, 8(3). https://doi.org/10.1089/fpd.2010.0730

Onning, G., Akesson, B., Oste, R., & Lundquist, I. (1998). Effects of consumption of oat milk, soya milk, or cow's milk on plasma lipids and antioxidative capacity in healthy subjects. Annals of Nutrition & Metabolism, 42(4), 211–220. https://doi.org/10.1159/000012736

Onning, G., Wallmark, A., Persson, M., Akesson, B., Elmståhl, S., & Oste, R. (1999). Consumption of oat milk for 5 weeks lowers serum cholesterol and LDL cholesterol in free-living men with moderate hypercholesterolemia. Annals of Nutrition & Metabolism, 43(5), 301–309. https://doi.org/10.1159/000012798

Onwulata, C. I., & Huth, P. J. (Eds.). (2008). Whey Processing, Functionality and Health Benefits (1st ed.). John Wiley & Sons, Inc.

Otani, H., Kihara, Y., & Park, M. (2000). The Immunoenhancing Property of a Dietary Casein Phosphopeptide Preparation in Mice. Food and Agricultural Immunology, 12(2), 165–173.

Pacheco, Y. M., López, S., Bermúdez, B., Abia, R., Villar, J., & Muriana, F. J. G. (2008). A meal rich in oleic acid beneficially modulates postprandial sICAM-1 and sVCAM-1 in normotensive and hypertensive hypertriglyceridemic subjects. The Journal of Nutritional Biochemistry, 19(3), 200–205. https://doi.org/10.1016/j.jnutbio.2007.03.002

Parodi, P. W. (2007). A role for milk proteins and their peptides in cancer prevention. Current Pharmaceutical Design, 13(8), 813–828. https://doi.org/10.2174/138161207780363059

Parrish, C. R. (2018). Moo-ove Over, Cow's Milk: The Rise of Plant-Based Dairy Alternatives. PRACTICAL GASTROENTEROLOGY, 7.

Payette, C., Blackburn, P., Lamarche, B., Tremblay, A., Bergeron, J., Lemieux, I., Després, J.-P., & Couillard, C. (2009). Sex differences in postprandial plasma tumor necrosis factor-alpha, interleukin-6, and C-reactive protein concentrations. Metabolism: Clinical and Experimental, 58(11), 1593–1601. https://doi.org/10.1016/j.metabol.2009.05.011

Pei, R., DiMarco, D. M., Putt, K. K., Martin, D. A., Gu, Q., Chitchumroonchokchai, C., White, H. M., Scarlett, C. O., Bruno, R. S., & Bolling, B. W. (2017). Low-fat yogurt consumption reduces biomarkers of chronic inflammation and inhibits markers of endotoxin exposure in healthy premenopausal women: A randomised controlled trial. The British Journal of Nutrition, 118(12), 1043–1051. https://doi.org/10.1017/S0007114517003038

Penberthy, W., & Kirkland, J. (2012). Niacin. In J. Erdman, I. MacDonald, & S. Zeisel (Eds.), Present Knowledge in Nutrition (10th ed., pp. 293–306). Wiley-Blackwell.

Pepe, J., Colangelo, L., Biamonte, F., Sonato, C., Danese, V. C., Cecchetti, V., Occhiuto, M., Piazzolla, V., De Martino, V., Ferrone, F., Minisola, S., & Cipriani, C. (2020). Diagnosis and management of hypocalcemia. Endocrine, 69(3), 485–495. https://doi.org/10.1007/s12020-020-02324-2

Perdijk, O., Splunter, M. van, Savelkoul, H. F. J., Brugman, S., & Neerven, R. J. J. van. (2018). Cow's Milk and Immune Function in the Respiratory Tract: Potential Mechanisms. Frontiers in Immunology, 9. https://doi.org/10.3389/fimmu.2018.00143

Pereira, P. C. (2014). Milk nutritional composition and its role in human health. Nutrition (Burbank, Los Angeles County, Calif.), 30(6), 619–627. https://doi.org/10.1016/j.nut.2013.10.011

Pessi, T., Isolauri, E., Sütas, Y., Kankaanranta, H., Moilanen, E., & Hurme, M. (2001). Suppression of T-cell activation by Lactobacillus rhamnosus GG-degraded bovine casein. International Immunopharmacology, 1(2), 211–218. https://doi.org/10.1016/s1567-5769(00)00018-7

Planet Oat. (2022). https://planetoat.com/

Poore, J., & Nemecek, T. (2018). Reducing food's environmental impacts through producers and consumers. Science, 360(6392), 987–992. https://doi.org/10.1126/science.aaq0216

Poppitt, S. D., Keogh, G. F., Lithander, F. E., Wang, Y., Mulvey, T. B., Chan, Y.-K., McArdle, B. H., & Cooper, G. J. S. (2008). Postprandial response of adiponectin, interleukin-6, tumor necrosis factor-alpha, and C-reactive protein to a high-fat dietary load. Nutrition (Burbank, Los Angeles County, Calif.), 24(4), 322–329. https://doi.org/10.1016/j.nut.2007.12.012

Rautiainen, S., Wang, L., Lee, I.-M., Manson, J. E., Buring, J. E., & Sesso, H. D. (2016). Dairy consumption in association with weight change and risk of becoming overweight or obese in middle-aged and older women: A prospective cohort study. The American Journal of Clinical Nutrition, 103(4), 979–988. https://doi.org/10.3945/ajcn.115.118406

Raziani, F., Tholstrup, T., Kristensen, M. D., Svanegaard, M. L., Ritz, C., Astrup, A., & Raben, A. (2016). High intake of regular-fat cheese compared with reduced-fat cheese does not affect LDL cholesterol or risk markers of the metabolic syndrome: A randomized controlled trial. The American Journal of Clinical Nutrition, 104(4), 973–981. https://doi.org/10.3945/ajcn.116.134932

Requena, P., Daddaoua, A., Guadix, E., Zarzuelo, A., Suárez, M. D., Sánchez de Medina, F., & Martínez-Augustin, O. (2009). Bovine glycomacropeptide induces cytokine production in human monocytes through the stimulation of the MAPK and the NF-kappaB signal transduction pathways. British Journal of Pharmacology, 157(7), 1232–1240. https://doi.org/10.1111/j.1476-5381.2009.00195.x

Reyes-Garcia, R., Mendoza, N., Palacios, S., Salas, N., Quesada-Charneco, M., Garcia-Martin, A., Fonolla, J., Lara-Villoslada, F., & Muñoz-Torres, M. (2018). Effects of Daily Intake of Calcium and Vitamin D-Enriched Milk in Healthy Postmenopausal Women: A Randomized, Controlled, Double-Blind Nutritional Study. Journal of Women's Health (2002), 27(5), 561–568. https://doi.org/10.1089/jwh.2017.6655

Rideout, T. C., Marinangeli, C. P. F., Martin, H., Browne, R. W., & Rempel, C. B. (2013). Consumption of low-fat dairy foods for 6 months improves insulin resistance without adversely affecting lipids or bodyweight in healthy adults: A randomized free-living cross-over study. Nutrition Journal, 12, 56. https://doi.org/10.1186/1475-2891-12-56

Ripple Foods. (2022). https://www.ripplefoods.com/

Rivlin, R. (2010). Riboflavin. In P. Coates, J. Betz, & M. Blackman (Eds.), Encyclopedia of Dietary Supplements (2nd ed., pp. 691–699). Informa Healthcare.

Rosa, D. D., Dias, M. M. S., Grześkowiak, Ł. M., Reis, S. A., Conceição, L. L., & Peluzio, M. do C. G. (2017). Milk kefir: Nutritional, microbiological and health benefits. Nutrition Research Reviews, 30(1), 82–96. https://doi.org/10.1017/S0954422416000275

Ross, A. (2006). Vitamin A and Carotenoids. In M. Shils, M. Shike, A. Ross, B. Caballero, & R. Cousins (Eds.), Modern Nutrition in Health and Disease (10th ed., pp. 351–375). Lippincott Williams & Wilkins.

Ross, C. (2010). Vitamin A. In P. Coates, J. Betz, & M. Blackman (Eds.), Encyclopedia of Dietary Supplements (2nd ed., pp. 778–791). Informa Healthcare.

Rotz, C. A. (2018). Modeling greenhouse gas emissions from dairy farms. Journal of Dairy Science, 101(7), 6675–6690. https://doi.org/10.3168/jds.2017-13272

Sacks, F. M., Lichtenstein, A. H., Wu, J. H. Y., Appel, L. J., Creager, M. A., Kris-Etherton, P. M., Miller, M., Rimm, E. B., Rudel, L. L., Robinson, J. G., Stone, N. J., & Van Horn, L. V. (2017). Dietary Fats and Cardiovascular Disease: A Presidential Advisory From the American Heart Association. Circulation, 136(3), e1–e23. https://doi.org/10.1161/CIR.0000000000000510

Sánchez, B., Delgado, S., Blanco-Míguez, A., Lourenço, A., Gueimonde, M., & Margolles, A. (2017). Probiotics, gut microbiota, and their influence on host health and disease. Molecular Nutrition & Food Research, 61(1). https://doi.org/10.1002/mnfr.201600240

Savage, J., Sicherer, S., & Wood, R. (2016). The Natural History of Food Allergy. The Journal of Allergy and Clinical Immunology. In Practice, 4(2), 196–203; quiz 204. https://doi.org/10.1016/j.jaip.2015.11.024

Scholz-Ahrens, K. E., Ahrens, F., & Barth, C. A. (2020). Nutritional and health attributes of milk and milk imitations. European Journal of Nutrition, 59(1), 19–34. https://doi.org/10.1007/s00394-019-01936-3

Schönfeld, P., & Wojtczak, L. (2016). Short- and medium-chain fatty acids in energy metabolism: The cellular perspective. Journal of Lipid Research, 57(6), 943–954. https://doi.org/10.1194/jlr.R067629

Schuster, M., Wang, X., Hawkins, T., & Painter, J. (2018). Comparison of the Nutrient Content of Cow's Milk and Nondairy Milk Alternatives. Nutrition Today, 53(4), 153–159.

Schwingshackl, L., Hoffmann, G., Lampousi, A.-M., Knüppel, S., Iqbal, K., Schwedhelm, C., Bechthold, A., Schlesinger, S., & Boeing, H. (2017). Food groups and risk of type 2 diabetes mellitus: A systematic review and meta-analysis of prospective studies. European Journal of Epidemiology, 32(5), 363–375. https://doi.org/10.1007/s10654-017-0246-y

Schwingshackl, L., Schwedhelm, C., Hoffmann, G., Knüppel, S., Laure Preterre, A., Iqbal, K., Bechthold, A., De Henauw, S., Michels, N., Devleesschauwer, B., Boeing, H., & Schlesinger, S. (2018). Food groups and risk of colorectal cancer. International Journal of Cancer, 142(9), 1748–1758. https://doi.org/10.1002/ijc.31198

Sebastian, R., Goldman, J., Cecilia Wilkinson Enns, & LaComb, R. (2010). Fluid Milk Consumption in the United States: What We Eat in America, NHANES 2005-2006. Food Surveys Research Group Dietary Data Brief, 3, 8.

Sethi, S., Tyagi, S. K., & Anurag, R. K. (2016). Plant-based milk alternatives an emerging segment of functional beverages: A review. Journal of Food Science and Technology, 53(9), 3408–3423. https://doi.org/10.1007/s13197-016-2328-3

Shannon, R., & Rodriguez, J. M. (2014). Total arsenic in rice milk. Food Additives & Contaminants: Part B, 7(1), 54–56. https://doi.org/10.1080/19393210.2013.842941

Silk. (2022). Silk. https://silk.com/

Simeone, D., Miele, E., Boccia, G., Marino, A., Troncone, R., & Staiano, A. (2008). Prevalence of atopy in children with chronic constipation. Archives of Disease in Childhood, 93(12), 1044–1047. https://doi.org/10.1136/adc.2007.133512

Singh, G. M., Micha, R., Khatibzadeh, S., Shi, P., Lim, S., Andrews, K. G., Engell, R. E., Ezzati, M., Mozaffarian, D., & Group (NutriCoDE), G. B. of D. N. and C. D. E. (2015). Global, Regional, and National Consumption of Sugar-Sweetened Beverages, Fruit Juices, and Milk: A Systematic Assessment of Beverage Intake in 187 Countries. PLOS ONE, 10(8), e0124845. https://doi.org/10.1371/journal.pone.0124845

Singhal, S., Baker, R. D., & Baker, S. S. (2017). A Comparison of the Nutritional Value of Cow's Milk and Nondairy Beverages. Journal of Pediatric Gastroenterology and Nutrition, 64(5), 799–805. https://doi.org/10.1097/MPG.0000000000001380

Siri-Tarino, P. W., Chiu, S., Bergeron, N., & Krauss, R. M. (2015). Saturated Fats Versus Polyunsaturated Fats Versus Carbohydrates for Cardiovascular Disease Prevention and Treatment. Annual Review of Nutrition, 35, 517–543. https://doi.org/10.1146/annurev-nutr-071714-034449

Slykerman, R. F., Hood, F., Wickens, K., Thompson, J. M. D., Barthow, C., Murphy, R., Kang, J., Rowden, J., Stone, P., Crane, J., Stanley, T., Abels, P., Purdie, G., Maude, R., Mitchell, E. A., & Probiotic in Pregnancy Study Group. (2017). Effect of Lactobacillus rhamnosus HN001 in Pregnancy on Postpartum Symptoms of Depression and Anxiety: A Randomised Double-blind Placebo-controlled Trial. EBioMedicine, 24, 159–165. https://doi.org/10.1016/j.ebiom.2017.09.013

So Delicious Dairy Free. (2022). So Delicious Dairy Free. https://sodeliciousdairyfree.com/

Soedamah-Muthu, S. S., Ding, E. L., Al-Delaimy, W. K., Hu, F. B., Engberink, M. F., Willett, W. C., & Geleijnse, J. M. (2011). Milk and dairy consumption and incidence of cardiovascular diseases and all-cause mortality: Dose-response meta-analysis of prospective cohort studies. The American Journal of Clinical Nutrition, 93(1), 158–171. https://doi.org/10.3945/ajcn.2010.29866

Soerensen, K. V., Thorning, T. K., Astrup, A., Kristensen, M., & Lorenzen, J. K. (2014). Effect of dairy calcium from cheese and milk on fecal fat excretion, blood lipids, and appetite in young men. The American Journal of Clinical Nutrition, 99(5), 984–991. https://doi.org/10.3945/ajcn.113.077735

Solomons, N. (2006). Vitamin A. In B. Bowman & R. Russell (Eds.), Present Knowledge in Nutrition (9th ed., pp. 157–183). International Life Sciences Institute.

Song, L. (2017). Calcium and Bone Metabolism Indices. Advances in Clinical Chemistry, 82, 1–46. https://doi.org/10.1016/bs.acc.2017.06.005

Stancliffe, R. A., Thorpe, T., & Zemel, M. B. (2011). Dairy attenuates oxidative and inflammatory stress in metabolic syndrome. The American Journal of Clinical Nutrition, 94(2), 422–430. https://doi.org/10.3945/ajcn.111.013342

Stone, M. S., Martyn, L., & Weaver, C. M. (2016). Potassium Intake, Bioavailability, Hypertension, and Glucose Control. Nutrients, 8(7), E444. https://doi.org/10.3390/nu8070444

Suchy, F. J., Brannon, P. M., Carpenter, T. O., Fernandez, J. R., Gilsanz, V., Gould, J. B., Hall, K., Hui, S. L., Lupton, J., Mennella, J., Miller, N. J., Osganian, S. K., Sellmeyer, D. E., & Wolf, M. A. (2010). NIH consensus development conference statement: Lactose intolerance and health. NIH Consensus and State-of-the-Science Statements, 27(2), 1–27.

Sweetman, L. (2010). Pantothenic acid. In P. Coates, J. Betz, M. Blackman, G. Cragg, M. Levine, J. Moss, & J. White (Eds.), Encyclopedia of Dietary Supplements (2nd ed., pp. 604–611). Informa Healthcare.

Timon, C. M., O'Connor, A., Bhargava, N., Gibney, E. R., & Feeney, E. L. (2020). Dairy Consumption and Metabolic Health. Nutrients, 12(10), E3040. https://doi.org/10.3390/nu12103040

Tong, X., Dong, J.-Y., Wu, Z.-W., Li, W., & Qin, L.-Q. (2011). Dairy consumption and risk of type 2 diabetes mellitus: A meta-analysis of cohort studies. European Journal of Clinical Nutrition, 65(9), 1027–1031. https://doi.org/10.1038/ejcn.2011.62

Torres-Gonzalez, M., Cifelli, C. J., Agarwal, S., Fulgoni, V. L., & III. (2020). Association of Milk Consumption and Vitamin D Status in the US Population by Ethnicity: NHANES 2001–2010 Analysis. Nutrients, 12(12). https://doi.org/10.3390/nu12123720

Tripkovic, L., Lambert, H., Hart, K., Smith, C. P., Bucca, G., Penson, S., Chope, G., Hyppönen, E., Berry, J., Vieth, R., & Lanham-New, S. (2012). Comparison of vitamin D2 and vitamin D3 supplementation in raising serum 25-hydroxyvitamin D status: A systematic review and meta-analysis. The American Journal of Clinical Nutrition, 95(6), 1357–1364. https://doi.org/10.3945/ajcn.111.031070

Tucker, K. L., Rich, S., Rosenberg, I., Jacques, P., Dallal, G., Wilson, P. W., & Selhub, J. (2000). Plasma vitamin B-12 concentrations relate to intake source in the Framingham Offspring study. The American Journal of Clinical Nutrition, 71(2), 514–522. https://doi.org/10.1093/ajcn/71.2.514

Turkmen, N. (2017). Chapter 35—The Nutritional Value and Health Benefits of Goat Milk Components. In R. R. Watson, R. J. Collier, & V. R. Preedy (Eds.), Nutrients in Dairy and their Implications on Health and Disease (pp. 441–449). Academic Press. https://doi.org/10.1016/B978-0-12-809762-5.00035-8

Ulven, S. M., Holven, K. B., Gil, A., & Rangel-Huerta, O. D. (2019). Milk and Dairy Product Consumption and Inflammatory Biomarkers: An Updated Systematic Review of Randomized Clinical Trials. Advances in Nutrition (Bethesda, Md.), 10(suppl_2), S239–S250. https://doi.org/10.1093/advances/nmy072

Unger, A. L., Torres-Gonzalez, M., & Kraft, J. (2019). Dairy Fat Consumption and the Risk of Metabolic Syndrome: An Examination of the Saturated Fatty Acids in Dairy. Nutrients, 11(9), E2200. https://doi.org/10.3390/nu11092200

U.S. Department of Agriculture and U.S. Department of Health and Human Services. (2020). Dietary Guidelines for Americans, 2020-2025 (9th Edition; p. 164).

US Environmental Protection Agency. (n.d.). Ag 101: Dairy Production: Lifecycle production phases. EPA, 424.

U.S. Food and Drug Administration. (2016). Arsenic in Rice and Rice Products Risk Assessment Report. https://www.fda.gov/media/96071/download

US Food and Drug Administration. (2021, April 13). Bovine Somatotropin (bST). FDA; FDA. https://www.fda.gov/animal-veterinary/product-safety-information/bovine-somatotropin-bst

US Preventive Services Task Force, Grossman, D. C., Curry, S. J., Owens, D. K., Barry, M. J., Caughey, A. B., Davidson, K. W., Doubeni, C. A., Epling, J. W., Kemper, A. R., Krist, A. H., Kubik, M., Landefeld, S., Mangione, C. M., Silverstein, M., Simon, M. A., & Tseng, C.-W. (2018). Vitamin D, Calcium, or Combined Supplementation for the Primary Prevention of Fractures in Community-Dwelling Adults: US Preventive Services Task Force Recommendation Statement. JAMA, 319(15), 1592–1599. https://doi.org/10.1001/jama.2018.3185

USDA. (2018). FoodData Central. FoodData Central | U.S. Department of Agriculture, Agricultural Research Service. https://fdc.nal.usda.gov/

USDA Foreign Agricultural Service. (n.d.). Tree Nuts: World Markets and Trade. USDA Foreign Agricultural Service. Retrieved February 6, 2022, from https://www.fas.usda.gov/data/tree-nuts-world-markets-and-trade

USDA Natural Resources Conservation Service, Grazing Lands Technology Institute. (1996). Dairy Farmer Profitability Using Intensive Rotational Stocking: Better grazing management for pastures. USDA. https://www.nrcs.usda.gov/wps/PA_NRCSConsumption/download?cid=STELPRDB1257144&ext=pdf

Vanga, S. K., & Raghavan, V. (2018a). How well do plant based alternatives fare nutritionally compared to cow's milk? Journal of Food Science and Technology, 55(1), 10–20. https://doi.org/10.1007/s13197-017-2915-y

Vanga, S. K., & Raghavan, V. (2018b). How well do plant based alternatives fare nutritionally compared to cow's milk? Journal of Food Science and Technology, 55(1), 10–20. https://doi.org/10.1007/s13197-017-2915-y

Villegas, R., Gao, Y.-T., Yang, G., Li, H.-L., Elasy, T. A., Zheng, W., & Shu, X. O. (2008). Legume and soy food intake and the incidence of type 2 diabetes in the Shanghai Women's Health Study. The American Journal of Clinical Nutrition, 87(1), 162–167. https://doi.org/10.1093/ajcn/87.1.162

Vogiatzoglou, A., Smith, A. D., Nurk, E., Berstad, P., Drevon, C. A., Ueland, P. M., Vollset, S. E., Tell, G. S., & Refsum, H. (2009). Dietary sources of vitamin B-12 and their association with plasma vitamin B-12 concentrations in the general population: The Hordaland Homocysteine Study. The American Journal of Clinical Nutrition, 89(4), 1078–1087. https://doi.org/10.3945/ajcn.2008.26598

von Mutius, E., & Vercelli, D. (2010). Farm living: Effects on childhood asthma and allergy. Nature Reviews. Immunology, 10(12), 861–868. https://doi.org/10.1038/nri2871

Voth, K., & Gilker, R. (2017, November 14). What 30 Years of Study Tell Us About Grazing and Carbon Sequestration. On Pasture. https://onpasture.com/2017/11/13/what-30-years-of-study-tell-us-about-grazing-and-carbon-sequestration/

Wang, W. P., Iigo, M., Sato, J., Sekine, K., Adachi, I., & Tsuda, H. (2000). Activation of intestinal mucosal immunity in tumor-bearing mice by lactoferrin. Japanese Journal of Cancer Research: Gann, 91(10), 1022–1027. https://doi.org/10.1111/j.1349-7006.2000.tb00880.x

Warensjö, E., Jansson, J.-H., Cederholm, T., Boman, K., Eliasson, M., Hallmans, G., Johansson, I., & Sjögren, P. (2010). Biomarkers of milk fat and the risk of myocardial infarction in men and women: A prospective, matched case-control study. The American Journal of Clinical Nutrition, 92(1), 194–202. https://doi.org/10.3945/ajcn.2009.29054

Wennersberg, M. H., Smedman, A., Turpeinen, A. M., Retterstøl, K., Tengblad, S., Lipre, E., Aro, A., Mutanen, P., Seljeflot, I., Basu, S., Pedersen, J. I., Mutanen, M., & Vessby, B. (2009). Dairy products and metabolic effects in overweight men and women: Results from a 6-mo intervention study. The American Journal of Clinical Nutrition, 90(4), 960–968. https://doi.org/10.3945/ajcn.2009.27664

What is Yogurt? (n.d.). The Yogurt in Nutrition Initiative. Retrieved January 23, 2022, from https://www.yogurtinnutrition.com/what-yogurt/

Willett, W. C., & Ludwig, D. S. (2020). Milk and Health. The New England Journal of Medicine, 382(7), 644–654. https://doi.org/10.1056/NEJMra1903547

Woodford, K. (2009). Devil in the Milk—Illness, Health and the Politics of A1 and A2 Milk. Chelsea Green Publishing.

World Cancer Research Fund/American Institute for Cancer Research. (2018). Diet, Nutrition, Physical Activity and Cancer: A Global Perspective. Continuous Update Project Expert Report 2018. dietandcancerreport.org

Yalçin, A. S. (2006). Emerging therapeutic potential of whey proteins and peptides. Current Pharmaceutical Design, 12(13), 1637–1643. https://doi.org/10.2174/138161206776843296

Yao, X., Hu, J., Kong, X., & Zhu, Z. (2021). Association between Dietary Calcium Intake and Bone Mineral Density in Older Adults. Ecology of Food and Nutrition, 60(1), 89–100. https://doi.org/10.1080/03670244.2020.1801432

Yu, E., & Hu, F. B. (2018). Dairy Products, Dairy Fatty Acids, and the Prevention of Cardiometabolic Disease: A Review of Recent Evidence. Current Atherosclerosis Reports, 20(5), 24. https://doi.org/10.1007/s11883-018-0724-z

Zhang, K., Dai, H., Liang, W., Zhang, L., & Deng, Z. (2019). Fermented dairy foods intake and risk of cancer. International Journal of Cancer, 144(9), 2099–2108. https://doi.org/10.1002/ijc.31959

Zhu, G., & Xiao, Z. (2017). Creation and imitation of a milk flavour. Food & Function, 8(3), 1080–1084. https://doi.org/10.1039/c7fo00034k

Zimecki, M., & Kruzel, M. L. (2000). Systemic or local co-administration of lactoferrin with sensitizing dose of antigen enhances delayed type hypersensitivity in mice. Immunology Letters, 74(3), 183–188. https://doi.org/10.1016/s0165-2478(00)00260-1

THE SERIES

Culinary Medicine From Clinic to Kitchen: A Hands-on Guide to Transforming Nutrition Guidelines into Cooking Skills

- Book 1 – The Basics of Eating and Cooking
- Book 2 – The Essential Foods
- Book 3 – Maximizing Flavor
- Book 4 – Creating A Teaching Kitchen
- Book 5 – Common Diets

Join Dr. Deborah Kennedy, a pioneer in Culinary Medicine, on a flavorful journey from Clinic to Kitchen in this groundbreaking series. Through a scientifically based modular approach, Dr. Deb empowers clinicians, chefs, and food enthusiasts alike to revolutionize the way we support and guide others on their food journey.

In "Culinary Medicine From Clinic to Kitchen," each volume explores the art of transforming nutritional guidelines into delicious dishes, providing essential culinary skills for a healthier lifestyle. From mastering the basics of cooking to implementing a coaching model that empowers the individual to creating teaching kitchens, Dr. Deb's expertise bridges the gap between theory and practice, offering practical tips and insights for integrating nutritious foods seamlessly into daily life.

With contributions from leading experts in nutrition science, behavior change, and flavor exploration, this series offers a comprehensive guide to culinary medicine. Whether you're a healthcare professional seeking to enhance patient care, a chef looking to elevate your culinary creations, or simply passionate about healthy living and sharing that with others, these books will equip you with the knowledge and skills to make a difference in people's lives.

Embark on a journey to lifelong wellness with the "Culinary Medicine From Clinic to Kitchen" series and discover the transformative power of food in healing both body and soul one delicious bite at a time.

Series Features:
- Practical tips for behavior change, shopping, cooking, and menu planning;
- Exploration of the flavor potential of key food groups;
- Integration of culinary skills with nutritional science; and

- Contributions from leading experts in nutrition and culinary arts.
- Join the Culinary Medicine Movement today and become a catalyst for positive change in health and well-being!

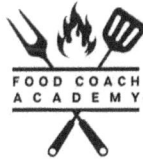

If you are interested in the Food Coach Academy, which was built from the science and culinary arts presented in the textbook series, scan the QR code above. The Food Coach Academy includes:

- Online cooking classes graded by professional chefs in real time
- A research-based modular approach for coaching others on their diet
- One on one motivational interviewing practice and assessment with an expert
- Menu planning based on the modular approach
- 510 continuing education hours for the American Culinary Federation
- A certification as a **Food Coach**

Take the **free** 42 task sample course here:
The Food Coach Academy Sample Course

If you would like to stay up to date, join our facebook group.
The Food Coach Academy Facebook Group

MEET DR. DEBORAH KENNEDY

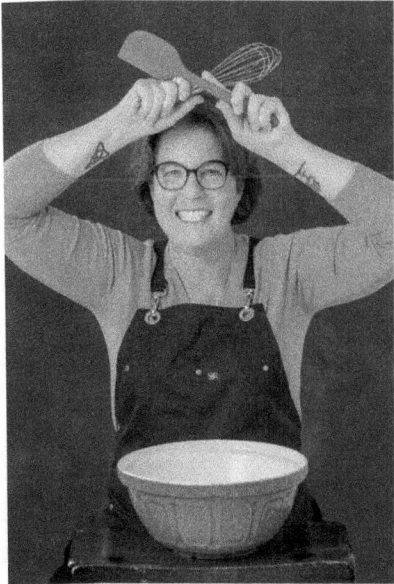

Dr. Deborah Kennedy, PhD and chef, brings nutrition science and the culinary arts together to heal people, communities, and our planet, one delicious bite at a time.

As the CEO of The Food Coach Academy™, Build Healthy Kids® and Culinary Rehab®; Director of Culinary Medicine at Rouxbe; Adjunct Professor at the University of New England, and consultant in Food is Medicine, Dr. Kennedy (or Dr. Deb as she prefers) is at the forefront of integrating food and health. She has published five books in the Culinary Medicine Textbook series, collaborating with a dozen chefs and over 40 nutrition experts. Dr. Deb has developed culinary competencies for nutrition recommendations and various diseases, building culinary medicine courses for institutions such as The New England Culinary Institute and DHMC Weight and Wellness Center

Dr. Deb holds a PhD in Nutritional Biochemistry from Tufts University. Her lifelong passion for food began at age 4, learning to cook in her parents' kitchen. Notably, she was the first Chair of Best Practices with the Teaching Kitchen Collaborative and serves as a subject matter expert in Food is Medicine for companies of all sizes. She believes that food can heal and prevent disease. Her mission is to help individuals, communities, businesses, and the healthcare sector to support culinary skill building in order to strengthen individuals in their capacity to heal themselves. In today's world, many people are paralyzed with confusion and need clarification about what to eat. Her mission is to help people discover that they can choose to walk on a path toward health based on their food decisions - just one bite at a time.

www.ingramcontent.com/pod-product-compliance
Lightning Source LLC
Chambersburg PA
CBHW080415030426
42335CB00020B/2455